HEALTH CARE IN TRANSITION

MEDICAID

FRAUD, PAYMENTS AND BENEFICIARIES

HEALTH CARE IN TRANSITION

Additional books and e-books in this series can be found on Nova's website under the Series tab.

HEALTH CARE IN TRANSITION

MEDICAID

FRAUD, PAYMENTS AND BENEFICIARIES

NADIA M. HEDEGAARD
EDITOR

New York

Library of Congress Cataloging-in-Publication Data

ISBN: 978-1-53617-666-7

Published by Nova Science Publishers, Inc. † New York

CONTENTS

PREFACE

Medicaid, a joint federal-state health care financing program, is one of the nation's largest sources of health care coverage for low-income and medically needy individuals. It provides vital health care to over 70 million Americans, regardless of preexisting conditions and must spend taxpayer dollars appropriately and efficiently. This book looks at current issues facing the Medicaid program.

Chapter 1 - This is an edited, reformatted and augmented version of Hearing before the Committee on Homeland Security and Governmental Affairs, United States Senate, One Hundred Fifteenth Congress, Second Session, Publication No. S. Hrg. 115–543, dated JUNE 27, 2018.

Chapter 2 - Medicaid, a joint federal-state health care financing program, is one of the nation's largest sources of health care coverage for low-income and medically needy individuals. A 2016 report published by the National Governors Association noted that high-expenditure Medicaid beneficiaries typically have poorly managed chronic conditions and a host of unmet social needs that result in potentially preventable use of costly services, such as emergency department visits. The report also noted that identifying and better managing those beneficiaries are key to reducing costs and improving outcomes. GAO was asked to examine state and federal efforts to manage costs and improve care coordination for high- expenditure Medicaid beneficiaries. This chapter describes (1) approaches selected states used to identify or predict high-expenditure Medicaid beneficiaries; (2) strategies selected states used to manage beneficiaries' health care costs while ensuring quality of care; and (3) resources CMS provided to states to help them identify, predict, or better manage high- expenditure beneficiaries. GAO interviewed officials from CMS, as well as Medicaid officials from a nongeneralizable sample of seven states (Indiana, Nevada, Pennsylvania, South Carolina, South Dakota, Vermont, and Washington) and five MCOs. States were selected for variation in their total Medicaid enrollment, enrollment in Medicaid managed care, percentage of state population living in rural settings, and percentage of state population with disabilities. MCOs were selected based on state suggestions, and varied in terms of whether they operated nationally or on a state or regional basis.

Chapter 3 - The Medicaid program is typically the payer of last resort. The Bipartisan Budget Act of 2018 changed the Medicaid third-party liability payment requirements for prenatal care services, pediatric preventive services, and services provided to CSE beneficiaries. Before the act, in the case of these three services, states were generally required to pay providers for services delivered to Medicaid beneficiaries and then obtain any payments from liable third parties. The Bipartisan Budget Act of 2018 also included a provision for GAO to study the potential effects of these changes. In this chapter, GAO (1) describes the status of selected states' implementation of Medicaid third-party liability changes; (2) evaluates CMS's implementation and oversight of the Medicaid third-party liability changes; and (3) describes stakeholders' views of the possible effects of these changes on providers and beneficiaries. GAO conducted interviews with state Medicaid agencies and provider associations in nine selected states, which were selected by taking into consideration Medicaid spending and stakeholder recommendations, among other factors. GAO also conducted interviews with national experts in Medicaid, national organizations representing beneficiaries and providers, and officials from CMS.

Chapter 4 - The EPSDT benefit is key to ensuring that Medicaid beneficiaries aged 20 and under receive periodic screening services, such as well-child screenings, and diagnostic and treatment services, such as physical therapy and eyeglasses, to correct or ameliorate conditions discovered during a screening. GAO was asked to examine the extent to which Medicaid beneficiaries aged 20 and under receive health care services under the EPSDT benefit. Among other things, GAO examined (1) what is known about the provision of EPSDT services based on CMS-required annual state reporting, and (2) CMS oversight of the EPSDT benefit. To do this, GAO analyzed annual state reporting data from fiscal years 2010 through 2017, the most current year data were available; CMS documentation; and federal internal control standards. GAO also interviewed CMS officials and Medicaid officials from 16 states selected, in part, on the variation in number of beneficiaries and geographic diversity.

Chapter 5 - The Medicaid statute requires states to make disproportionate share hospital (DSH) payments to hospitals treating large numbers of low-income patients. This provision is intended to recognize the disadvantaged financial situation of those hospitals because low-income patients are more likely to be uninsured or Medicaid enrollees. Hospitals often do not receive payment for services rendered to uninsured patients, and Medicaid provider payment rates are generally lower than the rates paid by Medicare and private insurance. (See CRS Report R42865, Medicaid Disproportionate Share Hospital Payments.) Whereas most federal Medicaid funding is provided on an open-ended basis, federal Medicaid DSH funding is capped. Each state receives an annual DSH allotment, which is the maximum amount of federal matching funds that each state is permitted to claim for Medicaid DSH payments. In FY2018, federal DSH allotments totaled $12.3 billion.

In: Medicaid: Fraud, Payments and Beneficiaries
Editor: Nadia M. Hedegaard
ISBN: 978-1-53617-666-7

Chapter 1

MEDICAID FRAUD AND OVERPAYMENTS: PROBLEMS AND SOLUTIONS*

Wednesday, June 27, 2018
U.S. Senate, Committee on Homeland Security and Governmental Affairs
Washington, DC.

The Committee met, pursuant to notice, at 10:30 a.m., in room SD–342, Dirksen Senate Office Building, Hon. Ron Johnson, Chairman of the Committee, presiding.

Present: Senators Johnson, Daines, McCaskill, Carper, Heitkamp, Hassan, Harris, and Jones.

OPENING STATEMENT OF CHAIRMAN JOHNSON

Chairman Johnson. Good morning. This hearing will come to order.

I want to thank Gene Dodaro and our witness from the Inspector General (IGs) office, Mr. Brian Ritchie, for taking the time and for preparing your testimony. I am looking forward to your answering our questions.

This hearing is on "Medicaid Fraud and Overpayments: Problems and Solutions." I am really looking for—solutions would be nice. Last week, in anticipation of this hearing, where we delayed it a week for a number of reasons, we did issue our staff report, primarily based on the Government Accountability Office (GAO) and IG findings, just kind of summarized all the good work you have done. And what I would like to do is

* This is an edited, reformatted and augmented version of Hearing before the Committee on Homeland Security and Governmental Affairs, United States Senate, One Hundred Fifteenth Congress, Second Session, Publication No. S. Hrg. 115–543, dated JUNE 27, 2018.

I have a series of charts. Members have paper copies at their desks. I just want to quick show why this is such an important issue.

The first chart[1] just shows who pays for health care as a percentage of total health care spending. You can see the trend since 1940 where patients were paying more than 80 cents out of every dollar. Today it is around 11 cents out of every dollar. And government has gone from not quite 20 percent to almost 50 percent. Insurance is the remaining 40 percent.

So what we have seen is a huge shift from patients being connected to the payment of the product to that disconnect. And when patients do not pay for products, they do not even know what they cost, and so there is not that discipline of a free market really disciplining the cost increase in health care. And from my standpoint, that is the root cause of our broken health care financing system, which is why health care costs have really risen dramatically.

The next chart[2] is who pays just in dollar terms. A little bit different-looking chart, but it basically makes the same point. We do have investment at the very bottom. But you can see what Americans spend totally pretty much has been the same dollar-wise—these are inflation-adjusted dollars—but government's role has dramatically increased and, again, the third-party payer in terms of insurance has also increased dramatically.

The result of all this is the next chart,[3] health care spending as a percent of GDP. When you remove the discipline of the free market system in terms of ensuring the highest possible quality, lowest possible cost, best possible level of customer service, you see costs rise dramatically.

Now, we also can do far more—and this is a good thing—in terms of our medical system. We have so many miracles. So that also drives costs. But I have to believe the fact that consumers really do not care—they do not know what things cost, and they really do not care, other than their insurance. They really care about how much they pay for insurance, but the individual health care items, they really do not care. And so as a result, we have gone from in the 20s, 3.1 percent of grodd domestic product (GDP) being spent on health care, to in 2016 17 percent, and there is really no relief from that in sight.

Now, what I would say, truthfully, if Americans are spending their own money and in freedom were deciding to spend 17 percent of their disposable income on improving their health, I would not have a problem with that. But because they are not spending their own money directly for this, I think this is a real distortion of the marketplace.

---

[1] The chart referenced by Senator Johnson appears in the Appendix on page 85.
[2] The chart referenced by Senator Johnson appears in the Appendix on page 86.
[3] The chart referenced by Senator Johnson appears in the Appendix on page 87.

The next chart[4] is total Medicaid spending, which is really the subject of the hearing today in terms of why we have to be very careful with taxpayer dollars. You can see going back to 1965—and, again, these are just nominal dollars. They are not inflation-adjusted. But I did a chart inflation-adjusted, and it looks the exact same. Medicaid was not even mentioned by Lyndon Johnson when he unveiled Medicare, but you can see the dramatic increase in Medicaid spending. Just in the last 10 years, it has more than doubled, from right around $200 billion to $430 billion. That is just Federal Government spending.

Now, in our report we show that total taxpayer spending on Medicaid in 2017 was $554 billion. I think it is 2017, correct? Which, when you take a look at what the Federal Medicaid percentages should be, somewhere between 58 and 60 percent, we are only seeing $124 billion spent by the States versus $430 billion spent by the Federal Government. That is a 22/78 percent split. So I am going to dig more into those numbers. What happens—and it drives me nuts being an accountant—numbers come from different sources, and it is very difficult to reconcile. That is something, as I am preparing for the hearing, that just jumped off the page for me. Why is that such a disconnect from, let us say, the 60 percent Federal match to this thing shows almost 78 percent? Maybe, General Dodaro can comment on that.

Our final chart[5] is, again, really the highlight of what GAO and the IG have uncovered in terms of improper payments. You can see in 2013 improper payments in Medicaid was $14.4 billion. In 2017 it was $37 billion, the largest percentage of any agency, any program in the Federal Government in terms of improper payments. Coming into this role, I always thought the term "improper payment" was a little odd because it covered both underpayment and overpayment. In this case, only 0.8 percent of the improper payment is underpayment, which means 99.2 percent is overpayment. So this is payments that should not be made, whether they are to ineligible recipients, what percent of that is fraud. It is kind of hard to understand all that, which is another problem as well.

So we will be talking about a letter we got from Administrator Verma yesterday announcing increased action on this, audits, those types of things. I will probably ask General Dodaro to kind of speak to his comments on that when he makes his opening remarks. But, anyway, this is an important issue. We are spending hundreds of billions of dollars. We want this money spent well. We certainly want to support individuals, help them gain access to quality care, those that cannot afford it. And when we have $37 billion of improper payments in a program that large, it is something that we need to pay attention to and we need to provide oversight of.

So, with that, I will turn it over to Ranking Member McCaskill.

---

[4] The chart referenced by Senator Johnson appears in the Appendix on page 88.

[5] The chart referenced by Senator Johnson appears in the Appendix on page 89.

OPENING STATEMENT OF SENATOR MCCASKILL

Senator McCaskill. I have a formal statement that I would ask be made part of the record.[6] I want to make a couple of comments.

First of all, the Chairman and I agree totally that we need to go after improper payments, and so does Senator Carper, who has been working on this for many years. All of us think we can find efficiencies in these programs, and we should find the fraudsters up front so we are not chasing payment. We should be more efficient with the technology, which we have struggled with in terms of improper payments. But there are a couple of things that I think need to be pointed out.

I certainly agree with the Chairman that transparency on costs would help a great deal. Americans are great shoppers. You give me a coupon off on a cheeseburger, and I can go online and figure out where the very best cheeseburger is and compare the coupons available, and I can do that in 2 or 3 minutes within a 1-mile radius of anywhere I am in this country. But me getting my knee replaced, as a U.S. Senator, I could not get a straight answer on what it cost. So we cannot be good shoppers if we do not know what things cost, and that is all hidden behind the curtain. Anybody who says we have a free market in health care is deluding themselves. It is not a free market. All you have to look at is the pharmaceutical costs and what is happening in this country.

We did an investigation and determined that the 20 most prescribed drugs in the Medicare Part D program have gone up consistently 10 times the rate of inflation 5 years running. That is because most of them do not have competition. That is because the system is rigged with a bogus patent system and with a barrier to entry for generics and, frankly, the fact that we are refusing to use free market principles by negotiating for volume discounts or allowing reimportation of drugs. It is ridiculous that we are handcuffing Americans with higher costs because we are protecting profits of the pharmaceutical industry, to say nothing of what has happened with the insurance industry.

And I do not believe, frankly, Mr. Chairman, that the out-of-pocket costs for the American citizen has not gone up in the last several years. I believe the out-of-pocket costs for insurance have gone up and for health care have gone up. I do not believe it is any longer on a downward trajectory. And the government spending, I think it is really important that the government number on this chart shows 49 percent. The majority of that is Medicare. So are we going to suggest that we privatize Medicare? I am absolutely opposed to privatizing Medicare.

I think there are a lot of things we can do to put incentives in the right places in the system. I think we have done a little of that in the Affordable Care Act (ACA) where we punished hospitals for readmission. So now when you get out of the hospital, I mean, you

---

[6] The prepared statement of Senator McCaskill appears in the Appendix on page 35.

have to sit and listen to—I know because when my husband had to check out of the hospital, it took us three times, four different people coming in, and telling us all the after-care and setting up the next appointment. That did not used to happen. But these hospitals know now if they are not paying attention to after-care and this patient comes back in, they are going to get financially dinged. It is working. Readmission is down, and that is a very expensive part of our health care delivery system.

So if we can change where the incentives are, rewarding quality not quantity, this fee-for-service (FFS) thing has gotten our system all out of whack. A Medicare doctor cannot even bill for taking time with patients to explain end-of-life care so that someone has the opportunity to say to their loved ones, "Do not keep me on a ventilator. I do not want to be on a ventilator." And most of these costs are in the last 6 months of someone's life.

So there are a whole lot of things we can do to bring down these costs, and I am all in on improper payments. But this notion that we are going to go after the Medicaid or Medicare programs or that somehow the private sector is a shining example of good free market behavior in this country, we have set up all kinds of ways to make sure they have guaranteed profits. That is not the way the free market is supposed to work.

So I just wanted to make those points, and I do want to spend some time today talking about the issues, especially the enrollment of providers and how badly that is going, and the digital systems and how badly that is going in terms of cutting down on improper payments. But I also want to spend some time today talking about a previous report you did, Mr. Dodaro, on preexisting conditions and the behavior of insurance companies before we had the protections for people with preexisting conditions.

Thank you, Mr. Chairman. I appreciate the hearing.

Chairman JOHNSON. Let me just qualify that the chart showing what consumers were paying, patients, that is just directly paid to the provider. We pay the bill, whether it is our taxes to fund the government funding or whether it is insurance premiums to fund the insurance portion. All I am saying is direct payment by the patient to the provider, which that is where you know what things cost in general. And even that is generally done as co-pays, and you still do not even know what you are really buying. We have a broken health care financing system, and that drives up all these costs.

So, again, I do not think we really disagree on a lot of these things. There are a lot of details. This $37 billion of Medicaid improper payments is just one small little chunk but one that I think we need to take a look at.

OPENING STATEMENT OF SENATOR CARPER

Senator CARPER. Mr. Chairman, I do not have a statement. I would like to say something. These are interesting charts. I am glad you provided them. One of the things I am just sitting here thinking, it would be interesting to know what is going on in terms of the amount of money that is being spent in uncompensated care by hospitals. As the government has spent more, has uncompensated care come down? It would be interesting to know that.

Thank you.

Chairman JOHNSON. We did issue a larger report with a lot more charts and graphs to try to answer that. One thing I did find—again, I always find it really aggravating—it is hard to get the information. It really is. How much do we really spend on drugs? What is the profitability of the entire health care system? It is far less than I think people imagine. So I would love to get more and more accurate information across the board on these things because in order to solve a problem, you need to start with information, problem definition, acknowledging we have the problem.

So, anyway, I do want to ask consent to have my written atatement entered into the record[7] and the letter I received from Seema Verma as well entered into the record.[8]

With that, it is the tradition of this Committee to swear in witnesses, so if you will both stand and raise your right hand. Do you swear that the testimony you will give before this Committee will be the truth, the whole truth, and nothing but the truth, so help you, God?

Mr. DODARO. I do.

Mr. RITCHIE. I do.

Chairman JOHNSON. Please be seated.

Our first witness absolutely deserves but does not really need an introduction, not before this Committee, but we have the Honorable Gene Dodaro, the Comptroller General of the United States and head of the U.S. Government Accountability Office. General Dodaro.

TESTIMONY OF THE HONORABLE EUGENE L. DODARO,[9] COMPTROLLER GENERAL OF THE UNITED STATES, U.S. GOVERNMENT ACCOUNTABILITY OFFICE

Mr. DODARO. Thank you very much, Mr. Chairman. Good morning to you, Ranking Member McCaskill, and Senator Carper. I am very pleased to be here today to talk about this important topic.

---

[7] The prepared statement of Senator Johnson appears in the Appendix on page 33.
[8] The letter referenced by Senator Johnson appears in the Appendix on page 121.
[9] The prepared statement of Mr. Dodaro appears in the Appendix on page 39.

The Medicaid program, serving over 73 million Americans, is a very critical part of our health care system as currently configured. But I have been very concerned about the payment integrity in this program for a number of years, for three main reasons: number one, as both of you have mentioned, Senator Johnson and Senator McCaskill, in your opening statements, improper payments are an issue. There were over $36 billion in overpayments for the Medicaid program for 2017. And this does not represent what I believe to be the full risk of the program.

There are three components of the improper payment rate. One is fee-for-service, and right now that is over a 12 percent rate and is a problem. But there are two other components. One is managed care. That are measured by the Centers for Medicare and Medicaid Services (CMS) is 0.3 percent. About half of total Medicaid spending now is in managed care. So the efforts to estimate the improper payment rate do not fully represent the risk in the managed care portion of Medicaid, which is growing every year.

Also, the beneficiary eligibility component of the improper payment rate has been frozen at 3.1 percent since 2014, so they have not really gone back in since the Affordable Care Act and checked on States' determination of beneficiary eligibility.

While $36 billion of overpayments is an issue in and of itself and that component has been growing in fee-for-service, there really is not a full measure of the payment issues and payment integrity in the Medicaid program, number one.

Number two are supplemental payments. These are payments made for uncompensated care or high concentrated rates of Medicaid recipients. They have been growing as well. In 2017 it was up to $48 billion. There are two types. One type is capped by statute. The other has not been capped and is discretionary. That has almost doubled over the years. There is no transparency over supplemental payments, and CMS does not have accurate reporting. Also it is not clear to payments are efficient and economical, which is one of the requirements. And they are potentially shifting, with the lack of transparency, shifting some of the costs from the States to the Federal Government without CMS even knowing that it is occurring. So that is problem number two.

Problem number three is demonstrations where the law allows CMS to permit States to experiment with different approaches in Medicaid. Three-quarters of the States have approved demonstrations. Right now demonstration spending accounts for one-third of the total Medicaid costs. What we have found, though contrary to CMS policy, the approved demonstrations are not budget neutral. They are actually costing more money because they have been very liberal in how they have allowed States to set spending limits.

And the evaluations of the demonstrations have serious limitations that have prevented anyone from learning what is happening with the demonstrations that could be used by others.

Now, CMS recently took action on one aspect of this based on our recommendations, which is to limit the amount of excess spending capacity that could be carried over from one year to the next year. They put some limits on that. So from 2016 to 2018, that one change that was based on our recommendations will save Medicaid costs of over $100 billion, and the Federal share will be $62.9 billion that would be saved. But that still does not fully respond to all our recommendations.

Mr. Chairman, you mentioned the plan that CMS released yesterday. That addresses some but not all of the recommendations we have made. We have 83 recommendations we have made over the years. Only 25 have been fully implemented. We think the plan is a step in the right direction, and I can elaborate more on what we see as some of the limitations in the plan. But I would say, in order to stay within my limits here in the opening statement, that much more urgent and aggressive action is needed by CMS in this area, because the CMS Actuary estimates that Medicaid spending will be growing at 5.7 percent annually. And as you pointed out in your chart, the Federal share, the total estimated spending for Medicaid by 2025 is estimated to be $958 billion. So it will be knocking on the door of $1 trillion a year.

So based upon that expected growth, known problems of the current system, I think it calls for a much more aggressive action plan on the part of CMS in order to deal effectively with payment integrity issues in the program.

Thank you very much. I look forward to responding to questions at the appropriate time.

Chairman JOHNSON. You said $1 trillion in 2028, correct?

Mr. DODARO. 2025.

Chairman JOHNSON. 2025?

Mr. DODARO. Yes. 2025.

Chairman JOHNSON. OK. In 2008 we were about $200 billion. It has gone from $200 billion in not even 20 years. That is rather shocking.

Mr. DODARO. This is one of the fastest-growing parts of the Federal Government budget. Interest is becoming a problem, too, on our debt, but that is a different hearing.

Chairman JOHNSON. Yes, a large subject in and of itself.

Our next witness is Brian Ritchie. Mr. Ritchie is the Assistant Inspector General for Audit Services in the Office of Inspector General (OIG) of the Department of Health and Human Services (HHS). Mr. Ritchie oversees audits of Medicare, Medicaid, and the Children's Health Insurance Program (CHIP) Mr. Ritchie.

TESTIMONY OF BRIAN P. RITCHIE,[10] ASSISTANT INSPECTOR GENERAL FOR AUDIT SERVICES, OFFICE OF INSPECTOR GENERAL, U.S. DEPARTMENT OF HEALTH AND HUMAN SERVICES

Mr. RITCHIE. Good morning, Chairman Johnson, Ranking Member McCaskill, and distinguished Members of the Committee. Thank you for inviting me here today, and thank you for your longstanding commitment to ensuring that the Medicaid program's 67 million beneficiaries are well served and the taxpayers' more than half trillion dollar investment is well spent. I appreciate the opportunity to discuss the Office of Inspector General's work and what more can be done to ensure that this important program operates as intended.

OIG shares your commitment to protecting Medicaid from fraud, waste, and abuse and has an extensive body of work in this area. Our oversight work has identified high improper payment rates, inadequate program integrity safeguards, and beneficiary health and safety concerns.

I will use my time today to focus on three critical areas: first, the need for accurate beneficiary eligibility determinations; second, curtailing inappropriate State financing mechanisms; and, third, improving national Medicaid data. My written testimony also notes the importance of provider screening, fiscal controls, quality of care, and our valuable partnerships.

A strong program integrity strategy starts with prevention. Correctly determining beneficiary eligibility prevents Medicaid from making improper payments for people that are not eligible for the program. However, recent OIG audits in three States estimated that more than $1.2 billion in Federal payments were made on behalf of beneficiaries that were not eligible or may not have been eligible for Medicaid. These three States did not comply with requirements to verify applicants' income, citizenship, identity, and other eligibility criteria.

The second area that I want to discuss is the need to curtail inappropriate State financing mechanisms. Over the years OIG has identified a number of State policies that may have improperly shifted costs by inflating the Federal share of Medicaid expenditures. States have misused provider taxes, intergovernmental transfers, supplemental payments, and inflated payment rates to increase the Federal funding that States receive. While CMS has tried to limit the inappropriate financing mechanisms, more needs to be done. CMS should closely review State Medicaid plans and amendments to identify any potentially inappropriate cost shifting.

And, finally, I want to discuss a consistent impediment to effective prevention, detection, and enforcement within the Medicaid program. The lack of complete, accurate, and timely national Medicaid data hampers the ability for CMS, States, managed care

---

[10] The prepared statement of Mr. Ritchie appears in the Appendix on page 73.

entities, providers, OIG and GAO, and others to quickly identify and address problems in the program. Enhanced national Medicaid data would also promote value and improve quality of care by allowing OIG and others to leverage advanced data analytics to identify vulnerabilities to avoid and best practices to replicate. Congress has recognized the value of enhanced Medicaid data, but more needs to be done to achieve this goal. CMS must ensure that States consistently report and uniformly interpret the same data elements. In addition, with a large part of the Medicaid population receiving part or all of their services through managed care, CMS needs to ensure that States report encounter data for all managed care entities.

So, in conclusion, OIG will continue prioritizing Medicaid oversight to prevent and detect fraud, waste, and abuse and take appropriate action when it occurs. We are committed to ensuring that Medicaid pays the right amount for the right provider, for the right service, on behalf of the right beneficiary.

Thank you for your ongoing leadership and for affording me the opportunity to testify on this important topic.

Chairman JOHNSON. Thank you, Mr. Ritchie.

I do want to quick correct the record. The numbers I was using, the reason I was confused, is we got the 2016 actuarial report in 2017, but it was on 2015 spending, the 554, versus the Congressional Budget Office (CBO) 2017. So I was conflating both the 2017—but one—so never mind on the one. But, again, it is just part of the problem here. You just do not have a consistent set of numbers and trying to get to the bottom of these things is like pulling teeth.

But, again, I appreciate our other colleagues here showing up for the hearing, so I will defer my questions to the end and be respectful of their time. Senator McCaskill.

Senator MCCASKILL. I am happy to defer also to my colleagues. Chairman JOHNSON. Senator Carper.

Senator CARPER. Thanks so much. It is great to see both of you. Thank you for your long-time service and for being here. I said to some of the staff sitting behind me, Gene, I said if we had to pay you by the visit, we would be broke, because you come a lot and we are grateful here for your appearances.

My colleagues have heard me saying and you have probably heard me say before that we talk about Matthew 25, the least of these, we have a moral imperative to those who are hungry, thirsty, naked, people who are sick and in prison, we have a moral imperative to those who are strangers in our land. And while we have a moral imperative to the least of these, there is also a fiscal imperative that is involved. Matthew 25 does not say anything about when they did not have any health care. My only access to health care was showing up at the emergency room of a hospital. They had to give me some kind of care. But there is a fiscal imperative to finding a way to meet those moral imperatives in a fiscally responsible way.

One of the things that I learned a long time ago when I was new on this Committee was that this Committee, as hard as we might work, we can only do so much in terms of oversight over the Federal Government. But if we could somehow work with GAO, if we could work with the Inspectors General, if we could work with the Office of Management and Budget (OMB) and other watchdog organizations, we can actually make some progress.

One of my first questions would be: Where do you think is the basis agreement between the two? Where do you see some areas of just really strong agreement that you both embrace and think we should?

Mr. DODARO. Well, I think in listening to Brian's statement, we are in almost total agreement on all issues. I think on the improper payment issue, there is strong agreement that the current approach does not fully account for program risk. The supplemental payments that Brian mentioned have not gotten enough oversight. There is not enough accurate reporting, and as a result it is not clear where costs may be inappropriately being shifted from the States to the Federal Government and not really based upon actual Medicaid spending in those areas. And then the demonstration projects I am not sure where we agree or disagree on that area because I did not hear him mention that. But the last comment he made was on the need for more and better, accurate, and timely data.

One of the problems that has hindered us all in the past in the oversight community has been the fact that Medicaid data has been 2 and 3 years old, and that has been very problematic. So they have a big effort underway to address this issue, but it has to be done properly.

So I do not see too much disagreement between the two of us on the analysis of the problems, and I will let Brian speak for himself.

Senator CARPER. OK. Thank you. Mr. Ritchie.

Mr. RITCHIE. Yes, I agree. I cannot recall ever picking up a GAO report and disagreeing. And I think we coordinate up front because we are both watchdogs over the program, and with the health care side of GAO, we coordinate on the Medicare and Medicaid work. We did not mention the demonstrations, but we have certainly had the body of work ongoing, and in the past on different waiver programs where we have seen issues. I think we just try not to duplicate each other's efforts but yet complement it, because the dollars are so valuable and rare that we do not want to be doing the same thing.

I know with Mr. Dodaro's staff, with Carolyn Yocom and others, we will coordinate, and we will have our staff coordinating to make sure, but I do think the data is the key to a lot of this, and national data especially would really be helpful. Quality oversight comes at a cost, and you do need that data, and both the age of the data and then just the consistency of it.

Some of the things we have found—I think two examples really drive it home—are investigators going out on the opioid crisis. They had a lead of a provider prescribing drugs, and they went and they checked one State. They knew the prescriber was abusing drugs in one State. They checked another State. They looked at the national provider identifier, and they did not find any hits in the claims data and thought, OK, they are not prescribing drugs in that State. Later they found out this cannot possibly be, and they looked and they found out they were using the Drug Enforcement Administrator number. So they were interpreting it differently and it did not work. And then on the beneficiary health and abuse side, we have a series of group home audits where we are looking at potential abuse and neglect in group homes. And to do that, we are starting at the emergency room, and we are looking at diagnosis codes that indicate potential abuse and neglect and backing up. And in one of the States, when we looked, the primary diagnosis code was not there. So we had to take steps to get around it, but it is not there to allow us to quickly do the job. So I think it would help all of us, including CMS, States, and the entities themselves.

Senator CARPER. Going back to the charts that the Chairman shared with us earlier today, they show an increasing commitment by the Federal Government, up to now 49 percent of the costs of health care are paid by the Federal Government or by some government. The charts do not show the number of people who are uncovered now, and I think it would probably look a good deal different, because back in 1940, 1950, and 1960, we had a whole lot of people who did not have coverage, any kind of coverage. What we have tried to do is to reduce that, and reducing that uncompensated care for providers.

One of the questions I oftentimes ask when we have oversight hearings is: What would you do if you were in our shoes? And time and again over the last 17 years the witnesses have said, "I would do more oversight." At almost every hearing, they say, "Do more oversight. Keep us honest," that sort of thing.

If you were in our shoes, given what we are facing here in terms of continued growing costs in Medicaid, what would you do if you were in our shoes? Give us three things that you would be doing if you were on this side of the dais.

Mr. DODARO. Well, I do not want to break the string of saying you need more oversight, but I believe that to be the case here. I think CMS needs to take much more aggressive and assertive action in these areas.

We have some recommendations to the Congress where we have had disagreements with CMS in the past, and I think Congress could pass legislation. For example, on the budget neutrality issue, they have had a policy that when they approve demonstrations, it should be budget neutral. And we have repeatedly found that that is not the case. They approve demonstrations, and they end up costing the Federal Government more. And then when we looked at whether we are learning anything from the demonstrations, it is not clear.

I think we have called for Congress to pass a law to require CMS to make sure that there are clear criteria for approving demonstrations that are budget neutral so it does not add to the costs of the Federal Government without any measurable benefits.

In addition, on supplemental payments, the criteria for the use of approving these and how they distribute the supplemental payments is a problem, particularly in what is called the "non-disproportionate share." The disproportionate share is mandated by Congress. That is, for uncompensated care for hospitals or where they have high concentrations of Medicaid payments. These are payments over and above reimbursing them for the services. But there are also a lot of these non-disproportionate share payments. They have doubled over the past several years, and what we have seen is that—and Brian mentioned this in his comment—they can meet the State share by having provider taxes and other intergovernmental transfers so that the local governments and provider provide more money. That requires the Federal Government to then match, and it does not increase the State share at all in that process. And it is not clear that the money is going to the people who were giving the greatest service or the people who have given more in provider taxes and payments up front. So there are questions of equity. We have some matters for Congress there.

So there is oversight and legislative fixes that you could do.

Senator CARPER. Thank you. My time has expired. Could we get just maybe two quick points from Mr. Ritchie, just really quick? Same question. Give us two. If you were us, what would you be doing to follow on what Gene said? Very briefly.

Mr. RITCHIE. I think that is the answer, more oversight. Our focus is very much focused on prevent, detect, and enforce. I think specifically for Congress, I noticed in the report that was issued last week, touching on Mr. Dodaro's last point, you mentioned maybe limiting the safe harbor on the financing mechanisms. I think that is something in Congress' wheelhouse that could be done. That is something that States, we have seen where they have manipulated it and just shifted. I think any financing mechanism that is considered or in place now, I just think you need to ask: Are these dollars being well spent, and are they providing additional quality care for beneficiaries? And in these cases, when we are looking at it, it often seems like the intent is really to sort of shift the burden, not to provide additional care. And another one, again, prevent, detect, and enforce. On the enforcement side we partner with the Medicaid Fraud Control Units (MFCUs) a lot, and I know—I am not a MFCU expert, so I will throw that out there, but I know with our office they work closely with our investigators, and MFCUs enforce fraud and then they enforce the beneficiary abuse and neglect. And they have a limitation on that side where they can only do it in facilities. So on the home and community-based services side, they do not have the authority to go after those cases. So I think pursuing that, especially as the population moves more there. In some of the group home work I mentioned before, we have certainly seen a lot of potential abuse and neglect. To protect these beneficiaries, the MFCUs could play a part to enforce that and ensure the safety, and that is something the Congress could help with.

Senator CARPER. Thank you.

Mr. Chairman, it always comes back to the MFCUs.

Chairman JOHNSON. Apparently. Senator Hassan.

OPENING STATEMENT OF SENATOR HASSAN

Senator HASSAN. Thank you, Mr. Chair and Ranking Member McCaskill, and thank you, Mr. Dodaro and Mr. Ritchie, for being here today.

Thousands of Granite Staters rely on Medicaid for really critical care. They use it to stay healthy, and they also use it to access substance use disorder services. As you know, New Hampshire has been particularly hard-hit by the opioid epidemic, and Medicaid has been a true lifeline for those suffering from addiction, which is why Granite Staters were so adamant last year in their opposition to Republican attempts to dismantle the Medicaid program.

Last year Granite Staters and people from all across America raised their voices and spoke out against Republican attempts to cut and cap Medicaid. They recognized the importance of the Medicaid program for kids, for families, for older adults. I will note that after we expanded Medicaid in New Hampshire, the number of cases in which people got health care and then could return to work, having been sidelined by chronic illness, were substantial. So protecting Medicaid's integrity is critical to protecting the Medicaid program for vulnerable populations.

I agree with your findings that CMS should be doing more to ensure that States are doing all they can to ensure the integrity of the Medicaid program because millions of Americans rely on Medicaid for care. From the reports that form the basis of your testimony, it appears that improving provider screening and analyzing claims data for patterns of fraud would go a long way toward reducing improper payments because most improper payments stem from the conduct of providers rather than from Medicaid beneficiaries.

Do both of you agree with that assessment? I will start with you, Mr. Dodaro.

Mr. DODARO. I think so far the data indicates that, but that is because most of the focus has been on the providers. They really have not focused on the beneficiary eligibility area. That rate has been frozen since 2014. They are planning now to start looking at that in 2019 through 2022, so that we would learn more about the beneficiary area. So I think both need to be attended to.

Senator HASSAN. OK. Thank you. Mr. Ritchie.

Mr. RITCHIE. I am sorry. Could you repeat the question?

Senator HASSAN. So the reports that form the basis of the testimony that you provided, it appears that it is critical to improve provider screening and analyzing claims data for patterns of fraud, because most improper payments stem from the conduct of providers rather than Medicaid beneficiaries.

Mr. RITCHIE. Yes, I do not know that we really have work specifically targeting that, but I would say our beneficiary eligibility concerns are—our three recent eligibility reports that I referred to in our testimony, those were cases where the State systems did not work, and beneficiaries that did not meet the criteria were enrolled. So it was not a case of intentional fraud or anything like that, but they were improper payments that were made to beneficiaries who——

Senator HASSAN. But I also just do not want to take the eye off the ball that there are providers who are engaged in——

Mr. RITCHIE. Oh, absolutely.

Senator HASSAN [continuing]. Fraud and abuse, and I do not want to be scapegoating beneficiaries who may think they are eligible, even if they are not.

Mr. RITCHIE. I totally agree. And when I mentioned before our prevent, detect, and enforce, I mean, prevention to us is by far the key. If you can up front get an enrollment system, get an eligibility system that keeps bad actors out, that does a thorough job of knowing who you are doing business with, we have seen cases where States are not collecting the correct ownership information, cases where someone gets terminated in one State and another State does not have the data to tell so they can enroll there. So just a consistent—again, back to the data theme, sorry, but to know that these people are not there and keep the bad players out, it can prevent a lot of improper payments up front so you are not paying and chasing them down.

Senator HASSAN. Well, thank you.

I do want to change to a different topic, Mr. Ritchie, because of recent events. Like my colleagues who have spoken already about this, I am outraged at the humanitarian crisis that President Trump has created on our Southern Border. Pediatricians, psychologists, and health professionals have been raising the alarm about the irreparable harm, including brain development and long-term behavioral health issues, that forcibly separating children from their parents can cause. We must strengthen border security, but we have to do that in a way remaining true to our American values. And I think we all agree here that this is not about politics. It is about our moral obligation to stand up and act in the face of clear and absolute injustice.

The President created this crisis, and, unfortunately, his Executive Order (EO) seems to have created even more confusion at HHS and other agencies scrambling to implement it. And then, frankly, Secretary Azar yesterday further confused things by testifying that in order for children to be reunited with parents who have asylum claims, the parents have to give up the asylum claims, which is a violation of so many fundamental American values that it is just hard to grasp.

So, Mr. Ritchie, I am participating in formal requests to your office to review the Office of Refugee Resettlement's (ORR) response to the Administration's practice of separating children and parents. I know this is not your specific area, but as a representative of your office, do you know whether you plan to investigate the response to this issue of family separation?

Mr. RITCHIE. Yes, so you are correct, it is not my area. But I do know a bit about this. I know it is a high priority within our office, and I did—knowing, obviously, that this is such a high priority there and that I was coming here today, I asked the people that were doing it a little bit about it, so I can tell you what I do know. We obviously have some past work on the ORR. Since 2006, OIG has provided oversight of the unaccompanied alien children (UAC) program operated by the Office of Refugee Resettlement. And what we have ongoing right now and planned, we are planning nationwide work that is going to focus on the health and safety of the children in the facilities. It is underway so the plan is in place. In fact, we had sort of boots-on-the-ground investigators and auditors last week at four facilities, and they are back now in the office planning the work. We could certainly set up a briefing for you or anyone else that is interested as soon as that work is ready, because we are concerned and want to have the oversight of that and see how things are going.

We also are wrapping up some work at 11 facilities and looking at the health and safety controls that were in place. That actually is prior to 2018, but it is going to serve as the launching point for new work but the data is prior to 2018, so it may not reflect the current condition, but it will reflect some of the current work that we will be doing.

Senator HASSAN. Well, thank you for the response, and thank you for thinking ahead to this hearing and anticipating that we may be interested in it and asking about it. What I would ask is that you bring a message back to Mr. Levinson and the rest of the IG's office. This issue, what is happening to these children today, now, every minute, every hour, every day, every week, month that they are separated from their parents is doing them irreparable harm, and I would hope and expect that the Department reprioritize as necessary to get not only boots on the ground to find out what is happening, but also to develop a policy that is consistent and reflects the urgency and the priority that the American people place on reuniting these children.

Certainly the government of the United States of America can reunite 2,000 children—and it is a little bit over 2,000 children if Secretary Azar's testimony yesterday was correct. Certainly the U.S. Government can find a way to reunite these children, even if it means reorganizing and reprioritizing resources. So I hope you will take that message back. I thank you for your testimony today.

Thank you, Mr. Chair.

Chairman JOHNSON. Senator Heitkamp.

OPENING STATEMENT OF SENATOR HEITKAMP

Senator HEITKAMP. Thank you, Mr. Chairman. And I apologize I was not here during your testimony, but I can only imagine it did not escape your notice that CMS, who is not here today even though they have been invited, actually issued a couple press releases yesterday with some ideas on how they could better facilitate stopping fraud, waste, and abuse. It is really unfortunate that they are not here to have that conversation.

Chairman JOHNSON. Senator Heitkamp, let me just clarify. I did speak with Administrator Verma, and she is happy to come in, whenever we do a follow up hearing on this. So she is more than willing to testify. So I just want to put that on the record. She offered to do that, and we will certainly——

Senator HEITKAMP. Well, is there a reason why she is not here today?

Chairman JOHNSON. I just do not think she was prepared.

Senator HEITKAMP. That is even more frightening than she is not here today.

Chairman JOHNSON. From my standpoint, I was happy to first hear the testimony from GAO and the IG, and then we will follow up on it. Again, it was a press release. I said it was a letter. It was a press release and there is a fact sheet, and this is going to be ongoing oversight.

Senator HEITKAMP. Well, time is wasting. —

Senator MCCASKILL. I think we need to be clear. She was invited and declined to come and, instead of coming, issued a press release. I think that is fair, and that is what the facts are, and I think it is important to put those facts out there.

Chairman JOHNSON. I understand, but also the fact is she is willing to come and testify in the future, and it will be the reasonably near future.

Senator HEITKAMP. I get it, and I voted for her, and I think that she is competent. But the bottom line is if she was not prepared to testify in front of us, she should not have been prepared to send out a press release.

And so if I can just ask, have you had a chance, Mr. Dodaro or Mr. Ritchie, to review her statements?

Mr. DODARO. My staff has, and they briefed me on it.

Senator HEITKAMP. And do you believe that this is a good start, a finished product, or needs some work and collaboration to try and create a network and a consistent amount of accountability for trillions of Federal dollars and State dollars that are being spent so that we can avoid fraud, waste, and abuse no matter who is committing it?

Mr. DODARO. Yes, we think it is a step in the right direction, but much more neededs to be done. There are details that are not in there that I would have expected to be included, some milestones. There are some areas not covered, like supplemental payments and demonstrations that I would have expected to be covered. We have, as I mentioned, 83 recommendations that we have made to them. They have implemented 25 so far. And the plan does not address all of our recommendations.

So much more needs to be done. I think there needs to be more aggressive and urgent oversight.

Senator HEITKAMP. I think that my point that I am getting at is that when we look at this, we need a structure because if we just deal with taking care of the waste, fraud, and abuse of today, there are going to be other opportunities for waste, fraud, and abuse, and we need to know who is accountable and how we are going to hold people accountable for making payments that are inappropriate, putting people on Medicaid rolls or Medicare rolls that is not appropriate. We have to get a handle on this.

I do not disagree with the looming problem, and the low-hanging fruit in taking care of our health care costs on the Federal Government is stopping waste, fraud, and abuse. And, I can tell you, when I was the Attorney General (AG), there was this collaborative process with State Attorneys General. Where did that go? What do we know about a structure that is in place, working with the State, auditors with the State Inspectors General, to try and get an overall plan so that we can have meaningful accountability?

The frustration that I have is that we come here and we are picking around the edges and getting distracted without really thinking about the overall structure of oversight. And, it is not acceptable that the recommendations from GAO have not been responded to. This is a big-ticket item, behind national defense and is probably going to loom bigger than national defense. We have to get ahead of this. And to me, the frustration that the American people have is that they are willing to give people some help. They are willing to recognize that providers needs to pay the bills. But they do not want this money wasted.

And so, when you look at structure, Mr. Dodaro, and you think, OK, we have these State agencies, they have responsibility as well. Fifty percent in North Dakota of this money that is spent on Medicaid is State-based money. Where have been historically the gaps? Who have you seen on the State side do an excellent job in holding people accountable? And has the Federal Government learned from State audit programs on what we could do more effectively?

Mr. DODARO. Yes, well, one of the biggest gaps has been that the State auditors have not been involved on a regular basis. This is one of the points that I have made. In fact, I have brokered meetings between State auditors and CMS in order to make sure that they are brought into the program. A lot has been focused on the Attorneys General and the fraud units in the States, but not the State auditors. The State auditors need to be involved much more in this program. They are willing to do it, but they need to be brought into the structure. They need to be compensated. They can have a big effect on this issue.

Senator HEITKAMP. And another place where we share revenue in Minerals Management Service, we have an audit program that is pretty robust to try and make sure that people are paying the appropriate royalty, there is a great example of Federal-State collaboration where you know who has the lines of authority and who has oversight over those lines of authority. So it is not like we are without examples on how we could do this better.

Mr. DODARO. Right.

Senator HEITKAMP. The problem that you have with AGs is that assumes automatically all fraud, waste, and abuse is criminal or that you are going to take it criminal.

Mr. DODARO. Right.

Senator HEITKAMP. Do you think there is appropriate civil penalties for fraud, waste, and abuse to provide a substantial deterrent?

Mr. DODARO. I do not know offhand to be able to answer that right now. I could provide something for the record.[11]

Senator HEITKAMP. Maybe, Mr. Ritchie, you know if instead of just having to go the very aggressive action of filing an indictment and prosecuting people versus, no, do not do that, repay the money, is there an effective system of civil penalties?

Mr. RITCHIE. That is not my area of expertise. I do know our office works with the MFCUs who can pursue cases, and I know our office has civil remedies, civil monetary penalties and exclusions and things like that available. So I believe they can do some of that, but I could get you a better answer and consult with my colleagues and get back to you.

Senator HEITKAMP. I think it is important that we not ignore some additional legislative tools, whether it is additional incentives to work with the States, additional incentives, and then putting together with the recommendations at HHS a robust and very clear line of authority on audit responsibility so that we are not picking around the edges here, that we are actually creating a program that will solidify the frustration that the American public has and the frustration that we have, that we are not getting at waste, fraud, and abuse as effectively as what we should.

Mr. DODARO. I agree. I think the other biggest gap in this whole area—and I mentioned this in my opening statement—is the managed care portion of Medicaid. The managed care contractors have not been audited on a regular basis. There is rule out to start auditing them, but that is half of Medicaid spending. So the known overpayments right now are mostly in the fee-for-service area, and the beneficiary eligibility audits have been frozen since 2014. So there are huge gaps in knowledge about the extent of the program integrity issues in the Medicaid program, and much more needs to be done.

I agree with you, they need an overall plan, and they need to be held accountable for it. And there are more resources that need to be available, including the State auditors.

Senator HEITKAMP. And if I can just make one final comment, when you do not do those audits, you do not see the patterns in behavior that either could be deterred or they could be, in fact, prosecuted and deterred. And so that is why it is really important that

---

[11] The information submitted by Mr. Dodaro appears in the Appendix on page 170.

these audits be current, that these audits see trend lines, and that we actually take the appropriate action to do prevention, whether it is on the benefit side, whether it is on the provider side. This is incredibly frustrating to me because it should be the most robust audit program in the Congress and in the Administration, and it seems to me it is not.

Mr. DODARO. Well, that is why it has been on our High-Risk List since 2003. It is also why I am here today instead of sending another GAO witness because I am personally concerned about the program integrity issues of Medicaid and its expected continued growth of 5.7 percent a year. As I mentioned earlier, by 2025 the estimated total government spending, Federal and State, on this is knocking on the door of $1 trillion a year. And it is a very important program. I agree it is a critical service that needs to be delivered. But we need to get a better handle on the integrity of the program to make sure that we are not wasting money that could be better used to provide legitimate health care services.

Senator HEITKAMP. I appreciate so much what the IGs do and what you do, Mr. Dodaro. You guys are doing work. We hope you are just not hollering into the empty well, that someone is actually listening to you and taking your advice, and that is why we are here.

Chairman JOHNSON. Let me clarify because I do not want to be putting words into Administrator Verma's mouth. She was not available. OK? About a month ago, she had to go to her child's graduation. My assumption is that when I say "not prepared," not far enough along in the process to really have the testimony be all that particularly valuable at this point.

Now, trust me, I wish years ago, whoever the CMS Director or Administrator was further along in the process. So from my standpoint, this is progress. She has agreed to testify in the future. We are holding this hearing to define the problem, to put pressure on CMS to come up with—OK, we got the fact sheet. We have a little bit of a game plan. We are going to want to see more meat on the bones of that fact sheet.

So this is why we do this. We do put hopefully cooperative pressure on the agency to finally start doing this, and it has not been done since 2003.

Senator HEITKAMP. Mr. Chairman, if I can just say, I would be more sympathetic if she had not conveniently released a press release yesterday. I would be more sympathetic. I would say, "Fine, she is taking this seriously. She wants to come up with a robust plan." Instead, it seems to me that what happened here was, "Oh, this is going to get talked about, so I need to have some talking points about this," instead of actually sitting down with us. She inherited this mess. I get that. But this has to be a priority. I talked to her about this as a priority. And so my frustration is then do not issue a press release.

Chairman JOHNSON. Again, I appreciate the heat you are putting on CMS. I am putting on the same heat, OK? And so this is good. This is exactly what we should be doing. We are providing oversight, and it will be interesting when she does come to testify, and it will be a matter of do we want it in a month, do we want it in 2 months. We will work together with you on that.

Senator HEITKAMP. I want a plan.

Chairman JOHNSON. So do I.

Senator HEITKAMP. And I want it sooner rather than later.

Chairman JOHNSON. Right. I want a lot of meat on the bones of that plan. I think our witnesses do as well. Senator Jones.

OPENING STATEMENT OF SENATOR JONES

Senator JONES. Thank you, Mr. Chairman. And thank you to both the witnesses for being here. I apologize for having to attend another hearing on health care costs in the Health, Education Labor and Pension (HELP) Committee.

I want to just follow up a couple of things. One, I want to echo what Senator Hassan said about what is going on at the border and families. I do not need to repeat all of that. I share every concern that she expressed. I really appreciate that she did that. And, Mr. Ritchie, I appreciate, as she said, your anticipating some of these questions.

My one quick question to you on that is: Will any of your follow up work on that issue with what is going on down there, will that also be looking to see whether or not the Administration is complying with the injunction that was issued yesterday concerning the time limits given to bring these families back together?

Mr. RITCHIE. That I am not sure because, again, they were just out last week looking, and they are developing the plan now. They are probably meeting back in the office as we speak. So, again, they can provide a briefing in the very near future, as they do it, but the plan is being developed, so we can certainly take that into consideration as they go. I know they want to do as thorough of an approach as they can. It is a plan in development, because the work that they have completed is based on prior to 2018. And the other thing that I did not mention before is we do have reports that come in from ORR—we have been getting them since 2014—of serious incidents of abuse and neglect that occur, and we meet with ORR leadership on an as-needed basis on those. But, some of that could factor into it, too.

But, again, I am sorry, not my area. I am not part of the planning, and so I am not well informed enough to answer that. But the plan is being developed as we speak.

Senator JONES. All right. Mr. Dodaro?

Mr. DODARO. Yes, Senator Jones, Senator Hassan, we have been asked at GAO as well to look at the process for tracking these children in custody. We got the request this week. We immediately are starting the work in that area. So we will be happy as that work proceeds to follow up with you as well.

Senator JONES. All right. Great. I appreciate that from both of you and urge you to do that. I think that that is one of the top priorities that we ought to have as a country, and the Administration and Congress ought to both have there.

I want to then just briefly follow up from Senator Heitkamp's speeches, because I share those same concerns. I am a former prosecutor in Alabama. I have also had to defend cases of fraud and abuse. And so the whole issue of fraud and abuse is an important one.

Mr. Dodaro, you said, in response to the letter that CMS issued yesterday, that you would have liked to have seen more details, that you would have expected to see more detail. You also mentioned something about aggressive oversight, and I would like for you, if you could, for the record today just expand on that a little bit, of what you would have expected to see in that letter, the details, and I know you have a lot of recommendations, you cannot go through them all. And then also kind of expand on your comments about aggressive oversight.

Mr. DODARO. Yes. First, there is a section in the plan that talks about improving the quality of information—accuracy and completeness of information. I would expect to see more on how they are planning to make sure that it is comparable across the States, how they are going to use it for oversight and some milestones for when these things will occur over a period of time. As I mentioned earlier, and Brian has mentioned several times, the lack of complete and accurate information is an impediment to oversight. So it is important that it be done on an aggressive schedule going forward.

I would have expected to see more in the plan about the supplemental payments which are payments, made for uncompensated care and other things, to respond to our recommendations about making sure they are economical and efficient payments based on good data from the States. And, that the money is actually going to the right people as it is demonstrated within the area.

I would have expected to see more on the demonstration projects that we have said have not been budget neutral, and the evaluations have not been thorough. We are not learning a lot from the demonstrations, even though they are costing more Federal money than they were supposed to in those areas.

I would have expected to see more on use of State auditors. I have had this discussion. They have had some discussions with the State auditors, but there is no plan to use the State auditors. In some of the States, as I am sure you are well aware of, Medicaid is over a third of the total spending for the States. The State auditors should be involved on a robust basis, and it is in the Federal Government's interest to encourage them to do that and provide some resources for them. I think it will be a great return on investment.

One other thing is beneficiary eligibility determinations, which they have had on hold. By the time they start it, it will be 5 years since they have really done any audits of beneficiary eligibility determinations. They are planning to do it over a 3-year cycle.

There is no reason that this cannot be done on a faster basis if they apply additional resources. I think waiting until 2021 to finish all the States is too long, given the fact that Medicaid spending during that period of time is going to grow 15, 20 percent, and still be on the rise.

So these are the things that I mean about being more aggressive, and with the actions that they have said, including other actions and moving faster.

Senator JONES. OK. Well, thank you very much for that. My time is winding down. Mr. Chairman, I may have some other questions for the record. I would like to just make two points.

One—and I continue to do this every time I get a chance—my State did not expand Medicaid. We left a lot of money on the table, and I have people in my State—we have a very poor State. We have a very unhealthy State. We have a lot of people in my State, 200,000 or so by every estimate, that could have benefited from the expansion of Medicaid, not to mention the economic value that would have been brought by bringing those dollars in and expanding those health care deliveries in the areas of my State that need it so badly. We are losing health care providers in my rural Alabama left and right.

The last thing—and, Mr. Chairman, I appreciate the charts here. Those are always very helpful. You are very good at that, by the way. I would note an interesting comment from the hearing that is going on in the HELP.

Committee on the same issue about driving down health care, that these charts and all at the end of the day on who pays, it is the American taxpayer. That is why it is so important. That is why Senator Heitkamp was so animated about the fraud and abuse and the way we do this and why we should be involved, because at the end of the day, whether it is government, whether it is insurance or out-of-pocket, it is our constituents who are paying for the health care and everything we are doing.

So, with that, I will yield the remaining 27 seconds. Actually, I am over.

Chairman JOHNSON. Trust me, I understand we all pay it. It is just the form of payment. That first chart was really talking about what you pay directly to the provider.

By the way, I actually should have brought our more extensive report on just health care spending where we have a lot more charts. So we will make sure you have that in your office. Senator Daines.

OPENING STATEMENT OF SENATOR DAINES

Senator DAINES. Chairman Johnson, thank you, and Ranking Member McCaskill for having this hearing and compiling this very important report. I am very appreciative of the dedication of the Committee to uncover these areas for improvement in the Administration of Medicaid, which, as we know, is experiencing skyrocketing costs.

Mr. Chairman, this chart here, this reminds me of a steep ski jump in Montana, looking at not only where we are at but where we are going to be in the next 10 years.

Chairman JOHNSON. One I would not want to go down.

Senator DAINES. This would be one that my boys would be excited about in a terrain park. I can tell you that.

Taken by itself, the waste and fraud of the Medicaid program nearly exceeds the entire budgets of the Department of Agriculture (USDA), the Department of Commerce, and the Department of Interior (DOI) combined. I think about how we battle here for, for example, the full funding of Land and Water Conservation Fund (LWCF) with some $37 billion of overpayments. So the interest on that alone could fund LWCF fully. I hope we could make some progress on addressing Medicaid's soaring expenses so that we can protect taxpayers and safeguard the program, this important safety net for those who truly need it the most.

Mr. Ritchie, Homeland Security and Governmental Affairs Committee (HSGAC's) oversight report pointed to structural incentives in Obamacare and Medicaid expansion for States to enroll as many people on the program as possible. The report cites the ACA State reimbursement formula, which is driven by the number of enrollees, and Medicaid's 100 percent cost coverage in the first 3 years.

Do you agree with the report's assessment that these financial incentives may result in States adding people to Medicaid who do not truly meet eligibility requirements?

Mr. RITCHIE. We have not done anything looking at the incentive, but I would say we have done the recent eligibility reports that we mentioned in our testimony and that I mentioned earlier, and with those eligibility reports, we found that people were certainly enrolled that were not eligible. So there is a concern there.

Also, with the increased 100 percent Federal Medical Assistance Percentages (FMAP), or Federal matching funds we have done, this is not the first time that Medicaid has been set up where they have paid at one level for a service versus another level, and we have a history of work where we have looked to see if the payments have been appropriate. We have seen where they have offered those increased payments, there have been inappropriate payments where things have been submitted at the higher level versus the other level. So certainly the past has shown work where an increased Federal participation has led to improper payments. So from our perspective, we follow a risk assessment. We see that there is certainly risk there. And from an eligibility perspective, regardless of the policy decision of whether it is 100 percent of Federal poverty level or 138 percent, we think the rules need to be followed, that the right beneficiaries need to be enrolled, and that is clearly not happening right now.

Senator DAINES. Well, I mean, just look at it. If you are a State and you are held accountable, like most States are for balancing their budget, which we are not held accountable for here, I just testified in front of the Select Committee on Budget Reform that needs to be done. It just continues to baffle me that Washington, DC., is not held accountable for a balanced budget but the States are. And because the States are, if you give an incentive to the State where they can offload for that FMAP, in Montana, 67 percent FMAP, take either that number covered by the Federal Government or move to 100 percent, what is the incentive? Do you think that could maybe factor into a State's decision to move more folks in Medicaid expansion because it is not costing the State any money for a period of time, at least for 3 years? And then it is 90 percent after that.

Mr. RITCHIE. Right. But, again, I mean, we do not look at the political decision of doing that, but we do look at the criteria, and——

Senator DAINES. And I am not saying it is a political decision. It is just, if you are looking at the math——

Mr. RITCHIE. Right, but there is different criteria for each category, so people that—like when we did our eligibility determination reviews, we found cases where people would have qualified for the standard Medicaid, but they were determined to be in the higher Medicaid, so that was an issue. We did not find it was outright fraud. We found it was system and human data entry errors that led to it. But our audit also was not designed to do that. But if they meet that 138 percent and they qualify for one category, the 100 percent, they meet the other category.

Senator DAINES. Mr. Ritchie, for fiscal year (FY) 2017 GAO found that Medicaid overpayments were $36.4 billion. If Medicaid grows at its current expected pace to $900 billion by 2025, overpayments, kind of using the rough percentages there, it could be as high as $55 billion. I applaud CMS for yesterday announcing initiatives designed to improve the Medicaid program integrity by taking a more active role in auditing the program.

As Administrator Verma's Medicaid Integrity Initiative begins, Mr. Ritchie, what do you believe are the keys to its success?

Mr. RITCHIE. Well, I agree with GAO that I think it is a step in a positive direction. I have not had a lot of time to sort of go through, and it did not have a lot of the details there, but I know in working with CMS it is reflecting some of the work that we have done and that we have recommended. I think they are taking positive steps there. I think a lot more needs to happen and more details need to be there. But, again, our key issues and the key things they need to do, the most important is prevent, is up front making sure that the fraudulent providers, providers that should not be in the program are prevented from getting in, and then you have prevented improper payments up front, making sure along the lines of the prior question that eligible beneficiaries are in and the dollars are being spent on the people that need to and deserve to be in the program. And then data has been a big theme of our discussion today and what I brought up, having improved data is it allows everyone that is providing program oversight to actually identify and detect the issues of fraud, waste, and abuse quickly; and then once you find them, enforce it, deal with it quickly, recover the money, and put added safeguards in place to prevent additional future payments.

Senator DAINES. Thank you.

I want to ask a question of Mr. Dodaro here before I run out of time. In fiscal year 2013, Federal and State Medicaid cost tax-payers about $287 billion, just a little less than that. But the program double its expenses to $596 billion.

Are you concerned that there has been an increased overpayment and fraud following the States' expansion of Medicaid?

Mr. DODARO. I am concerned that the full extent of program risks in the Medicaid program have not been adequately determined, and by that I mean that part of the growth has been in the managed care portion of the program, and there have been no audits of the managed care providers except a few that the State auditors have done and some other ones, and the IG. The beneficiary eligibility determination rate, improper payment rate, has been frozen at 3.1 percent since 2004. So there is no real good information about whether or not the beneficiaries' determinations have been done properly under the expansion program, because that program has been suspended. So I am concerned about this. That is why I am here today urging greater attention to this very important issue. And the growth in Medicaid is expected, by the CMS Actuary, to be 5.7 percent a year. And as you mentioned and we have in our report, by 2025 it will be knocking, total costs, on the door of about $1 trillion.

So there must be greater attention to this program to ensure the integrity of it and its sustainability over a long period of time.

Senator DAINES. Thank you, Mr. Dodaro, and thank you for remaining concerned, and I ask that you continue to remain concerned. I appreciate it.

Mr. DODARO. Thank you.

Chairman JOHNSON. I want to pick up on two lines of Senator Daines' questioning, first of all, the beneficiary eligibility. I think, General Dodaro, you said something, we have really not looked at it. Isn't it basically true one of the reasons we have not really dug into the eligibility is because that match with the States, we pretty well relied on the States having the incentive to police that themselves because they are spending money as well. Is that kind of one of the dynamics? And then, of course, when you expand Medicaid and it is a 100 percent match, now you literally have given them a great incentive to sign up people that necessarily are not eligible, which is why in the IG report and we have highlighted in our report, for example, in California, about $1 billion worth of Medicaid funds for 445,000 ineligible—isn't that kind of dynamic going on here? In the past we just really relied on the States spending money. They are not going to want to spend money on ineligible individuals because they are having to pick up about 40 percent of the tab. But now with Medicaid expansion, they have every incentive to sign as many people up as possible. Do you want to comment on that?

Mr. DODARO. Yes. The Affordable Care Act required greater screening of both providers and there were new eligibility determinations for beneficiaries as well.

Now, from my perspective, when you introduce new requirements, there is every reason to believe that there needs to be a greater oversight during that period, not less. CMS took the approach that basically the States need time to adjust to these new requirements over time, so CMS was not going to go in and take a look until States have had time to adjust. I do not agree with that. I do not think that was the right approach. When you make changes, you should be looking more at the internal controls that are in place to make sure that those new changes are implemented properly so you can take timely action. But that is water under the bridge at this point. And so this is why I am saying that when they startin 2019 they are going to take one-third of the States over a 3-year period until they cover all the States.

My belief is we should do more, have a more aggressive strategy. During that 3-year or 4-year period, by the time everything is done costs are going to increase over the period of time.

So that is the reason that we are where we are at this point, from what I understand.

Chairman JOHNSON. When I talked to Administrator Verma, I had asked her who is going to be doing the auditing, and my bias would be engage private sector auditors. There are plenty of them there in every State and in every community. So she said they were going to do that. Let us hope so. And if they are doing that, they can cover all 50 States immediately.

Mr. DODARO. They should use the State auditors. I mean, you are sitting next to a former State auditor over here, and——

Senator MCCASKILL. And it would not be that hard to put into the single audit protocol.

Mr. DODARO. Right. They are already auditing it and the State auditors know this program better than anybody.

Senator MCCASKILL. Yes.

Mr. DODARO. And I have dealt with the State auditors for Louisian, Mississippi, and Massachusetts. They have started on their own, because I have been encouraging them to get more involved. But if they are given proper support and resources, you could help prevent a lot of these program integrity problems. And I would encourage the Congress to——

Chairman JOHNSON. But the bottom line, there is no reason to do a third, a third, a third. There is really no reason to wait. Let us do now and do all 50 States.

Mr. DODARO. Yes, well, they are doing it based upon their own resources, not figuring how you could deploy resources and expertise that is already there resident in each State. And each State's program is different.

Chairman JOHNSON. So clarify the managed care point. You are saying we are frozen. Describe what you are talking about. What is frozen at 3.1 percent?

Mr. DODARO. The beneficiary eligibility determination is frozen; there are three components of the improper payment rate. There is a fee-for-service component, and I think the latest is about 12.9 percent error rate. And that is where most of the $36 billion in overpayments come from.

Chairman JOHNSON. That is what you can measure?

Mr. DODARO. Yes. The second part has been in place for a number of years.

The second component is managed care. The managed care component of this is set at 0.3 percent, which is what they figure, because nobody is really auditing the managed care providers on how they are providing services. They just have been looking at whether or not the States are providing the money to the managed care providers, the organizations, but not the actual provision—delivery of services, whether the services were medically necessary, whether they are following all the right rules or procedures. So no one knows.

Chairman JOHNSON. So, again, what set—I mean, describe what is the set point. What does that that do?

Mr. DODARO. The set point is in the beneficiary eligibility at 3.1 percent. The managed care rate they do every year, but they are not measuring everything that needs to be measured. That is the difference between the two. They froze the beneficiary eligibility determination at 3.1, which is what it was in 2013, I believe, or 2014. For the medicare managed care portion, they do an estimate every year, but it does not measure everything that needs to be measured for half of the program expenditures.

Chairman JOHNSON. So another thing I wanted to clarify—and I am going to dig into that further. You talked about demonstration spending, not budget neutral. It is about a third of spending. From 2016 to 2018, you said there was a carryover of $100 billion. Just again make me understand that.

Mr. DODARO. Yes, because they are not going to allow them to carry over the expenditures. When they approve a demonstration, they agree in a State of what the spending limit could be. So if the State, let us say, just for theoretical purposes, sets the limit at $20 billion, but they really only spend $18 billion, they get to carry over the $2 billion into the next year. Now they are not going to allow them to accumulate all that and you cannot carry over all of it, and so they are limiting it. As we said that that it is raising the costs of the program to the Federal Government without a good basis. So they have stopped this practice.

Chairman JOHNSON. So it really is use it or lose it, which creates its own incentives. But that is better than having this simply not being able to spend the money and then just banking it in the future.

Mr. DODARO. Yes, particularly if the spending limit that they set was based in some cases on hypothetical services and hypothetical costs that was not the actual costs that they had before.

Chairman JOHNSON. OK. I do want to get into State gimmicks before we close out this hearing, but I will turn it over to Senator McCaskill.

Senator MCCASKILL. I would like to first briefly talk about the fact that we are not doing screening and enrollments, even though we passed a law requiring it. It began to be a requirement in 2011, and the States are supposed to be screening and looking at enrollment requirements for the providers.

Comptroller, your colleagues previously testified in the House that the requirement for screening and enrollment for Medicaid providers prevents improper payment and reduces fraud. Your colleague Ms. Yocom stated, "If you can screen and enroll and ensure your providers act in good faith, you have managed most of the fraud. A beneficiary alone trying to commit fraud needs a complicit provider. So focusing attention on ensuring good screening and enrollment process is critical."

Do you agree with her statement? And what we can be doing, what can CMS be doing to require these States to do a better job on screening and enrollment of various providers that are looking to be able to collect Medicaid dollars?

Mr. DODARO. Yes, first of all, I agree with Ms. Yocom. She is sitting right behind me.

Senator MCCASKILL. Thank you, Ms. Yocom.

Mr. DODARO. She is my best adviser on this issue and is very knowledgeable of the program. She is absolutely right. We have made many recommendations to CMS to make more databases available to the States.

Now, one novel thing that is in the plan CMS—or the press release from yesterday is the offer for them to do some screening for the States on the providers as well, and I think that could be helpful if implemented properly as well, because they can access more databases. So we have been trying to make sure that they give more databases to the States for screening purposes.

For example, on Medicare, there are some of the same providers in both programs, and you can use the experience with the Medicare screening to help Medicaid as well. So that has been one of our recommendations: to improve the accuracy of the databases. We have been trying for a while to get better, more accurate Death Master File (DMF) information to the States as well. And it is particularly important that CMS help because beneficiaries may move from State to States.

Senator MCCASKILL. Correct.

Mr. DODARO. So those are some of our recommendations. I can provide a detailed list for the record.[12]

Senator MCCASKILL. That would be terrific.

And since you spoke of Medicare, it is my understanding that the improper payment percentage is higher in the Medicare program than it is in the Medicaid program.

Mr. DODARO. That is because they have better measurement techniques. I think the Medicare program has good methodologies. They do regular reviews. They check on

[12] The information submitted by Mr. Dodaro appears in the Appendix on page 171.

whether or not the service was medically necessary and take samples. They take national samples every year. So they have a much more robust program than the Medicaid program, and it is a little easier because it is a national program as opposed to each State having its own different design for the Medicaid program.

So to be fair, it is more complicated to do it in Medicaid, but Medicare has a very good program. In fact, what we did, we looked at the TRICARE program at the Department of Defense (DOD) and compared what they were doing to measure their improper payment rate to Medicare and found that DOD was not doing anywhere close to what Medicare is doing, so we recommended they improve their methodology.

Senator MCCASKILL. Well, the fact that the States all have different programs and that we have the high improper payment number that we have and it is growing, it certainly would be one point that you would want to make if we were going to be block-granting the money, because if we block-grant the money, then we lose all controls, not just dealing with perhaps different scenarios or provider taxes based on the State but, rather, a situation where we would just send the money out and trust them.

Mr. DODARO. Yes, it depends on how you design it. If you capped it and said, OK, this is all the money that you are going to get, then there is an incentive—part of the issue here has been an incentive issue because of the Federal match.

Senator MCCASKILL. Right.

Mr. DODARO. Senator Daines pointed this out, and he is exactly right.

Senator MCCASKILL. Right.

Mr. DODARO. The incentives have not all been aligned properly, and I think a lot of the State attention to this has increased, particularly in the expansion States, as they see it is rapidly growing, being a bigger portion of the budget, the Federal match is going to start tapering off from 100 percent——

Senator MCCASKILL. To 90, though. It never goes below 90.

Mr. DODARO. Right.

Senator MCCASKILL. Assuming the law does not change.

Mr. DODARO. Right, but they still see that they need to do more in this area. That is why the State auditors are beginning to step up.

Senator MCCASKILL. That would be great.

I want to turn to a report you did back in 2011, and what you did at the GAO in 2011 is you looked at application and coverage denials in the individual health and insurance market. And I have gone back and looked at that because we now have this Administration going to court along with the Attorney General of my State asking the courts to do away with the preexisting condition protection along with many of the others—capped payments and the ability to charge women more for insurance just because they are women. There is a variety of protections that we have in there for consumers that this Administration is now actively, along with these Attorneys General, trying to get rid of and make sure that they completely go away.

I would like you to talk about the sources of information you used for your 2011 report, if you could give us that. What data did you use to determine the level of coverage denial in the years before, immediately before we put the ACA protections in?

Mr. DODARO. As I recall, and I will provide the details for the record,[13] but we used data that HHS had been collecting. We also went to a few States to see if they had better information since they have delegated responsibility for a lot of insurance issues. And then we also had information from the American health insurance industry as well. So we had those three sort of data sources.

Senator MCCASKILL. And your review found there were two kinds of denials. There is an application denial.

Mr. DODARO. Right.

Senator MCCASKILL. And I put into the record and I would ask it be put into the record in this hearing also Humana's document[14] that listed 400 diseases that required application denial, along with a number of occupations, including air traffic controller, steel-worker.

So there is an application denial and then there is a policy they were writing that allowed them to do a coverage denial. So if you had, for example, a heart condition, they might insure you, but you would have to pay out of your own pocket for anything having to do with your heart condition—in other words, completely incomplete insurance, and that was called "coverage denial."

So on the application denial, do you recall what the denial rate was on average for people who were trying to get insurance?

Mr. DODARO. Yes, the national figure we had was 19 percent, but it varied among insurers.

Senator MCCASKILL. OK. So some insurers it was higher, some——

Mr. DODARO. Some of it was up to 40 percent or more. Others were 0 to 15 percent. So there was a lot of variation, but the overall national average I believe was 19 percent denial.

Senator MCCASKILL. So one in five people that tried to get insurance were denied the opportunity to get insurance because they had been sick before. Is that an accurate finding of your report prior to the ACA protections?

Mr. DODARO. Yes, that is, with certain limitations. I mean, we do not know whether or not they applied somewhere else and got coverage or whether they actually ended up getting coverage but had a higher premium rate. So there was not a lot of good data available. We had what was available, and it is appropriately caveated in the report. But that is what we said.

Senator MCCASKILL. And what about the denial of coverage? What did you find as it related to the denial of coverage?

---

[13] The information submitted by Mr. Dodaro appears in the Appendix on page 179.

[14] The Humana document referenced by Senator McCaskill appears in the Appendix on page 127.

Mr. DODARO. That was very detailed, very specific. I do not have a good answer for that at an aggregate level as well. But what I recall on the application denial side, the 19 percent, it was not really clear why they denied it. So the only other data that was available at that point was from the America's Health Insurance Plans and what they said was that the denial rate was much higher for medical reasons than non-medical reasons, for example, you were not in the right geographic area. So that was abouyt 1 percent. About 13 percent of the denials were because of medical conditions and their underwriting status.

I can give you for the record the coverage denial detail from that report.[15]

Senator MCCASKILL. I just wanted to bring it out because I think people forget—I mean, there was not an effort to pass the ACA because all of us were trying to make people's lives miserable. The effort was to try to give consumers some protections from some gross abuses that had grown up in the industry, and people were really searching for coverage and could not find it, could not get it. So I think it is important that we remember that in context and that we not throw out the preexisting condition protection unless and until we can come up with something that will replace it with the same level of protection.

Thank you, Mr. Chairman.

Chairman JOHNSON. And we will enter that Humana report in the record.[16]

Senator MCCASKILL. Yes.

Chairman JOHNSON. Not a problem.

I have only really got one more line of questioning here. It really does have to do with what sometimes is referred to as "State gimmicks." We refer to it in our report. I am talking about, for example—perfectly legal but it ends up costing the Federal Government more money and certainly increased the percentage of the Federal Government's match to the States. I am talking about, for example, State sales taxes or loans the State makes to cities that they claim—they get reimbursement at their match rate, and then they pay the loan back to the State.

Do you have a sense of how much those and other, I would call them, "gimmicks" really cost in terms of additional Federal spending?

Mr. DODARO. We have had some examples that we did in reports over the years, but no one really knows because CMS does not really collect the type of information necessary to make those determinations. That is part of our recommendations, is to have more information about what the sources of those funds are every year. There are supposed to be limits on how much they need to raise from local governments. For example, the State share is supposed to only gather up to 60 percent of their fair share from local providers or other sources, and no one knows whether that limit is really met on a regular basis. And that is one of our recommendations.

---

[15] The information submitted by Mr. Dodaro appears in the Appendix on page 180.

[16] The Humana report appears in the Appendix on page 127.

I know Brian has done some work in that area, too. I am sure he has something to add.

Mr. RITCHIE. Again, we do not have it quantified either, I think for the same reasons. We have reports out on a few States. Recently we have some ongoing work looking at the safe harbor and it is mentioned in your report. But I think the same issues, that it is just not being tracked, that we see this, and that the safe harbor may be met, but then that still allows the general process of the shifting of funds. And back to a point I made earlier, I think just for us the general intent is the dollars are spent. We just think—asked the question: Is this leading to better care for beneficiaries or is this leading to a shift in resources? And it is hard as an IG because it is not necessarily violating rules. The rule in place right now is it is up to the 6 percent. But if you look at it we are able to track it from an audit standpoint look and see a provider paid taxes, then the Federal share came in, and when the additional resources were sent, the supplemental payments went back; and the net effect is the Federal Government paid and the State really did not sort of come out any worse. It was sort of a net zero effect.

Mr. DODARO. Yes, the other thing——

Chairman JOHNSON. The States actually come out quite a bit better.

Mr. DODARO. Oh, yes.

Chairman JOHNSON. Yes. So is it measurable?

Mr. DODARO. If you have the data, you could measure it. And they should have the information to check.

Chairman JOHNSON. So is that something if I wrote either one of your gentlemen or both of you a letter, would you commit to doing a study on that to try and quantify it?

Mr. DODARO. We could see——

Chairman JOHNSON. Who wants to volunteer?

Mr. DODARO. Yes, we could see if it is feasible to do.

Chairman JOHNSON. OK.

Mr. DODARO. We can go back in and look at a sample of States, for example, and try to measure it that way. But it will take a while to do it because the data is not readily available, and you would have to go in and take a look at it. But I think we could do a study, but we have also got open recommendations that you could support, have CMS collect this information, because unless they collect it and do something with it, our study is really not going to change the outcome of this situation.

Chairman JOHNSON. I was struck in your answer on other audits in comparison to—again, CMS runs both Medicare and Medicaid, correct?

Mr. DODARO. Right.

Chairman JOHNSON. And I am really giving them praise in terms of how they are managing Medicare and doing the audits, that type of thing. The fact they are not dog it on Medicaid, with some caveats, do you almost get the sense that it is willful ignorance?

Mr. DODARO. Well, there has always been a deference to States, and that can go too far in terms of balancing the Federal interest versus States' flexibility. That has been an issue historically in our intergovernmental system. You see it in many different programs over time. Temporary Assistance for Needy Families (TANF) is another example. But, this program, as it started out, according to your chart really did not have much in expenditures, and letting the States have flexibility made sense. But now the stakes are higher, and the costs are not sustainable over the long term, and CMS need to change their paradigm. And they have been slow to do that.

Chairman JOHNSON. But, also, when both parties have skin in the game, there literally is an incentive to try and keep down the cost. But as one partner has more skin and the other partner does not—and that is exactly what Medicaid expansion does—it is what these State gimmicks do. It reduces the amount of skin in the game the States have, and it now starts shifting the incentive to, for example, sign up people that are ineligible because you get more Federal money.

The bottom line is oversight is critical, auditing this is critical. Designing the program so you actually have the incentives—and I would say the block grant would give every incentive to the State for efficient spending because they are going to have—according to Graham-Cassidy-Heller-Johnson, it would be money block-granted on the basic number of people in your State, the poverty rates, those types of things. That is not incentivizing you to sign more people up. You are going to get a set amount, and you better spend that as efficiently and as flexible as possible and do the best for your citizens. So to me that completely puts the incentive back where it belongs, at the State level where it will be a little more efficient, a little more effective, hopefully more accountable versus this one-size-fits-all model, which a $37 billion improper payment amount shows it is not being done very efficiently and effectively.

Anyway, so you will expect that letter just in terms of the feasibility of that study. I think we might be shocked at how much money that actually costs us.

Again, I want to thank both the witnesses for your great testimony and for taking the time. General Dodaro, you realize we are never going to let you retire. [Laughter.]

Mr. DODARO. Well, I have 7½ years left on my term, and then we can negotiate.

Chairman JOHNSON. I am amazed at—we are talking about— Senator McCaskill was asking about a study from 2011, and you have that at the tip of your fingers. I am always amazed at your ability to recall these things and provide detailed testimony off the top of your head.

And, Mr. Ritchie, again, thank you for all of your work. This Committee depends on the good work of Inspectors General and the Government Accountability Office. So thank you both for your testimony.

The hearing record will remain open for 15 days until July 12th at 5 p.m. for the submission of statements and questions for the record.

This hearing is adjourned.

[Whereupon, at 12:07 p.m., the Committee was adjourned.]

"MEDICAID FRAUD AND OVERPAYMENTS: PROBLEMS AND SOLUTIONS" OPENING STATEMENT OF CHAIRMAN RON JOHNSON, JUNE 27, 2018

Good morning and welcome.

The U.S. health care financing system is broken and increasingly is dominated by the government. By transitioning to a third-party payment system, we have separated the consumer of health care products and services from the direct payment for them. Most consumers don't know what treatments costs, and except for the cost of insurance or copays, they really don't care. We have removed the benefit of free market competition from health care, and costs have predictably soared. Since 1960, the share of all health care spending paid by government has more than doubled, from about one-fifth to just under half. The result: Overall health spending now consumes nearly 20 percent of the nation's GDP.

Central to this unsustainable growth is Medicaid. When President Lyndon Johnson signed Medicaid into law in 1965, he extolled the new Medicare program—but didn't even mention Medicaid. That first year, Medicaid enrolled just four million people, at a cost of $222 per enrollee.

Today, Medicaid is the nation's largest health insurer. It covers about 70 million people—one in five Americans—at a total cost to taxpayers of $554 billion per year. Per enrollee, Medicaid now costs nearly $8,000, a 3,491 percent increase over 1966. This strain on the American taxpayer will only continue to grow. Federal Medicaid spending is expected by 2025 to rise 96 percent above its 2014 level, in significant part because of Obamacare's Medicaid expansion. The Centers for Medicare & Medicaid Services, which runs Medicaid with the states, significantly understated its projections for how much that expansion would cost.

With federal Medicaid spending growing at an alarming rate, it is more important than ever that each Medicaid dollar is spent on someone in need. But we know that is far from the case. The Medicaid program doles out $37 billion a year of improper payments, a 157 percent increase since 2013. Medicaid accounted for 26 percent of all the improper payments made by the federal government in fiscal year 2017.

Medicaid's financial problems were highly predictable. The Government Accountability Office first deemed Medicaid a "high risk" program in 2003. Since then, the GAO has consistently reported on Medicaid's vulnerability to waste and fraud, and the need for the CMS to take proactive measures to reduce improper payments. The inspector general of the Department of Health and Human Services found that three states, principally California, spent over $1 billion in federal Medicaid funds on behalf of more than a half-million ineligible or potentially ineligible people. Apparently, CMS has no plans to recoup these funds.

The first steps in solving any problem are admitting you have one and then properly defining it. To that end, we are pleased to welcome Gene Dodaro, the comptroller general, who will testify about the GAO's work identifying Medicaid fraud and recommending solutions to CMS. We also welcome Brian P. Ritchie, the assistant HHS inspector general for audit services.

Last week, I also released a staff report that finds that CMS has failed to adequately police Medicaid fraud and overpayments. We look forward to having CMS Administrator Verma testify in the near future about the report's conclusions and the steps CMS is taking to tackle Medicaid fraud and overpayments. I thank our witnesses for their service, and I look forward to your testimony.

U.S. Senate Homeland Security and Governmental Affairs Committee, "Medicaid Fraud and Overpayments: Problems and Solutions," June 27, 2018, Ranking Member Claire McCaskill, Opening Statement

Thank you, Mr. Chairman. Mr. Chairman, I am happy to be here today with you, Mr. Dodaro, and Mr. Ritchie to discuss efforts to reduce improper payments in the Medicaid program.

Medicaid provides health care coverage to more than 70 million Americans, regardless of pre-existing conditions. In 2016, Medicaid spending totaled $565.5 billion and accounted for a full 17% of national health expenditures that year. Medicaid is a very important program, and it is this Committee's responsibility to ensure that the Medicaid program—and all government programs—are spending taxpayer dollars appropriately and efficiently.

According to CMS, Medicaid improper payments reached an estimated $37 billion in 2017. That is a full 10 percent of the total federal spending on Medicaid! That number is outrageous and CMS needs to find a way to bring that number way down. That is one of the reasons why just last week, we passed bipartisan legislation out of committee to cut down on improper payments made by the federal government. If enacted, our bill will require CMS and other agencies to undertake additional efforts and develop plans to prevent improper payments before they happen. These measures have the potential to save the government billions of dollars. Our bill is an important step to eradicate government waste and make important programs work for all Americans.

In addition to enacting the Stopping Improper Payments to Deceased People Act, there is no shortage of recommendations and concrete steps CMS can put into place today to enhance oversight efforts and prevent future improper payments. But let's be clear: Medicaid is an important program for Americans. And Medicaid expansion has been incredibly important as well, ensuring 12 million additional Americans were able to receive health care coverage under Medicaid for the first time. We need to make the program more efficient, but fixing its problems should not be confused with calling for an end to an important health program that millions of Americans rely upon for their medical care.

If a lawsuit against the Affordable Care Act brought by Republican Attorneys General is successful, insurance companies will once again be permitted to refuse health care coverage to vulnerable Americans with pre-existing health conditions. Workers will be locked in jobs just because it offers them insurance. And, once again, insurance companies will discriminate against millions of Americans based on their health status.

Mr. Chairman, I think we may need a reminder of what the world looked like before the passage of the Affordable Care Act. I seek unanimous consent to enter a document into the record. This memo was issued by the House Energy and Commerce Committee in 2010 following enactment of the ACA and the committee's investigation found the four largest for-profit health insurance companies denied over 600,000 individuals coverage because of pre-existing conditions in the three years before passage of health reform. The committee's investigation found that for certain medical conditions, companies routinely denied health insurance coverage without any further review. According to one internal memorandum created in 2006, one insurance company created a list of certain medical conditions that would result in an automatic denial of coverage. No further conversation necessary. No insurance for you. The categories included:

- "Any applicant who is a surgical candidate."
- "Any female applicant currently pregnant."
- Any applicant with a BMI [body mass index] of 39.0 or greater."

GAO also did important work documenting the rate at which insurance companies discriminated against people with pre-existing conditions. In a 2011 report, GAO found a quarter of insurers had denial rates of 40 percent or higher. I look forward to speaking to Mr. Dodaro about his findings on pre-existing conditions in more detail during my questions.

There are up to 130 million adults under the age of 65 with pre-existing conditions in the U.S. We cannot go back to a time when people were automatically denied health care coverage due solely to their health status.

Thank you, Mr. Chairman.

MEDICAID: ACTIONS NEEDED TO MITIGATE BILLIONS IN IMPROPER PAYMENTS AND PROGRAM INTEGRITY RISKS*

Gene L. Dodaro

Why GAO Did This Study

Medicaid, a joint federal-state health care program overseen by CMS, is a significant component of federal and state budgets, with total estimated expenditures of $596 billion in fiscal year 2017.

Medicaid allows significant flexibility for states to design and implement program innovations based on their unique needs. The resulting diversity of the program and its size, make the program particularly challenging to oversee at the federal level and also vulnerable to improper payments. In fiscal year 2017, estimated improper payments were $36.7 billion in Medicaid, up from $29.1 billion in fiscal year 2015. Further, the Medicaid program accounted for about 26 percent of the fiscal year 2017 government-wide improper payment estimate.

This testimony focuses on the (1) major risks to the integrity of the Medicaid program, and (2) actions needed to manage these risks. This testimony draws on GAO's reports issued between November 2012 and May 2018 on the Medicaid program.

What GAO Recommends

As a part of this body of work, GAO has made 83 recommendations to address shortcomings in Medicaid oversight and suggested four matters for congressional consideration. The Department of Health and Human Services and CMS have generally agreed with these recommendations and have implemented 25 of them.

GAO will continue to monitor implementation of the remaining recommendations.

---

* This is an edited, reformatted and augmented version of United States Government Accountability Office, Testimony, Before the Committee on Homeland Security and Governmental Affairs, U.S. Senate, Publication No. GAO-18-598T, dated June 27, 2018.

What GAO Found

GAO's work has identified three broad areas of risk in Medicaid that also contribute to overall growth in program spending, projected to exceed $900 billion in fiscal year 2025.

1) Improper payments, including payments made for services not actually provided. Regarding managed care payments, which were nearly half (or $280 billion) of Medicaid spending in fiscal year 2017, GAO has found that the full extent of program risk due to overpayments and unallowable costs is unknown.
2) Supplemental payments, which are payments made to providers—such as local government hospitals—that are in addition to regular, claims-based payments made to providers for specific services. These payments totaled more than $48 billion in fiscal year 2016 and in some cases have shifted expenditures from the states to the federal government.
3) Demonstrations, which allow states to test new approaches to coverage. Comprising about one-third of total Medicaid expenditures in fiscal year 2015, GAO has found that demonstrations have increased federal costs without providing results that can be used to inform policy decisions.

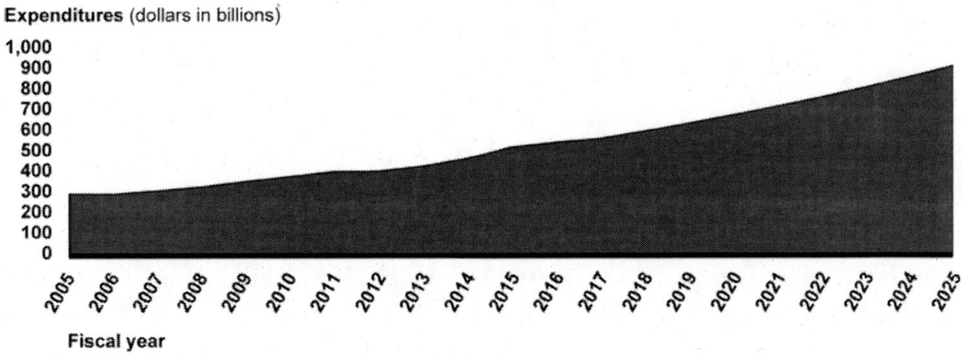

Source: 2016 Actuarial Report on the Financial Outlook for Medicaid. | GAO-18-598T.

Actual and Projected Growth Trends in Total Medicaid Spending.

GAO's work has recommended numerous actions to strengthen oversight and manage program risks.

- Improve data. The Centers for Medicare & Medicaid Services (CMS), which oversees Medicaid, needs to make sustained efforts to ensure Medicaid data are timely, complete, and comparable from all states, and useful for program oversight. Data are also needed for oversight of supplemental payments and ensuring that demonstrations are meeting their stated goals.

- Target fraud. CMS needs to conduct a fraud risk assessment for Medicaid, and design and implement a risk-based antifraud strategy for the program.
- Collaborate. There is a need for a collaborative approach to Medicaid oversight. State auditors have conducted evaluations that identified significant improper payments and outlined deficiencies in Medicaid processes that require resolution.

Chairman Johnson, Ranking Member McCaskill, and Members of the Committee:

I appreciate the opportunity to be here today to discuss areas of risk to the Medicaid program and oversight efforts that can help prevent improper payments and ensure the program's fiscal integrity.[17] The federal-state Medicaid program is one of the nation's largest sources of funding for medical and health-related services. In fiscal year 2017, the program covered acute health care, long-term care, and other services for over 73 million low income and medically needy individuals. In that same year, estimated federal and state Medicaid expenditures were $596 billion.

Medicaid has been on our high-risk list since 2003, in part, because of concerns about the adequacy of fiscal oversight and the program's improper payments—including payments made for people not eligible for Medicaid or services not actually provided.[18] The Medicaid program accounted for 26.1 percent of the fiscal year 2017 government-wide improper payment estimate.[19] While efforts to reduce improper payments have been made by the Centers for Medicare & Medicaid Services (CMS), the agency within the Department of Health and Human Services (HHS) that oversees Medicaid, overall improper payments continue to increase. In fiscal year 2017, improper payments accounted for $36.7 billion of Medicaid spending, up from $29.1 billion in fiscal year 2015. Of the $36.7 billion in improper payments, $36.4 billion were overpayments and $283 million were underpayments.

The size, complexity, and diversity of Medicaid make the program particularly challenging to oversee at the federal level. Medicaid allows significant flexibility for states to design and implement program innovations based on their unique needs; however, our prior work has found that these innovations have grown considerably over time, lack complete and accurate reporting, and do not always ensure the efficient use of federal dollars. It is critical that CMS and states take appropriate measures to reduce improper payments and ensure the fiscal integrity of Medicaid; as dollars wasted detract

---

[17] An improper payment is any payment that should not have been made or that was made in an incorrect amount (including overpayments and underpayments) under statutory, contractual, administrative, or other legally applicable requirements. It includes any payment to an ineligible recipient, any payment for an ineligible service, any duplicate payment, payment for services not received (except where authorized by law), and any payment that does not account for credit for applicable discounts. See 31 U.S.C. § 3321 note. Office of Management and Budget guidance also instructs agencies to report as improper payments any payments for which insufficient or no documentation is found.

[18] See GAO, *High-Risk Series: Progress on Many High-Risk Areas, While Substantial Efforts Needed on Others*. GAO-17-317 (Washington, D.C.: Feb. 15, 2017).

[19] See GAO, *Improper Payments: Actions and Guidance Could Help Address Issues and Inconsistencies in Estimation Processes*. GAO-18-377 (Washington, D.C.: May 31, 2018).

from the program's ability to ensure that the individuals who rely on Medicaid—including low-income children and individuals who are elderly or disabled—are provided adequate care.

My testimony today will focus on

1) major risks to the integrity of the Medicaid program, and
2) actions needed to manage these risks.

My remarks are based on our large body of work examining the Medicaid program, particularly reports issued and recommendations made from November 2012 to May 2018; these reports provide further details on our scope and methodology. (A list of related reports is included at the end of this statement.) For further context, my remarks also reference information reported by state auditors and the HHS Office of Inspector General (HHS-OIG), including information from two meetings with state auditors and Inspectors General we hosted in March and May 2018. We conducted all of the work on which this statement is based in accordance with generally accepted government auditing standards. Those standards require that we plan and perform the audit to obtain sufficient, appropriate evidence to provide a reasonable basis for our findings and conclusions based on our audit objectives. We believe that the evidence obtained provides a reasonable basis for our findings and conclusions based on our audit objectives.

Background

Among health care programs, Medicaid is the largest as measured by enrollment (over 73 million in fiscal year 2017) and the second largest as measured by expenditures ($596 billion in fiscal year 2017), second only to Medicare. The CMS Office of the Actuary projected that Medicaid spending would grow at an average rate of 5.7 percent per year, from fiscal years 2016 to 2025, with projected Medicaid expenditures reaching $958 billion by fiscal year 2025.[20] This projected growth in expenditures reflects both expected increases in expenditures per enrollee and in levels of Medicaid enrollment. Beneficiaries with disabilities and those who are elderly constitute the highest per enrollee expenditures, which are projected to increase by almost 50 percent from fiscal year 2016 to 2025. Medicaid enrollment is also expected to grow by as many as 13.2 million newly eligible adults by 2025—as additional states may expand their Medicaid

---

[20] Data are from the most recently issued CMS actuarial report. See Centers for Medicare & Medicaid Services, Office of the Actuary, *2016 Actuarial Report on the Financial Outlook for Medicaid* (Washington, D.C.: 2016).

programs to cover certain low-income adults under the Patient Protection and Affordable Care Act (PPACA).[21] (See Figure 1).

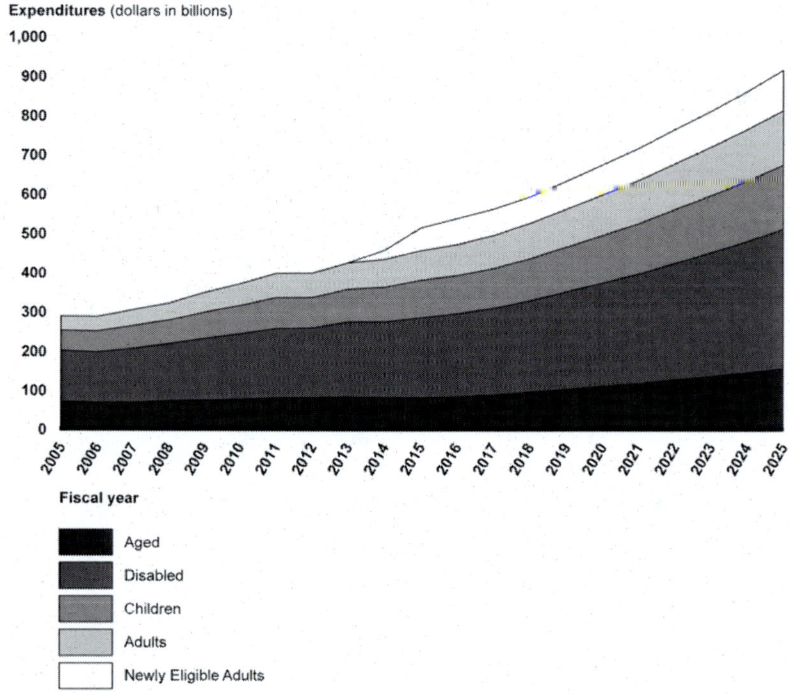

Source: GAO analysis of 2016 Actuarial Report on the Financial Outlook for Medicaid. | GAO-18-598T.

Note: Data after fiscal year 2012 are projected expenditures.

Figure 1. Growth Trends in Total Medicaid Spending by Eligibility Group.

The partnership between the federal government and states is a central tenet of the Medicaid program. CMS provides oversight and technical assistance for the program, and states are responsible for administering their respective Medicaid programs' day-to-day operations—including determining eligibility, enrolling individuals and providers, and adjudicating claims—within broad federal requirements. Federal oversight includes ensuring that the design and operation of state programs meet federal requirements and that Medicaid payments are made appropriately. (See Figure 2 for a diagram of the federal-state Medicaid partnership framework.) Joint financing of Medicaid is also a fixture of the federal-state partnership, with the federal government matching most state

[21] The Patient Protection and Affordable Care Act, enacted on March 23, 2010, permits states to expand their Medicaid programs to cover nonelderly, nonpregnant adults who are not eligible for Medicare, and whose income does not exceed 133 percent of the federal poverty level. Because of the way the limit is calculated, using what is known as an "income disregard," the level is effectively 138 percent of the federal poverty level. Pub. L. No. 111-148, 124 Stat. 119 (2010), as amended by the Health Care and Education Reconciliation Act of 2010 (HCERA), Pub. L. No. 111-152, 124 Stat. 1029 (2010).

Medicaid expenditures using a statutory formula based, in part, on each state's per capita income in relation to the national average per capita income.

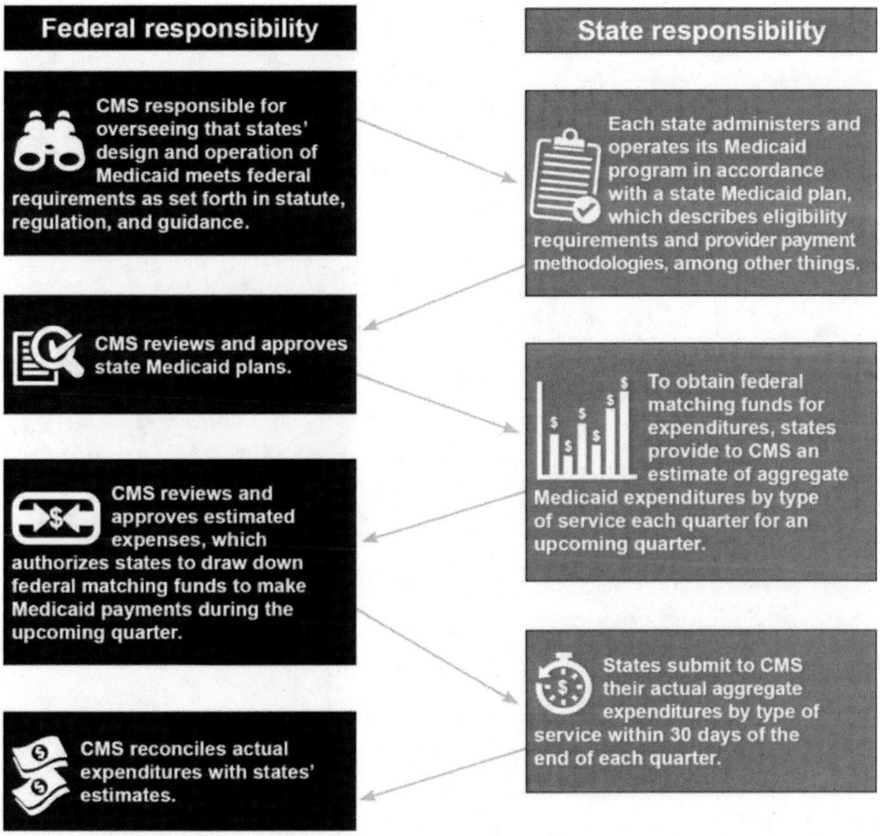

Source: GAO. | GAO-18-598T.

Note: If a state wishes to make amendments to its state Medicaid plan, it must seek approval from the Centers for Medicare & Medicaid Services (CMS). Similarly, a state that desires to change its Medicaid program in ways that deviate from certain federal requirements may seek to do so through a Medicaid demonstration waiver approved under section 1115 of the Social Security Act, which is outside of its state Medicaid plan. States must submit an application describing the proposed section 1115 demonstration to CMS for review. CMS will specify the special terms and conditions that encompass the requirements for an approved demonstration.

Figure 2. Federal-State Medicaid Partnership Framework.

States have flexibility in determining how their Medicaid benefits are delivered. For example, states may (1) contract with managed care organizations to provide a specific set of Medicaid-covered services to beneficiaries and pay the organizations a set amount, generally on a per beneficiary per month basis; (2) pay health care providers for each service they provide on a fee-for-service basis; or (3) rely on a combination of both delivery systems.[22] Managed care continues to be a growing component of the Medicaid program. In fiscal year 2017, expenditures for managed care were $280 billion, representing almost half of total program expenditures, compared with 42 percent in fiscal year 2015. (See Figure 3.)

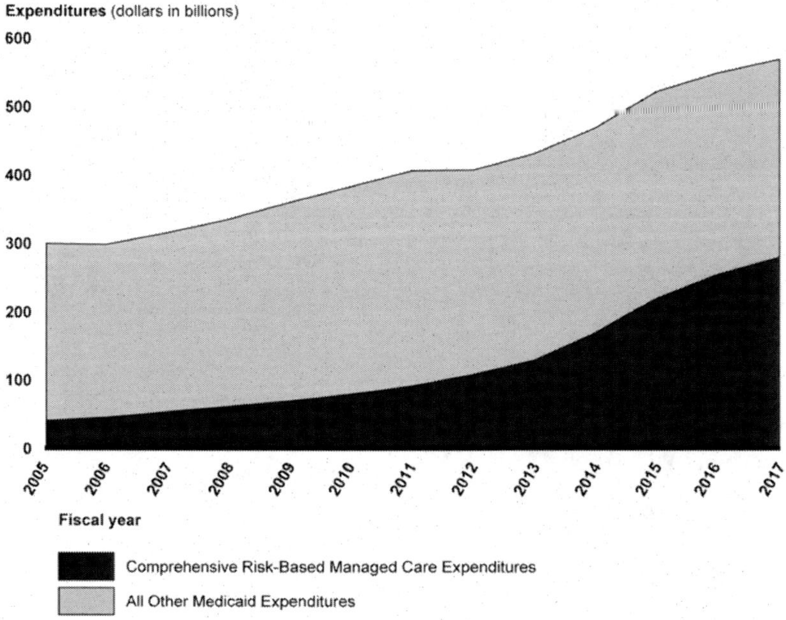

Source: GAO analysis of Centers for Medicare & Medicaid Services expenditures data. | GAO-18-598T.

Note: States may have different types of managed care arrangements in Medicaid; managed care expenditures in this figure include expenditures for comprehensive, risk-based managed care—the most common type of managed care arrangement.

Figure 3. Growth in Comprehensive Risk-Based Managed Care as a Share of Total Medicaid Expenditures, Fiscal Years 2005 through 2017.

States also have the flexibility to innovate outside of many of Medicaid's otherwise applicable requirements through Medicaid demonstrations approved under section 1115 of the Social Security Act.[23] These demonstrations allow states to test new approaches to

---

[22] CMS has also been developing and testing a variety of value-based payment models, under which physicians and other providers are paid and responsible for the care of a beneficiary for a long period and accountable for the quality and efficiency of the care provided. Examples of these models include accountable care organizations—groups of physicians and other health care providers who voluntarily work together to provide coordinated care—and bundled payment models, which provide a "bundled" payment intended to cover the multiple services beneficiaries receive during an episode of care for certain health conditions, such as hip replacements, congestive heart failure, and pregnancy.

[23] Under section 1115 of the Social Security Act, the Secretary of Health and Human Services may waive certain Medicaid requirements and approve new types of expenditures that would not otherwise be eligible for federal Medicaid matching funds for experimental, pilot, or demonstration projects that, in the Secretary's judgment, are likely to promote Medicaid objectives. See 42 U.S.C. § 1315(a). The Secretary has delegated the approval and administration of Medicaid section 1115 demonstrations to CMS, which requires that such demonstrations be budget neutral to the federal government; that is, the federal government should spend no more for

coverage and to improve quality and access, or generate savings or efficiencies. For example, under demonstrations, states have

- extended coverage to certain populations,
- provided services not otherwise eligible for federal matching funds, and
- made incentive payments to providers for delivery system improvements.

As of November 2016, nearly three-quarters of states have CMS-approved demonstrations. In fiscal year 2015, total spending under demonstrations represented a third of all Medicaid spending nationwide. (See Figure 4.)

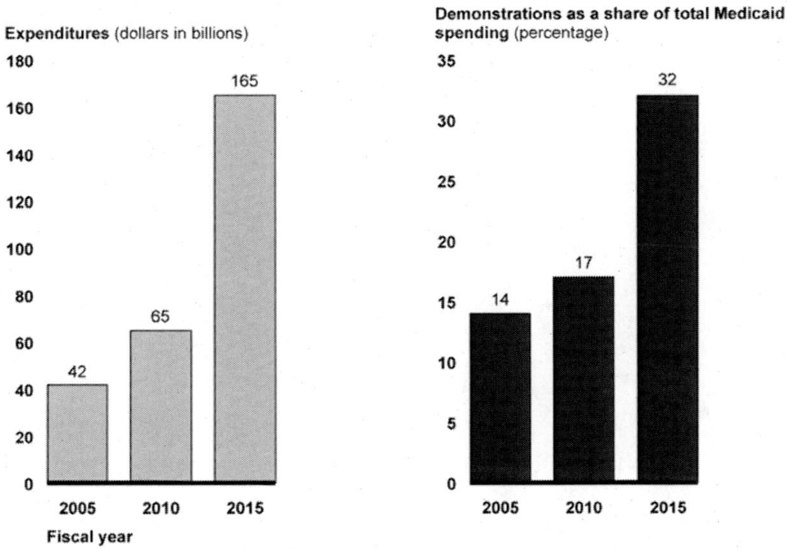

Source: GAO analysis of Centers for Medicare & Medicaid Services demonstration expenditures data. | GAO-18-598T.

Figure 4. Total Expenditures under Medicaid Section 1115 Demonstrations, Fiscal Years 2005, 2010, and 2015.

In addition to other types of improper payments, Medicaid presents opportunities for fraud, because of the size, expenditures, and complexities of the program—including the variation in states' design and implementation. Medicaid Fraud Control Units (MFCU)—state entities responsible for investigating and prosecuting Medicaid fraud—have reported on Medicaid fraud convictions and recovered monies, in their annual reports.[24] For example, over the past 5 years, MFCUs have reported an average of 1,072 yearly

Medicaid under a state's demonstration than it would have spent without the demonstration. There are other types of waivers that states can apply for and use, including those approved under section 1915(c) of the Social Security Act, which authorizes the Secretary of Health and Human Services to waive requirements that states providing home and community based services would otherwise need to meet in the absence of the waiver.

[24] Nearly all states have MFCUs responsible for investigating and prosecuting Medicaid fraud. MFCUs are funded jointly by the federal government and the states, and HHS-OIG provides oversight.

Medicaid fraud convictions. They also reported about $680 million in recoveries related to fraud in fiscal year 2017—almost double the recoveries from fiscal year 2016.[25]

Three Broad Areas of Risk Threaten the Fiscal Integrity of Medicaid

Our prior work has identified three broad areas of risk to the fiscal integrity of Medicaid: improper payment rates, state use of supplemental payments, and oversight of demonstration programs.

Estimated Improper Payments Exceed 10 Percent, and Do Not Fully Account for All Program Risks

CMS annually computes the national Medicaid improper payment estimate as a weighted average of states' improper payment estimates for three component parts—fee-for-service, beneficiary eligibility determinations, and managed care. The improper payment estimate for each component is developed under its own methodology.[26] The national rate in fiscal year 2017 was 10.1 percent, or $36.7 billion. Since 2016, Medicaid has exceeded the 10 percent criterion set in statute. As such, the program was not fully compliant with the Improper Payments Elimination and Recovery Act of 2010.[27]

In May 2018, we reported that the Medicaid managed care component of the improper payment estimate does not fully account for all program risks in managed care.[28] We identified 10 federal and state audits and investigations (out of 27 focused on Medicaid managed care) that cited about $68 million in overpayments and unallowable managed care organization costs that were not accounted for by the managed care improper payment estimate. Another of these investigations resulted in a $137.5 million settlement to resolve allegations of false claims.[29] We further noted that the full extent of overpayments and unallowable costs is unknown, because the 27 audits and investigations we reviewed were conducted over more than 5 years and involved a small fraction of the more than 270 managed care organizations operating nationwide as of September 2017.

---

[25] See Department of Health and Human Services, Office of Inspector General, *Medicaid Fraud Control Units Fiscal Year 2017 Annual Report*, OEI-09-18-00180 (Washington, D.C.: March 2018).

[26] CMS has not calculated the beneficiary eligibility determinations component estimate since 2014 and has held constant this component of the national rate at 3.1 percent.

Beginning in the 2019 reporting year, the agency plans to resume improper payment estimates for eligibility determinations.

[27] When an agency is determined to not be in compliance with one or more of the Improper Payments Elimination and Recovery Act criteria by its Inspector General, it must submit a plan to Congress describing the actions it will take to come into compliance.

[28] States may have different types of managed care arrangements in Medicaid; our findings apply to comprehensive, risk-based managed care, the most common type of managed care arrangement. See GAO, *Medicaid: CMS Should Take Steps to Mitigate Program Risks in Managed Care*, GAO-18-291 (Washington, D.C.: May 7, 2018).

[29] See GAO-18-291.

Some examples of the state audits that identified overpayments and unallowable costs include the following:

- The Washington State Auditor's Office found that two managed care organizations made $17.5 million in overpayments to providers in 2010, which may have increased the state's 2013 capitation rates.[30]
- The Texas State Auditor's Office found that one managed care organization reported $3.8 million in unallowable costs for advertising, company events, gifts, and stock options, along with $34 million in other questionable costs in 2015.[31]
- The New York State Comptroller found that two managed care organizations paid over $6.6 million to excluded and deceased providers from 2011 through 2014.[32]

To the extent that such overpayments and unallowable costs are unidentified and not removed from the cost data used to set managed care payment rates, they may allow inflated future payments and minimize the appearance of program risks in Medicaid managed care. This potential understatement of the program risks in managed care also may curtail investigations into the appropriateness of managed care spending. The continued growth of Medicaid managed care makes ensuring the accuracy of managed care improper payment estimates increasingly important.

In May 2018, we acknowledged that although CMS has increased its focus on and worked with states to improve oversight of Medicaid managed care; its efforts—for example, updated regulations and audits of managed care providers—did not ensure the identification and reporting of overpayments and unallowable costs.[33] In May 2016, CMS updated its regulations for managed care programs, including that states arrange an independent audit of the data submitted by MCOs, at least once every 3 years. We found that although this requirement has the potential to enhance state oversight of managed care; CMS was reviewing the rule for possible revision of its requirements.[34] We also noted that another effort to address program risks in managed care—the use of CMS program integrity contractors to audit providers that are paid by managed care

[30] Washington State Auditor, *Performance Audit: Health Care Authority's Oversight of the Medicaid Managed Care Program*, Audit No. 1011450 (April 14, 2014).

[31] Texas State Auditor, *An Audit Report on HealthSpring Life and Health Insurance Company, Inc., a Medicaid STAR+PLUS Managed Care Organization*, Report No. 17-025 (Austin, Tex.: February 2017).

[32] New York State Office of the State Comptroller, *Medicaid Managed Care Organization Fraud and Abuse Detection*, Report 2014-S-51 (Albany, N.Y.: July 15, 2016). HHS-OIG has the authority to exclude providers from federal health care programs, and maintains a list of all currently excluded providers called the List of Excluded Individuals/Entities. No payment may be made from any federal health care program for any items or services furnished, ordered, or prescribed by an excluded provider.

[33] GAO-18-291.

[34] CMS indicated it will issue a Notice of Proposed Rulemaking in 2018 to streamline Medicaid managed care regulations and reduce burden. See Department of Health and Human Services, Medicaid and CHIP Managed Care, *Spring 2018 Unified Agenda of Federal Regulatory and Deregulatory Actions*, (CMS-2480-P), RIN 0938-AT40, accessed in May 14, 2018, http://www.reginfo.gov.

organizations—has been limited. To address the program risks that are not measured as a part of CMS's methodology to estimate improper payments, in May 2018 we recommended that CMS take steps to mitigate such risks, which could include revising its methodology or focusing additional audit resources on managed care. HHS concurred with this recommendation.[35]

Table 1. Examples of GAO recommendations to address Medicaid program risks associated with managed care, provider enrollment, and beneficiary eligibility determinations

Program risks	GAO recommendations	Recommendation status
Addressing key risks, such as the extent of overpayments and unallowable costs, that are not measured in the managed care component of the Centers for Medicare & Medicaid Services' (CMS) improper payment estimate	One recommendation aimed at mitigating identified risks, such as revising the methodology to calculate the managed care component or focusing additional audit resources on managed care.[a]	CMS concurred with our recommendation, and indicated that it will review regulatory authority and audit resources to determine the best way to account for Medicaid program risks that are not accounted for in the managed care component.
Ensuring that only eligible providers are enrolled in Medicaid	Four recommendations aimed at assessing the databases used to screen providers, improve collaboration and coordination with other federal agencies on sharing databases and establishing a common identifier across databases, and providing guidance to state Medicaid agencies.[b]	CMS has addressed two of the four recommendations. To implement one remaining recommendation, CMS will need to determine whether the remaining databases (used by states and health plans to screen providers) that it has studied should be added to the agency's list of the databases used for screening purposes. For the other remaining recommendation, CMS needs to explore the use of a common identifier for screening providers across databases.
Ensuring that only eligible beneficiaries are enrolled in Medicaid	Two recommendations that CMS review federal determinations of Medicaid eligibility for accuracy, and take steps to increase assurance that expenditures for the different eligibility groups are correctly reported and appropriately matched.[c]	CMS established a more rigorous approach for verifying financial and nonfinancial information needed to determine Medicaid beneficiaries' eligibility. The agency stated that it would include reviews of federal eligibility determinations in states that have delegated that authority as a part of its review of states' eligibility determinations. The results of this effort will be reported in 2019.

Source: GAO | GAO-18-598T.

[a]See GAO, *Medicaid: CMS Should Take Steps to Mitigate Program Risks in Managed Care*, GAO-18-291 (Washington, D.C.: May 7, 2018).

[b]See GAO, *Medicaid Program Integrity: Improved Guidance Needed to Better Support Efforts to Screen Managed Care Providers*, GAO-16-402 (Washington, D.C.: April 22, 2016).

[c]See GAO, *Medicaid: Additional Efforts Needed to Ensure that State Spending is Appropriately Matched with Federal Funds*, GAO-16-53 (Washington, D.C.: Oct. 16, 2015). Under the Patient Protection and Affordable Care Act, state Medicaid expenditures for certain Medicaid enrollees are subject to higher federal matching percentages.

[35] GAO-18-291.

Our prior work on Medicaid has also identified other program risks associated with provider enrollment and beneficiary eligibility that may contribute to improper payments. In Table 1 above, we identify some examples of the previous recommendations we have made to address these types of program risks, and what, if any, steps CMS has taken in response to our recommendations.

Lack of Transparency and Federal Oversight of States' Use of Supplemental Payments Increase Program Risk

Supplemental payments are payments made to providers—such as local government hospitals and other providers—that are in addition to the regular, claims-based payments made to providers for services they provided.[36] Like all Medicaid payments, supplemental payments are required to be economical and efficient.[37]

Supplemental payments have been growing and totaled more than $48 billion in 2016. Our prior work has identified several concerns related to supplemental payments, including the need for more complete and accurate reporting, criteria for economical and efficient payments, and written guidance on the distribution of payments.[38]

Complete and Accurate Reporting

Our prior work has identified increased use of provider taxes and transfers from local government providers to finance the states' share of supplemental payments, which, although allowed under federal law, effectively shift Medicaid costs from the states to the federal government. In particular, we previously reported in July 2014 that states' share of Medicaid supplemental payments financed with funds from providers and local governments increased the federal share from 57 percent in state fiscal year 2008 to 70 percent in state fiscal year 2012.[39] The full extent of this shift in states' financing structure was unknown, because CMS had not ensured that states report complete and accurate data on the sources of funds they use to finance their share of Medicaid payments, and CMS's efforts had fallen short of obtaining complete data.[40] (See Table 2

---

[36] Two types of supplemental payments exist in Medicaid: (1) disproportionate share hospital (DSH) payments, which states are required to make to hospitals serving low- income and Medicaid patients to offset those providers' uncompensated care costs; and (2) non-DSH supplemental payments that states may, but are not required, to make to hospitals and other providers that, for example, serve high-cost Medicaid beneficiaries. Unless otherwise noted, our findings apply to both types of supplemental payments.

[37] Payments must also be sufficient to assure quality of care and to enlist enough providers so that care and services are available to Medicaid beneficiaries at least to the extent available to the general population in the geographic area. 42 U.S.C. § 1396a(a)(30)(A).

[38] See, for example, GAO, *Medicaid: Federal Guidance Needed to Address Concerns About Distribution of Supplemental Payments*, GAO-16-108 (Washington, D.C.: Feb. 5, 2016); and *Medicaid: CMS Oversight of Provider Payments Is Hampered by Limited Data and Unclear Policy*, GAO-15-322 (Washington, D.C.: April 10, 2015).

[39] See GAO, *Medicaid Financing: States' Increased Reliance on Funds from Health Care Providers and Local Governments Warrants Improved CMS Data Collection [Reissued on March 13, 2015]*, GAO-14-627 (Washington, D.C.: July 29, 2014).

[40] Federal law requires that no less than 40 percent of the state's share of Medicaid payments be state funds—which can include state general funds, health care provider taxes imposed by the state, and intra-agency funds from

below for our recommendation and actions CMS has taken.) For example, in July 2014, we reported that in one state, a $220 million payment increase for nursing facilities resulted in an estimated $110 million increase in federal matching funds to the state, and a net payment increase to the facilities of $105 million.[41] (See Figure 5.)

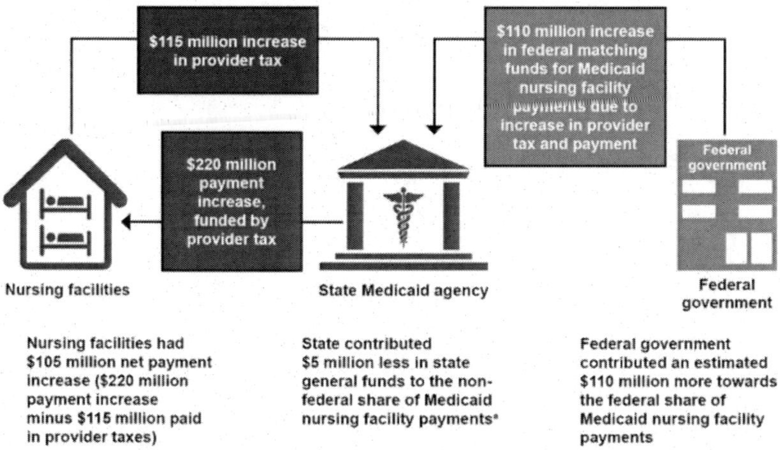

Source: GAO. | GAO-18-598T.

Figure 5. Example of How One State's Use of Non-State Sources to Fund Medicaid Payments to Nursing Facilities Shifted Medicaid Costs to the Federal Government in State Fiscal Year 2015.

Criteria for Economical and Efficient Payments

Our prior work has demonstrated that CMS lacks the criteria, data, and review processes to ensure that one type of supplemental payments—non-DSH supplemental payments—are economical and efficient.[42] For example, in April 2015, we identified public hospitals in one state that received such supplemental and regular Medicaid payments that, when combined, were hundreds of millions in excess of the hospitals' total Medicaid costs and tens of millions in excess of their total operating costs—unbeknownst to CMS.[43] Accordingly, we concluded that CMS's criteria and review processes did not ensure that it can identify excessive payments and determine if supplemental payments are economical and efficient. (See Table 2 below for our recommendations and actions CMS has taken.)

Written Guidance on the Distribution of Payments

According to CMS policy, Medicaid payments, including supplemental payments, should be linked to the provision of Medicaid services and not contingent on the

---

non-Medicaid state agencies— but up to 60 percent may be financed by local governments and local government providers. We have reported that, absent complete and accurate data, CMS cannot ensure that states' use of local funding sources does not exceed the 60 percent. See GAO-14-627.

[41] See GAO-14-627.

[42] Non-DSH supplemental payments that states may, but are not required to, make to hospitals and other providers that, for example, serve high-cost Medicaid beneficiaries.

[43] See GAO-15-322.

provision of local funds. However, in February 2016 we reported that CMS did not have written guidance that clarifies this policy. In February 2016, we found examples of hospitals with large uncompensated costs associated with serving the low-income and Medicaid population that received relatively little in supplemental payments, while other hospitals with relatively low uncompensated care costs—but that were able to contribute a large amount of funds for the state's Medicaid share— received large supplemental payments relative to those costs, raising questions as to whether CMS policies are being followed.[44] (See Table 2 for our recommendation and actions CMS has taken.)

Table 2. Examples of GAO recommendations to address Medicaid program risks associated with supplemental payments

Program risks	GAO recommendations	Recommendation status
Complete and accurate reporting	One recommendation aimed at the Centers for Medicare & Medicaid Services (CMS) taking steps to ensure states report accurate and complete information on all sources of funds they use to finance their share of Medicaid spending.[a]	CMS did not concur with GAO's recommendation, although the agency stated that it will examine efforts to improve data collection for oversight.
Criteria for economical and efficient payments	Two recommendations called for CMS to (1) develop a policy that establishes criteria for defining when payments made to individual providers are economical and efficient, and (2) subsequently develop a process for identifying and reviewing payments to individual providers in order to determine whether they meet the criteria.[b]	CMS told us in April 2018 that it is developing a proposed rule on supplemental payment financing and oversight that may address these recommendations, although it does not have a time frame for its release.
Written guidance on the distribution of payments	One recommendation aimed at CMS issuing written guidance for states clarifying its policy of the distribution of supplemental payments.[c]	CMS told us in April 2018 that it is developing a proposed rule on supplemental payment financing and oversight that may address this recommendation, although it does not have a time frame for its release.

Source: GAO | GAO-18-598T.

[a]See GAO, *Medicaid Financing: States' Increased Reliance on Funds from Health Care Providers and Local Governments Warrants Improved CMS Data Collection*, [Reissued on March 13, 2015], GAO-14-627 (Washington, D.C.: July 29, 2014).

[b]See GAO, *Medicaid: CMS Oversight of Provider Payments Is Hampered by Limited Data and Unclear Policy*, GAO-15-322 (Washington, D.C.: April 10, 2015).

[c]See GAO, *Medicaid: Federal Guidance Needed to Address Concerns About Distribution of Supplemental Payments*, GAO-16-108 (Washington, D.C.: Feb. 5, 2016).

Recognizing that Congress could help address some of the program risks associated with supplemental payments, in November 2012, we suggested that Congress consider requiring CMS to

[44] See GAO-16-108.

- improve state reporting of supplemental payments, including requiring annual reporting of facility-specific payment amounts;
- clarify permissible methods for calculating these supplemental payments; and
- implement annual independent certified audits to verify state compliance with methods for calculating supplemental payments.[45]

Subsequent to our work highlighting the need for complete and accurate reporting, in January 2017 a bill was introduced in the House of Representatives that, if enacted, would require annual state reporting of non-DSH supplemental payments made to individual facilities, require CMS to issue guidance to states that identifies permissible methods for calculating non-DSH supplemental payments to providers, and establish requirements for such annual independent audits.[46] Another bill was introduced in October 2017 that would require states to submit annual reports that identify the sources and amount of funds used to finance the state share of Medicaid payments.[47] As of May 2018, no action had been taken on either proposed bill.

Absent Better Oversight, Demonstrations May Increase Federal Fiscal Liability

Demonstration programs, comprising about one-third of total Medicaid expenditures in fiscal year 2015, can be a powerful tool for states and CMS to test new approaches to providing coverage and delivering services that could reduce costs and improve outcomes. However, our prior work has identified several concerns related to demonstrations, including the need for ensuring that (1) demonstrations meet the policy requirements of budget neutrality—that is, they must not increase federal costs—and (2) evaluations are used to determine whether demonstrations are having their intended effects.[48]

Budget Neutrality of Medicaid Demonstrations

Demonstration spending limits, by HHS policy, should not exceed spending that would have occurred in the absence of a demonstration. In multiple reports examining more than a dozen demonstrations between 2002 and 2017, we have identified a number of questionable methods and assumptions that HHS has permitted states to use when

---

[45] See GAO, *Medicaid: More Transparency of and Accountability for Supplemental Payments are Needed*, GAO-13-48 (Washington, D.C.: Nov. 26, 2012).

[46] The Improving Oversight and Accountability in Medicaid Non-DSH Supplemental Payments Act was introduced on January 13, 2017 and referred to the House Committee on Energy and Commerce. See H.R. 541, 115th Cong. § 2 (2017).

[47] The Medicaid Requiring Expenditures for Public Objectives to be Reflective of Total Spending Act (Medicaid REPORTS Act) was introduced on October 12, 2017 and referred to in the House Energy and Commerce Committee Subcommittee on Health. See H.R. 4054, 115th Cong. § 2 (2017).

[48] See, for example, GAO, *Medicaid Demonstrations: Evaluations Yielded Limited Results, Underscoring Need for Changes to Federal Policies and Procedures*, GAO-18-220 (Washington, D.C.: Jan 19, 2018); and *Medicaid Demonstrations: Federal Action Needed to Improve Oversight of Spending*, GAO-17-312 (Washington, D.C.: April 3, 2017).

estimating costs. We found that federal spending on Medicaid demonstrations could be reduced by billions of dollars if HHS were required to improve the process for reviewing, approving, and making transparent the basis for spending limits approved for Medicaid demonstrations.[49] The following are some examples of what we have previously found:

- In August 2014, we reported that HHS had approved a spending limit for Arkansas's demonstration—to test whether providing premium assistance to purchase private coverage through the health insurance exchange would improve access for newly eligible Medicaid beneficiaries—that was based, in part, on hypothetical, not actual, costs. Specifically, the spending limit was based on significantly higher payment amounts the state assumed it would have to make to providers if it expanded coverage under the traditional Medicaid program, and HHS did not request any data to support the state's assumptions. We estimated that by allowing the state to use hypothetical costs, HHS approved a demonstration spending limit that was over $775 million more than what it would have been if the limit was based on the state's actual payment rates for services under the traditional Medicaid program.[50]
- We also reported in August 2014 that HHS officials told us it granted Arkansas and 11 other states additional flexibility in their demonstrations in order to increase spending limits if costs proved higher than expected.[51] We concluded that granting this flexibility to the states to adjust the spending limit increased the fiscal risk to the federal government.
- More recently, in April 2017, we reported that two states used unspent federal funds from their previous demonstrations to expand the scope of subsequent demonstrations by $8 billion and $600 million, respectively. We concluded that inflating the spending limits in this way inappropriately increased the federal government's fiscal liability for Medicaid.[52]

We have previously made recommendations to improve oversight of spending on demonstrations, and HHS recently took action that partially responds to one of these recommendations. (See Table 3 for examples of the recommendations and actions HHS

---

[49] See, for example, GAO-17-312 and GAO, *Medicaid Demonstrations: HHS's Approval Process for Arkansas's Medicaid Expansion Waiver Raises Cost Concerns*, GAO-14-689R (Washington, D.C.: Aug. 8, 2014); *Medicaid Demonstration Waivers: Approval Process Raises Cost Concerns and Lacks Transparency*, GAO-13-384 (Washington, D.C.: June 25, 2013); *Medicaid Demonstration Waivers: Recent HHS Approvals Continue to Raise Cost and Oversight Concerns*, GAO-08-87 (Washington, D.C.: Jan. 31, 2008); and *Medicaid and SCHIP: Recent HHS Approvals of Demonstration Waiver Projects Raise Concerns*, GAO-02-817 (Washington, D.C.: July 12, 2002).

[50] See GAO-14-689R.

[51] In September 2014, the Chairman of the House Committee on Energy & Commerce and the Ranking Member of the Senate Committee on Finance sent a letter to CMS asking, among other things, how the agency planned to ensure that spending for those newly eligible under Arkansas's demonstration would not cost the federal government more than it would have cost under traditional Medicaid.

[52] See GAO-17-312.

has taken.) Specifically, under a policy implemented in 2016, HHS restricted the amount of unspent funds states can accrue for each year of a demonstration, and has also reduced the amount of unspent funds that states can carry forward to new demonstrations. For 10 demonstrations it has recently approved, HHS estimated that the new policy has reduced total demonstration spending limits by $109 billion for 2016 through 2018, the federal share of which is $62.9 billion. These limits reduce the effect, but do not specifically address all, of the questionable methods and assumptions that we have identified regarding how HHS sets demonstration spending limits.

Table 3. Examples of GAO recommendations to address Medicaid program risks associated with spending on medicaid demonstrations

Program risks	GAO recommendations	Recommendation status
Methods for determining budget neutrality	One recommendation that the Department of Health and Human Services (HHS) better ensure that valid methods are used to demonstrate budget neutrality.[a]	HHS has taken some steps in recent years to improve allowable methods for ensuring budget neutrality, but still needs written guidance on methodologies for demonstrating budget neutrality.
Lack of criteria for determining spending limits	One recommendation that HHS update its written budget neutrality policy to reflect the actual criteria and processes used to develop and approve demonstration spending limits.[b]	HHS announced and began implementing policy changes in 2016 that address some, but not all of our concerns, which it formalized in 2017. The agency expects to release additional guidance later in 2018. Once HHS provides additional written guidance on its criteria and processes, we will be in a position to consider closing this recommendation.

Source: GAO | GAO-18-598T.

[a]See GAO, *Medicaid and SCHIP: Recent HHS Approvals of Demonstration Waiver Projects Raise Concerns*, GAO-02-817 (Washington, D.C.: July 12, 2002).

[b]See *GAO, Medicaid Demonstration Waivers: Approval Process Raises Cost Concerns and Lacks Transparency*, GAO-13-384 (Washington, D.C.: June 25, 2013).

Evaluation of Medicaid Demonstrations

In a January 2018 report, we questioned the usefulness of both state-led and federal evaluations of section 1115 demonstrations, particularly with regard to how these evaluation results may inform policy decisions.[53]

- State-led evaluations. We identified significant limitations among selected state-led demonstration evaluations, including gaps in reported evaluation results for important parts of the demonstrations. (See Table 4.) These gaps resulted, in part, from CMS requiring final, comprehensive evaluation reports after the expiration of the demonstrations rather than at the end of each 3- to 5-year demonstration cycle. In October 2017, CMS officials stated that the agency planned to require

[53] See GAO-18-220.

final reports at the end of each demonstration cycle for all demonstrations, although it had not established written procedures for implementing this new policy. We concluded in January 2018 that without written procedures for implementing such requirements, gaps in oversight could continue.[54]

Table 4. Examples of gaps in states' evaluations of Medicaid section 1115 demonstrations GAO identified

State	Example of gaps in evaluations
Arizona	The state was required to evaluate whether providing long-term services and supports under a managed care delivery model improved access and quality of care. The evaluation report lacked information on important measures of access and quality.
Arkansas	The state was required to evaluate the effects of using Medicaid funds to purchase private insurance for more than 200,000 beneficiaries. The evaluation did not address a key hypothesis that using private insurance would improve continuity of coverage for these beneficiaries, who were expected to have frequent changes in income that could lead to coverage gaps.
Massachusetts	The state was required to evaluate the effectiveness of its approach of providing up to $690 million in incentive payments to seven hospitals to improve quality of care and reduce per capita costs. Evaluation reports submitted after 5 years provided no conclusions on the impact of the payments in these areas.

Source: GAO. | GAO-18-598T.

- Federal evaluations. Evaluations of federal demonstrations led by CMS have also been limited due to data challenges and a lack of transparent reporting. For example, delays obtaining data directly from states, among other things, led CMS to considerably reduce the scope of a large, multi-state evaluation, which was initiated in 2014 to examine the impact of state demonstrations in four policy areas deemed to be federal priorities.[55] In our January 2018 report, we found that although CMS had made progress in obtaining needed data, CMS had no policy for making the results public. By not making these results public in a timely manner, we concluded that CMS was missing an opportunity to inform important federal and state policy discussions.

In light of our concerns about state-led and federal demonstration evaluations, in January 2018, we recommended that CMS (1) establish written procedures for requiring final evaluation reports at the end of each demonstration cycle, (2) issue criteria for when it will allow limited evaluations of demonstrations, and (3) establish a policy for publicly

---

[54] CMS also planned to allow states to conduct less rigorous evaluations for certain types of demonstrations, but had not established criteria defining under what conditions these limited evaluations would be allowed, when we issued our January 2018 report.

[55] The policy areas are (1) delivery system reform incentive payment programs, which provide incentive payments to providers that engage in various improvement projects that align with state delivery system reform objectives; (2) premium assistance to purchase insurance coverage in the exchange under PPACA; (3) beneficiary engagement policies, such as requiring monthly contributions; and (4) use of managed care to deliver Medicaid long-term supports and services.

releasing findings from federal evaluations of demonstrations. HHS concurred with these recommendations.[56]

Fundamental Actions Needed to Strengthen Oversight and Manage Program Risks

Across our body of work, we have made 83 recommendations to CMS and HHS and suggested 4 matters for congressional consideration to address a variety of concerns about the Medicaid program. The agencies generally agreed with our recommendations and have implemented 25 of these recommendations to date, and CMS still needs to take fundamental actions in three areas—having more timely, complete, and reliable data; conducting fraud risk assessments; and strengthening federal-state collaboration—to strengthen Medicaid oversight and better manage program risks.

More Complete, Timely, Reliable Data for Oversight

An overarching challenge for CMS oversight of the Medicaid program is the lack of accurate, complete, and timely data. Our work has demonstrated how insufficient data have affected CMS's ability to ensure proper payments, assess beneficiaries' access to services, and oversee states' financing strategies.

As part of its efforts to address longstanding data concerns, CMS has taken some steps toward developing a reliable national repository for Medicaid data, most notably the Transformed Medicaid Statistical Information System (T-MSIS). Through T-MSIS, CMS will collect detailed information on Medicaid beneficiaries—such as their citizenship, immigration, and disability status—as well as any expanded diagnosis and procedure codes associated with their treatments. States are to report data more frequently—and in a timelier manner—than they have previously, and T-MSIS includes approximately 2,800 automated quality checks.[57] The T-MSIS initiative has the potential to improve CMS's ability to identify improper payments, help ensure beneficiaries' access to services, and improve program transparency, among other benefits.

As we reported in December 2017, implementing the T-MSIS initiative has been—and will continue to be—a multi-year effort. CMS has worked closely with states and has reached a point where nearly all states are reporting T-MSIS data. While recognizing the progress made, we noted that more work needs to be done before CMS or states can use these data for program oversight:

---

[56] See GAO-18-220.

[57] In particular, we found that the usefulness of CMS data on Medicaid is limited because of issues with completeness, accuracy, and timeliness. With regard to timeliness, we found that available data were reported up to 3 years late and were previously submitted on a quarterly basis. Under T-MSIS, data are to be reported monthly.

- All states need to report complete T-MSIS data. For our December 2017 report, we reviewed a sample of six states and found that none were reporting complete data.[58]
- T-MSIS data should be formatted in a manner that allows for state data to be compared nationally. In December 2017, we reported that state officials had expressed concerns that states did not convert their data to the T-MSIS format in the same ways, which could limit cross state comparisons.[59]

In our December 2017 report, we recommended that CMS take steps to expedite the use of T-MSIS data, including efforts to (1) obtain complete information from all states; (2) identify and share information across states to improve data comparability; and (3) implement mechanisms by which states can collaborate on an ongoing basis to improve the completeness, comparability, and utility of T-MSIS data. We also recommended that CMS articulate a specific plan and associated time frames for using T-MSIS data for oversight.[60] The agency concurred with our recommendations, but has not yet implemented them.

Our prior work has also noted areas where other data improvements are critical to program oversight:

- In July 2014, we found that there was a need for data on supplemental payments that states make to individual hospitals and other providers. In particular, our findings and related recommendation from July 2014 indicate that CMS should develop a data collection strategy that ensures that states report accurate and complete data on all sources of funds used to finance the states' share of Medicaid payments.[61]
- In January 2017, we found limitations in the data CMS collects to monitor the provision of, and spending on, personal care services— services that are at a high risk for improper payments, including fraud.[62] In particular, data on the provision of personal care services were often not timely, complete, or consistent. Data on states' spending on these services were also not accurate or complete. In January 2017, we recommended that CMS improve personal care services data by (1)

---

[58] The six selected states were not reporting complete data as of August 2017. See GAO, *Medicaid: Further Action* Needed *to Expedite Use of National Data for Program Oversight*, GAO-18-70 (Washington, D.C.: Dec. 8, 2017).

[59] See GAO-18-70.

[60] We concluded that absent a specific plan and time frames, CMS's ability to use these data to oversee the program, including ensuring proper payments, was limited. See GAO-18-70.

[61] Better data on supplemental payments could also help ensure that states comply with federal requirements regarding how much local governments may contribute to the state's share of Medicaid payments. See GAO-14-627.

[62] Personal care services are key components of long-term, in-home care, providing assistance with basic activities, such as bathing, dressing, and toileting, to millions of individuals seeking to retain their independence and to age in place.

establishing standard reporting guidance for key data, (2) ensuring linkage between data on the provision of services and reported expenditures, (3) ensuring state compliance with reporting requirements, and (4) developing plans to use data for oversight.[63] The agency concurred with two recommendations and neither agreed nor disagreed with the other two recommendations, and has not yet implemented any.

More Complete Fraud Risk Assessment and Better Fraud Targeting

In December 2017, we examined CMS's efforts managing fraud risks in Medicaid and compared it with our Fraud Risk Framework, which provides a comprehensive set of key components and leading practices that serve as a guide for agency managers to use when developing efforts to combat fraud in a strategic, risk-based way.[64] This framework describes leading practices in four components: commit, assess, design and implement, and evaluate and adapt. (See Figure 6.) The Fraud Reduction and Data Analytics Act of 2015, enacted in June 2016, requires the Office of Management and Budget (OMB) to establish guidelines incorporating the leading practices from our Fraud Risk Framework for federal agencies to create controls to identify and assess fraud risks, and design and implement antifraud control activities.[65] In July 2016, OMB published guidance, and among other things, this guidance affirms that managers should adhere to the leading practices identified in our Fraud Risk Framework.[66]

In a December 2017 report, we found that CMS's efforts partially aligned with our fraud risk framework. In particular, CMS had

- shown a commitment to combating fraud, in part, by establishing a dedicated entity—the Center for Program Integrity—to lead antifraud efforts, and offering and requiring antifraud training for stakeholder groups, such as providers, beneficiaries, and health-insurance plans; and
- taken steps to identify fraud risks, such as by designating specific provider types as high risk and developing associated control activities.

---

[63] See GAO, *Medicaid: CMS Needs Better Data to Monitor the Provision of and Spending on Personal Care Services,* GAO-17-169 (Washington, D.C.: Jan. 12, 2017).

[64] See GAO, *A Framework for Managing Fraud Risks in Federal Programs*, GAO-15-593SP (Washington, D.C.: July 28, 2015).

[65] Pub. L. No. 114-186, § 3, 130 Stat. 546 (2016).

[66] Office of Management and Budget, *Management's Responsibility for Enterprise Risk Management and Internal Control*, Circular No. A-123 (Washington, D.C.: July 15, 2016).

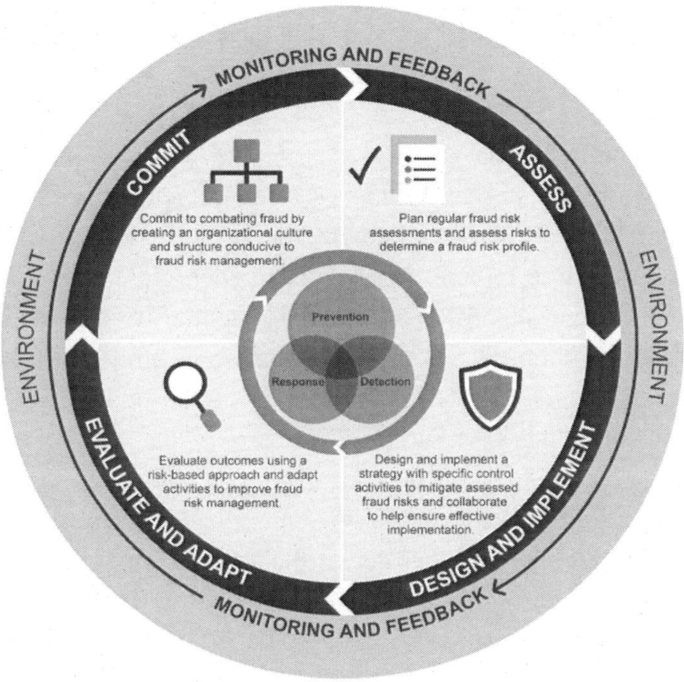

Source: GAO. | GAO-18-598T.

Figure 6. The Fraud Risk Management Framework.

However, CMS had not conducted a fraud risk assessment for Medicaid, and had not designed and implemented a risk-based antifraud strategy.[67] A fraud risk assessment allows managers to fully consider fraud risks to their programs, analyze their likelihood and impact, and prioritize risks. Managers can then design and implement a strategy with specific control activities to mitigate these fraud risks, as well as design and implement an appropriate evaluation. We concluded that through these actions, CMS could better ensure that it is addressing the full portfolio of risks and strategically targeting the most-significant fraud risks facing Medicaid. As a result, in December 2017 we made three recommendations to CMS, two of which were to conduct fraud risk assessments, and create an antifraud strategy for Medicaid, including an approach for evaluation.[68] HHS concurred with our recommendations, but has not yet implemented them.

Greater Federal-State Collaboration to Strengthen Program Oversight

The federal government and the states play important roles in reducing improper payments and overseeing the Medicaid program, including overseeing spending on Medicaid supplemental payments and demonstrations. Our prior work shows that oversight of the Medicaid program could be further improved through leveraging and

[67] See GAO, *Medicare and Medicaid: CMS Needs* to *Fully Align Its Antifraud Efforts with the Fraud Risk Framework*, GAO-18-88 (Washington, D.C.: Dec. 5, 2017).

[68] See GAO-18-88.

coordinating program integrity efforts with state agencies, state auditors, and other partners.

Collaborative Audits with State Agencies

As we have previously reported, CMS has made changes to its Medicaid program integrity efforts, including a shift to collaborative audits—in which CMS's contractors and states work in partnership to audit Medicaid providers. In March 2017, we reported that collaborative audits had identified substantial potential overpayments to providers, but barriers—such as staff burden or problems communicating with contractors—had limited their use and prevented states from seeking audits or hindered the success of audits.[69] We recommended that CMS address the barriers that limit state participation in collaborative audits, including their use in managed care delivery systems. CMS concurred with this recommendation and has taken steps to address them for a number of states, but has not yet made such changes accessible to a majority of states.

State Auditors and Federal Partners

We have found that state auditors and the HHS-OIG offer additional oversight and information that can help identify program risks. To that end, we routinely coordinate our audit efforts with the state auditors and the HHS-OIG. For example, we have convened and facilitated meetings between CMS and state audit officials to discuss specific areas of concern in Medicaid and future opportunities for collaboration. The state auditors and CMS officials commented on the benefits of such coordination, with the state auditors noting that they can assist CMS's state program integrity reviews by identifying program risks.

State auditors also have conducted program integrity reviews to identify improper payments and deficiencies in the processes used to identify them. We believe that these reviews could provide insights into program weaknesses that CMS could learn from and potentially address nationally. Coordination also provides an opportunity for state auditors to learn methods for conducting program integrity reviews. The following are recent examples of reviews conducted:

- In 2017, the Oregon Secretary of State Audits Division found approximately 31,300 questionable payments to Coordinated Care Organizations (which receive capitated monthly payments for beneficiaries, similar to managed care organizations), based on a review of 15 months of data. In addition, the state auditor found that approximately 47,600 individuals enrolled in Oregon's

[69] See GAO, *Medicaid Program Integrity: CMS Should Build on Current Oversight Efforts by Further Enhancing Collaboration with States*, GAO-17-277 (Washington, D.C.: March 15, 2017).

Medicaid program were ineligible, equating to $88 million in avoidable expenditures.[70]

- Massachusetts' Medicaid Audit Unit's recent annual report (covering the time period from March 15, 2017, through March 14, 2018) reported that the state auditor identified more than $211 million in unallowable, questionable, duplicative, unauthorized, or potentially fraudulent billing in the program.[71]
- A 2017 report released by the Louisiana Legislative Auditor's Office stated that the office reviewed Medicaid eligibility files and claims data covering January 2011 through October 2016, and found $1.4 million in questionable duplicate payments.[72]
- In fiscal year 2017, the Mississippi Division of Medicaid reported that they recovered more than $8.6 million through various audits of medical claims paid to health care providers. The division also referred seven cases to the state's attorney general's office, in which the division had identified $3.1 million in improper billing.[73]

At a May 2018 federal and state auditor coordination meeting that we participated in, the HHS-OIG provided examples of the financial impact of its work related to improper payments, including

- one review of managed care long term services and supports that identified $717 million potential federal savings,
- three reviews of managed care payments made after beneficiaries' death that identified $18.2 million in federal funds to be recovered, and
- two reviews of managed care payments made for beneficiaries with multiple Medicaid IDs that identified $4.3 million in federal funds to be recovered.

Healthcare Fraud Prevention Partnership

The Healthcare Fraud Prevention Partnership (HFPP) is an important tool to help combat Medicaid fraud. In 2012, CMS created the HFPP to share information with public and private stakeholders, and to conduct studies related to health care fraud, waste, and abuse. According to CMS, as of October 2017, the HFPP included 89 public and private partners—including Medicare—and Medicaid-related federal and state agencies, law

---

[70] State of Oregon, Secretary of State, Dennis Richardson and Oregon Audits Division Director, Kip Memmott, *Oregon Health Authority Should Improve Efforts to Detect and Prevent Improper Medicaid Payments* Report 2017- 25 (Salem, Ore.: November 2017).

[71] Commonwealth of Massachusetts, Office of the State Auditor Suzanne M. Bump, *Office of the State Auditor—Annual Report Medicaid Audit Unit, March 15, 2017-March 14, 2018* (Boston, Mass.: March 15, 2018).

[72] Louisiana Legislative Auditor, State of Louisiana, *Duplicate Payments for Medicaid Recipients with Multiple Identification Numbers* (Baton Rouge, La.: March 29, 2017).

[73] Mississippi Division of Medicaid, *Medicaid Recovers $8.6 Million in Fiscal Year 2017* (Jackson, Miss.), accessed May 29, 2018, https://medicaid.ms.gov/medicaid-recovers-8-6- million-in-fiscal-year-2017/.

enforcement agencies, private health insurance plans, and antifraud and other health care organizations. The HFPP has conducted studies that pool and analyze multiple payers' claims data to identify providers with patterns of suspect billing across private health insurance plans. In August 2017, we reported that the partnership participants separately told us the HFPP's studies helped them identify and take action against potentially fraudulent providers and payment vulnerabilities of which they might not otherwise have been aware, and fostered both formal and informal information sharing.[74]

Chairman Johnson, Ranking Member McCaskill, and Members of the Committee, this concludes my prepared statement. I would be pleased to respond to any questions you may have.

Medicaid Fraud and Overpayments: Problems and Solutions, Testimony of: Brian P. Ritchie, Assistant Inspector General for Audit Services, Office of Inspector General, U.S. Department of Health and Human Services

Testimony before the United States Senate Committee on
Homeland Security and Governmental Affairs
June 27, 2018
10:00 a.m.
Dirksen Senate Office Building, Room 342

Good morning, Chairman Johnson, Ranking Member McCaskill, and distinguished Members of the committee. I am Brian P. Ritchie, Assistant Inspector General for Audit Services, U.S. Department of Health and Human Services. Thank you for your longstanding commitment to ensuring that the Medicaid program's 67 million beneficiaries are well served and the taxpayers' approximately $600 billion investment is well spent. I appreciate the opportunity to discuss the Office of Inspector General's work to combat fraud, waste, and abuse in Medicaid and what more can be done to secure the future of this important program.

Introduction

Medicaid spending represents one-sixth of the national health care economy, and Medicaid serves more people, including some of the Nation's most vulnerable

[74] See GAO, *Medicare: CMS Fraud Prevention System Uses Claims Analysis to Address Fraud*, GAO-17-710 (Washington, D.C.: Aug. 30, 2017).

individuals, than any other Federal health care program. Congress created the Office of Inspector General (OIG) for the U.S. Department of Health and Human Services (HHS or the Department) in 1976 as an independent body to oversee HHS programs. A key component of my office's mission is to promote integrity and efficiency in Medicaid and other Federal health care programs. While OIG does not directly operate the Medicaid program, through a nation-wide program of audits, evaluations, inspections, investigations, and enforcement actions, OIG has identified numerous vulnerabilities to program operations and offered specific recommendations to the Centers for Medicare & Medicaid Services (CMS) and its State partners for how to mitigate or eliminate those vulnerabilities and enhance the economy and efficiency of the Medicaid program going forward.

OIG shares the committee's commitment to protecting Medicaid from fraud, waste, and abuse and has an extensive body of oversight work in this area. Persistent challenges include high improper payment rates, inadequate program integrity safeguards, and beneficiary health and safety concerns. In our extensive experience combating various types of vulnerabilities in all regions of the country, across all provider types, regarding all classes of items and services, one program administration shortcoming has emerged as a consistent impediment to effective oversight. That shortcoming is the lack of a robust national Medicaid dataset that is complete, accurate, and timely. A complete, accurate, and timely Medicaid dataset would greatly facilitate Medicaid program operations and promote economy and efficiency.

Much program integrity work seeks to recover improper payments already made and reduce improper payments going forward. In FY 2017, projected improper Medicaid payments totaled about $59 billion. CMS must do more to ensure that Medicaid payments are made to the right provider, for the right amount, for the right service, on behalf of the right beneficiary.

My testimony addresses how to protect Medicaid and its program beneficiaries through the lens of OIG's core program integrity principles of prevention, detection, and enforcement. Enhanced data functionality offers cross-cutting benefits that would enhance prevention, detection, and enforcement to correct problems and prevent future harm.

Oversight of CMS's Efforts to Address Fraud and Overpayments in Medicaid

Complete and Reliable National Medicaid Data Are Necessary for Effective Program Oversight and Management and to Detect Bad Actors

The ability to detect problems in real time, or as close to real time as possible, enables effective oversight and can protect patients and help prevent improper payments.

CMS, States, Medicaid managed care entities, and providers share the responsibility for detecting and addressing problems in the Medicaid program. The lack of national Medicaid data hampers the ability to quickly detect and address improper payments, fraud, waste, or quality concerns, both within States and across the Nation.

CMS Must Ensure the Completeness and Reliability of Data in the Transformed Medicaid Statistical Information System

Congress has recognized the value of enhanced Medicaid data, but more needs to be done to achieve the goal. Through the Balanced Budget Act of 1997, Congress mandated that States submit data to provide for a national Medicaid dataset. The Transformed Medicaid Statistical Information System (T-MSIS) is a joint effort by CMS and the States to address previously identified problems with national Medicaid claims and eligibility data. CMS's goals for T-MSIS are to improve the completeness, accuracy, and timeliness of Medicaid data.

CMS began testing T-MSIS with 12 volunteer States in 2011. T-MSIS builds on and replaces the Medicaid Statistical Information System. CMS initially set a goal for all States to submit T-MSIS data by July 2014. CMS subsequently extended that deadline several times. After multiple missed implementation deadlines, technological problems, competing priorities, and other implementation delays, as of May 2018, 49 States (all States except Wisconsin) and the District of Columbia had begun reporting data to T-MSIS, but concerns remain about the quality and completeness of the data reported.

OIG is concerned about whether the data will be actionable, as our work has identified numerous issues with the completeness and quality of the data. We found that States are not consistently submitting the same T-MSIS data elements, limiting the ability to make comparisons across all States. Despite CMS's attempts to further standardize meaning through a revised standard data dictionary, T-MSIS data elements may not mean the same thing across States. Different interpretations across States could result in data that is not comparable across different States.

Until CMS and States achieve full implementation, the Department must prioritize obtaining complete and reliable T-MSIS data. CMS must ensure that the same data elements are consistently reported and uniformly interpreted across States to best inform program management and oversight. To accomplish this, OIG recommends that CMS establish a deadline for when national T-MSIS data will be available for multi-State program integrity efforts. Without the prioritization motivated by a fixed deadline, some States and CMS may delay full implementation of T-MSIS to the detriment of Medicaid program integrity.

CMS Should Ensure That States Report Encounter Data for All Managed Care Entities

Eighty percent of all Medicaid beneficiaries receive part or all of their services through managed care. For CMS and States to operate Medicaid effectively at both the Federal and State level, it is vital that T-MSIS include complete and accurate managed care encounter data. State Medicaid agencies contract with managed care entities to deliver health care services and perform certain administrative functions such as data collection and reporting. Most importantly, managed care entities are required to report medical claims data, known as encounter data, to States that then report the data to CMS via T-MSIS. Encounter data include detailed information about the services provided to Medicaid beneficiaries enrolled in managed care. Like fee-for-service Medicaid claims, encounter data are the primary record of services provided to Medicaid beneficiaries enrolled in managed care. The Society of Actuaries calls encounter data "the single most important analytical tool for health plans and health programs. Without accurate and timely data, it is not possible to analyze costs, utilization or trends; evaluate benefits; or determine the quality of services being provided."

OIG found that States' Medicaid managed care encounter data were incomplete. Reasons that States cited for their failure to report complete information included the inability to collect encounter data from some managed care entities and limitations in the State's data systems. CMS has made some progress in addressing this problem, including regulatory requirements, guidance, and an ongoing data quality monitoring review of submissions of encounter data through T-MSIS. However, the Department must do more to ensure that the data necessary to support program integrity in Medicaid managed care are complete, accurate, and timely. Thus, OIG continues to recommend that CMS ensure that States report encounter data for all managed care entities.

The Lack of Quality National Medicaid Data Hampers Enforcement Efforts

States and the Federal Government need a high-quality Medicaid dataset to effectively administer the Medicaid program. National data can be used to identify fraud schemes and other vulnerabilities that cross State lines. Even localized schemes are more easily concealed absent national data. Aberrant utilization or spending patterns may not appear problematic until compared against another State's experience or national averages. Identifying such schemes in one State can alert other States to patterns of fraudulent or abusive practices that may be occurring in their jurisdiction. This information can generate referrals to State law enforcement agencies like the State Medicaid Fraud Control Units or joint investigations across State lines. Complete and reliable data are critical to identifying improper payments and to enable Federal and State enforcement efforts to keep fraudulent and harmful providers out of Medicaid and hold bad actors accountable. National Medicaid data holds the promise of supporting and amplifying enforcement efforts. We have seen this potential for data to strengthen the effectiveness of enforcement efforts. For example, in July 2017, OIG and its law enforcement partners conducted the largest ever National Health Care Fraud Takedown.

Sophisticated data analytics played an indispensable role in enabling the success of this takedown. The end result—charges against more than 400 defendants across 41 Federal districts for their alleged participation in health care fraud schemes involving about $1.3 billion in false billings—protected the programs and sent a strong signal that theft of taxpayer funds will not be tolerated. Notably, 120 defendants, including doctors, were charged for illegally prescribing and distributing opioids and other dangerous drugs, and 295 providers were served with exclusion notices for conduct related to opioid diversion and abuse. A concurrent data brief underscored the magnitude of the opioid problem, identifying concerns about extreme use and questionable prescribing of opioids in Medicare Part D. That is the potential of data— leveraged by skilled auditors, investigators, and analysts—to protect the program, to protect beneficiaries, and to bring bad actors to justice.

Unfortunately, we currently cannot replicate this type of analysis in Medicaid. Development of a national Medicaid dataset would promote economy and efficiency in Medicaid by facilitating timely detection of and rapid response to improper payments and fraud. Quality national Medicaid data provide visibility into payments and offer the transparency necessary to determine whether Medicaid is paying the right amount, to the right provider, for the right service, on behalf of the right beneficiary. OIG can harness the power of accurate, timely, and complete data not only to support enforcement efforts, but also to identify vulnerabilities to avoid, and best practices to replicate with the ultimate goal of promoting value and improving quality of care. While CMS and States have made important strides to improve Medicaid data, more can be done to ensure T-MSIS achieves its full potential. Ultimately, T-MSIS will be only as useful as the data it receives. This is why CMS must ensure the completeness and reliability of T-MSIS data and improve provider enrollment data to prevent unscrupulous providers from enrolling in Medicaid and gaining access to Medicaid funds and beneficiaries. Such data are essential to the efficiency, effectiveness, and integrity of Medicaid. Savings achieved through improved program integrity and reduced improper payments could fund improved services for beneficiaries.

Leveraging Tools to Prevent Fraud

Although OIG has extensive experience conducting investigations and enforcement actions to recoup improper payments and exclude fraudulent providers, the first pillar of our program integrity strategy is prevention. Keeping bad actors and ineligible beneficiaries out of the program on the front end prevents improper payments. Complete and reliable data can help States achieve this front-end integrity. By knowing with whom they are doing business, States can enroll trusted providers and avoid paying, or having their beneficiaries endure subpar services from, providers who do not deserve such trust.

States Have Not Fully Enacted Enhanced Provider Screening

To ensure that Medicaid pays the right provider, the program must be able to identify the providers with whom it does business, and keep bad actors out of the program. Preventing bad actors from entering the Medicaid program not only reduces improper payments, but also protects patients from harm.

States must screen providers commensurate with the potential risk for fraud, waste, and abuse that they pose to Medicaid, with high-risk providers requiring more intense scrutiny. However, States often fail to effectively screen high-risk providers, including key safeguards like conducting fingerprint-based criminal background checks and site visits. Previous OIG work found that many States had yet to implement fingerprint-based criminal background checks and site visits. OIG made recommendations to CMS to assist States with implementing these activities. CMS concurred with OIG's recommendations and has provided assistance to States. However, CMS has extended the deadline for implementation of fingerprint-based criminal background checks, indicating that States have not yet resolved the vulnerability inadequate background check procedures pose for provider enrollment. OIG has ongoing work to provide a status update on implementation of fingerprint-based criminal background checks.

CMS must ensure that States timely and fully implement these critical safeguards lest bad actors defraud Medicaid of millions of dollars and endanger beneficiaries. For example, in Virginia two individuals conspired to defraud a special caregiver program covered under Medicaid by submitting timesheets for payment for services that were never rendered. One of the conspirators was actually incarcerated on the days when he falsely claimed to have provided Medicaid services. Better compliance with criminal background check requirements can help prevent similar fraud schemes.

In another example, in North Carolina a mental health facility operator submitted fraudulent Medicaid claims for services for beneficiaries with developmental disabilities. The operator submitted at least $2.5 million in fraudulent claims using stolen beneficiary information from a defunct company that he previously co-owned, and he received more than $2 million in reimbursements from Medicaid. State site visits could have revealed that the beneficiaries never actually received services.

These cases exemplify why OIG recommends that CMS improve provider screening by working with States to implement fingerprint-based criminal background checks and site visits for high- risk providers.

For provider screening to be truly effective, States need timely, complete, and accurate data to identify the providers seeking access to Medicaid monies and patients. OIG has issued several recommendations to reduce duplicate provider enrollment data collection by sharing data across States or creating central repositories. Sharing data across States and with Medicare data systems would streamline the Medicaid enrollment process and reduce the chance for error within any one database. A joint enrollment system would provide a "one-stop shop" for State Medicaid officials and providers—reducing provider burden and duplication in reporting, verifying, and updating information. This could reduce data-collection duplication and burdens on States and providers and improve the completeness and accuracy of the data available to Medicaid. The President's FY 2019 Budget request includes a proposal to consolidate provider enrollment screening for Medicare, Medicaid, and the Children's Health Insurance Program.

Reducing Improper and Wasteful Payments and Ensuring Compliance with Fiscal Controls

Ensuring Compliance with Fiscal Controls

Reducing improper payments to providers is a critical element in protecting the financial integrity of Medicaid. In FY 2017, HHS reported a Medicaid improper payment rate of 10.1 percent. CMS has engaged with State Medicaid agencies to develop corrective action plans that address State-specific reasons for improper payments as a part of CMS's Payment Error Rate Measurement program, which measures Medicaid improper payments. CMS has facilitated national best practices calls to share ideas across States, provided State education through the Medicaid Integrity Institute, offered ongoing technical assistance, and provided additional guidance as needed to address the root causes of improper payments. CMS has indicated that it continues to provide guidance to States on their procedures for calculating and claiming costs under waiver programs for home and community-based services.

OIG audits have identified substantial improper payments to providers across a variety of Medicaid services, including school-based services, nonemergency medical transportation, targeted case management services, and personal care services. OIG has also identified several States that made improper payments to Medicaid managed care entities. More specifically, we found that several States made monthly capitated payments on behalf of deceased Medicaid beneficiaries, and we identified several States that made duplicate monthly capitated payments for the same beneficiary. CMS should continue to engage with State Medicaid agencies to develop corrective action plans and provide specific guidance to States regarding services and benefits most vulnerable to improper payments.

OIG audits have identified billions of dollars in Medicaid overpayments that States should pay back. OIG has conducted extensive work looking at how much of this money CMS has collected. One OIG study found that CMS had collected about 80 percent of

$1.2 billion in Medicaid overpayments identified in certain audits. OIG plans continued work in this area to ensure the program effectively reclaims overpayments.

At times, States may exploit the Federal-State partnership for Medicaid financing to improperly shift costs to the Federal Government. OIG has identified a number of State policies that may inflate the Federal share of Medicaid expenditures. States have misused provider taxes, intergovernmental transfers, supplemental payments, and inflated payment rates to increase the Federal Medicaid funding that States receive. Such practices may distort the statutorily defined Federal share of Medicaid expenditures and undermine the Federal-State partnership.

CMS has tried to curtail inappropriate State financing mechanisms that inflate the Federal share of Medicaid costs. For example, CMS issued guidance to State Medicaid directors and State health officials to clarify the rules for health care provider taxes.

But more needs to be done. CMS should closely review State Medicaid plans and plan amendments to identify any potentially inappropriate cost-shifting from States to the Federal Government.

Oversight of Eligibility Determinations

States Are Not Always Correctly Determining Medicaid Eligibility for Beneficiaries

Correctly determining beneficiary eligibility is vital to the accuracy of Medicaid payments. To ensure that Medicaid makes payments on behalf of the right beneficiary, it is critical to determine whether the beneficiary receiving services is actually eligible for Medicaid. Recent OIG audits of three States estimated that more than $1.2 billion in Federal Medicaid payments has been made on behalf of potentially ineligible and ineligible beneficiaries. Lack of enrollment data systems functionality was a key contributor to these payments.

OIG recently reviewed whether certain States were correctly determining eligibility, following changes made by the Affordable Care Act (ACA) to Medicaid eligibility rules. ACA allowed States to expand Medicaid eligibility for certain low-income adults and claim a higher Federal Medical Assistance Percentage for those who are newly eligible under the expansion. As a result of States incorrectly determining beneficiaries' eligibility, payments made on behalf of those beneficiaries could be incorrect, resulting in the improper shift of costs from the State to the Federal Government. OIG reviews of Medicaid eligibility determinations by California, New York, and Kentucky reveal that these States did not always comply with Federal and State requirements to verify applicants' income, citizenship, identity, and other eligibility criteria. In total, across these three States, OIG estimated that more than $580 million in Federal Medicaid payments were made on behalf of 183,579 potentially ineligible beneficiaries, and about $655 million in payments made on behalf of 413,349 ineligible beneficiaries—over $1.2

billion in total for more than 596,000 beneficiaries. Both human and system errors contributed to these payments, with some enrollment data systems lacking the ability to (1) deny or terminate ineligible beneficiaries; (2) properly redetermine eligibility when a beneficiary aged out of an eligibility group; (3) maintain records, per Federal requirements, relating to eligibility determinations and verifications; and (4) retrieve and use information from other Government databases, such as those managed by the Social Security Administration and Department of Homeland Security.

To ensure compliance with Federal and State requirements for determining Medicaid eligibility, we recommended that States ensure that enrollment data systems are able to verify eligibility criteria, develop and implement written policies and procedures to address vulnerabilities, and undertake redeterminations as appropriate.

Medicaid Is Overpaying for Prescription Drugs due to Underpaid Rebates

To help contain the costs of prescription drugs in Medicaid, manufacturers are generally required to pay rebates to the States for covered outpatient drugs under the Medicaid Drug Rebate Program. As part of the rebate agreements, manufacturers must report product and pricing information to CMS that is used to calculate the rebates owed. CMS and States share responsibility for ensuring that manufacturers pay all rebates to which the States and Federal Government are entitled.

Ensuring that manufacturers report product and pricing information correctly is a challenge for HHS. Manufacturer misreporting can result in manufacturers' underpaying rebates, which inappropriately increases Federal and State Medicaid costs. We found that from 2012 to 2016, Medicaid may have lost $1.3 billion in base and inflation-adjusted rebates for 10 potentially misclassified drugs.

Overseeing States' collection of manufacturer rebates is also a challenge for HHS. OIG has identified instances in which States failed to bill for or collect Medicaid rebates for physician- administered drugs, forgoing money owed to those States and the Federal Government. OIG has ongoing work assessing CMS's oversight of the Medicaid Drug Rebate Program to identify opportunities for improvement.

Quality of Care

Medicaid must know with whom it is doing business, not only to prevent improper payments to ineligible providers, but also to protect beneficiaries from low-quality care. OIG has raised concerns about the varying standards, and in some cases, minimal vetting, for Medicaid personal care services (PCS) providers, potentially exposing the Medicaid program to financial fraud and Medicaid beneficiaries to abuse and neglect. For example, an elderly woman in Idaho was found dangerously malnourished and dehydrated after her Medicaid-funded caregiver failed to provide her with water and food. Investigators found the woman living in filth, when Medicaid was paying a PCS attendant to care for her everyday needs. OIG continues to recommend that CMS improve States' ability to monitor billing and care quality by requiring States to either enroll PCS attendants as providers, or require them to register with their State Medicaid agencies, and assign each attendant a unique identifier.

Group Homes

In response to reports of abuse and neglect of developmentally disabled residents in group homes, OIG launched a series of audits examining how States responded to critical incidents in group homes. OIG found that up to 99 percent of these critical incidents were not reported to the appropriate law enforcement or State agencies as required. To address these troubling findings, we worked with experts from HHS Administration for Community Living, HHS Office for Civil Rights, CMS, the Department of Justice, and State stakeholders to create a joint report entitled *Ensuring Beneficiary Health and Safety in Group Homes Through State Implementation of Comprehensive Compliance Oversight.* This chapter contains workable, holistic solutions that States can use to protect the health and safety of their residents living in group homes. Building on State efforts to protect people with disabilities in group homes, the report features suggested Model Practices for States and offers suggestions on the Federal level for CMS. These Model Practices focus on four main aspects of handling critical incidents: investigation, reporting, correction, and transparency and accountability. The joint report contains detailed suggestions, including what actions States should take when group homes repeatedly fail to report incidents.

Partnerships with MFCUs and Law Enforcement and Using Data to Protect Programs

Medicaid Fraud Control Units (MFCUs), the State agencies authorized to fight fraud and prevent patient abuse and neglect, are key partners in battling fraud and abuse in Medicaid. In FY 2017, MFCUs reported more than 1,500 convictions, nearly 1,000 civil settlements and judgements, and more than $1.8 billion in criminal and civil recoveries. OIG partners with MFCUs in joint investigations to hold wrongdoers accountable, recover stolen taxpayer dollars, and send a strong message to deter would-be fraudsters.

OIG provides oversight and administers the grants that fund the MFCUs. In this role, OIG continually strives to maximize the effectiveness of State MFCUs, thereby empowering States to better serve their populations. OIG actions to drive the effectiveness of MFCUs include enhancing OIG oversight using a data-driven risk assessment to target engagement, improving MFCUs' capabilities through training, increasing law enforcement collaboration between MCFUs and OIG, and working to help the MFCU program obtain resources consistent with an evolving Medicaid program.

Although Medicaid has grown substantially since 2010, the fraud-fighting resources of the State MFCUs have not kept pace. The 50 existing MFCUs receive 75 percent of their funding on a matching basis from the Federal Government but often they encounter severe restrictions on their ability to maintain or expand staff. In addition to the challenges of securing State- appropriated dollars for the MFCU match, some Units have difficulty in recruiting and retaining staff because of salary limitations.

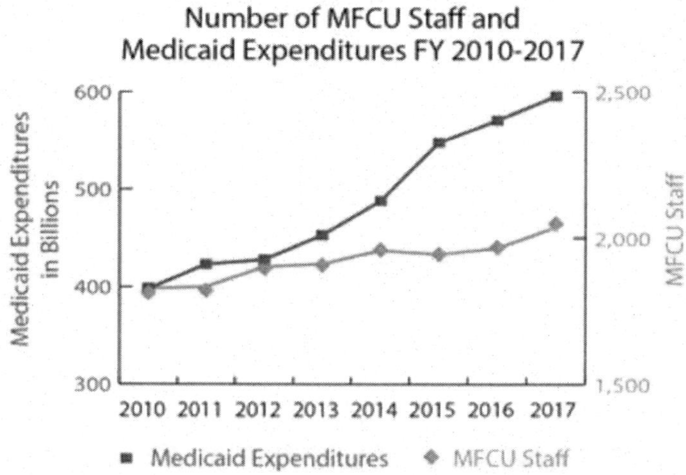

Between FY 2010 and 2017, while total MFCU staff resources increased 11.5 percent, total Medicaid expenditures for both Federal and State Governments increased 50 percent. In 2010, each MFCU employee had oversight responsibility for nearly $218 million in program expenditures, but by FY 2017 that ratio increased, and each MFCU employee was responsible for overseeing nearly $293 million. MFCUs are a wise investment, offering an estimated return of $6.52 for every $1 invested.

Conclusion

Effectively overseeing Medicaid remains a top management challenge for HHS. OIG has offered several suggestions to improve Medicaid program operations, including the following unimplemented recommendations:

- CMS should ensure that national Medicaid data are complete, accurate, and timely.
- CMS should facilitate State Medicaid agencies' efforts to screen new and existing providers by ensuring the accessibility and quality of Medicare's enrollment data.
- CMS should pursue a means to compel manufacturers to correct inaccurate classification data reported to the Medicaid Drug Rebate Program.
- CMS should require States to either enroll PCS attendants as providers or require PCS attendants to register with their State Medicaid agencies and assign each attendant a unique identifier.

OIG plans to continue prioritizing Medicaid oversight to prevent and detect fraud, waste, and abuse, and take appropriate action when fraud, waste, or abuse occur.

OIG has the capacity to leverage advanced data analytic techniques to detect potential vulnerabilities and fraud and better target our resources to those areas and individuals most in need of oversight. However, to date, this innovative way to enhance and strategically target our oversight efforts cannot be accomplished in Medicaid without better quality, national Medicaid data. This is the consistent cross-cutting impediment to effective prevention, detection, and enforcement within the Medicaid program. While neither CMS nor State Medicaid agencies presently command the data necessary to optimally support a 21st century Medicaid program, we believe this committee's continued oversight will help achieve this goal. Thank you for your ongoing leadership and for affording me the opportunity to testify on this important topic.

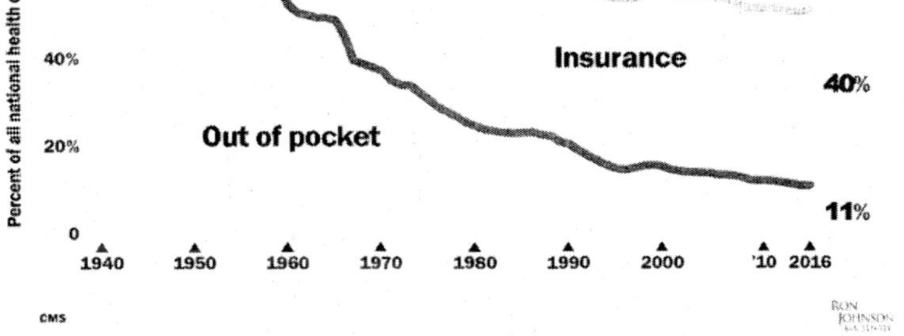

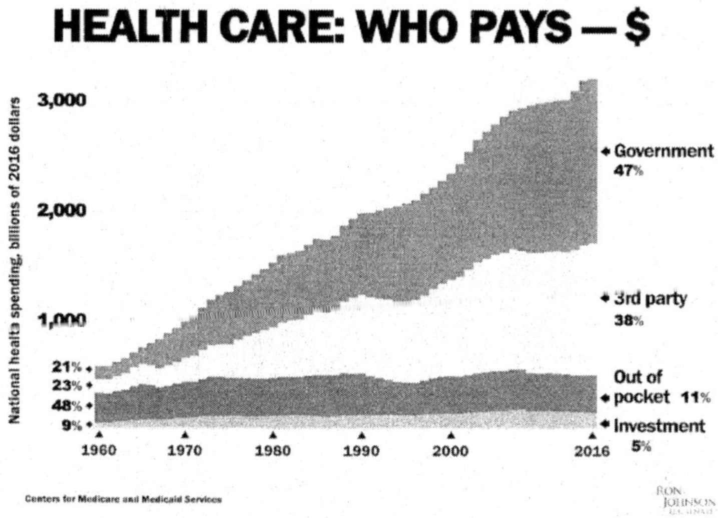
HEALTH CARE: WHO PAYS — $
National health spending, billions of 2016 dollars
3,000
2,000
1,000
21%
23%
48%
9%
1960
1970
1980
1990
2000
2016
Government 47%
3rd party 38%
Out of pocket 11%
Investment 5%
Centers for Medicare and Medicaid Services

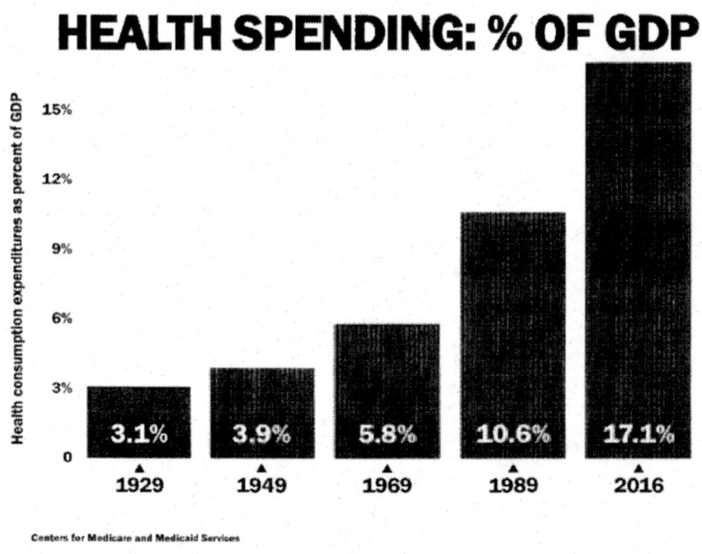
HEALTH SPENDING: % OF GDP
Health consumption expenditures as percent of GDP
15%
12%
9%
6%
3%
0
3.1%
3.9%
5.8%
10.6%
17.1%
1929
1949
1969
1989
2016
Centers for Medicare and Medicaid Services

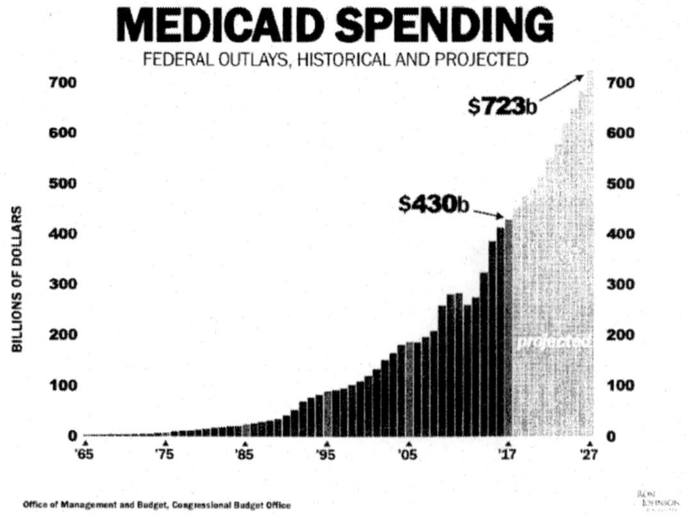
MEDICAID SPENDING
FEDERAL OUTLAYS, HISTORICAL AND PROJECTED
BILLIONS OF DOLLARS
700
600
500
400
300
200
100
0
$723b
$430b
projected
'65
'75
'85
'95
'05
'17
'27
Office of Management and Budget, Congressional Budget Office

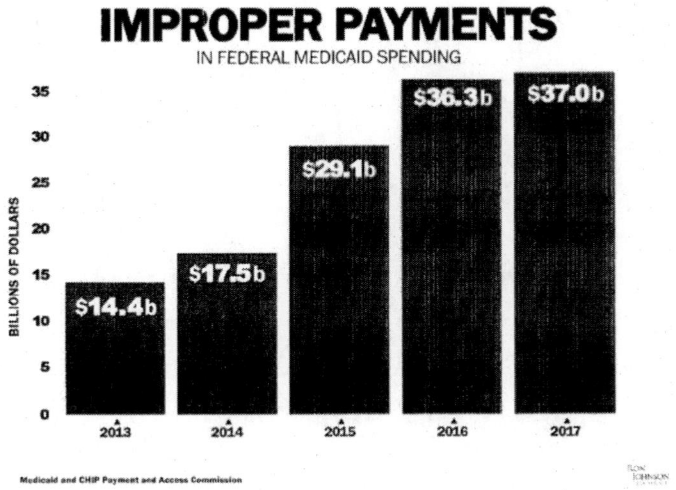

The Centers for Medicare & Medicaid Services Has Been a Poor Steward of Federal Medicaid Dollars

A Majority Staff Report of the Committee on Homeland Security and Governmental Affairs United States Senate,
Senator Ron Johnson, Chairman
June 20, 2018

Executive Summary

The U.S. health care financing system is broken and increasingly is dominated by the government. By transitioning to a third-party payment system, we have separated the consumer of health care products and services from the direct payment for them. Most consumers do not know what treatments costs, and except for the cost of insurance or copays, they really do not care.

As the benefit of free market competition from health care has been removed, the costs have predictably soared. Since 1960, the share of all health care spending paid by government has more than doubled, from about one-fifth to just under half. The result: Overall health spending now consumes about 17 percent of the nation's gross domestic product.

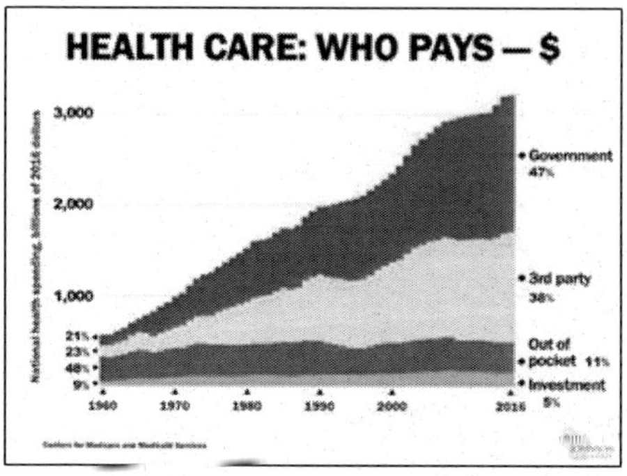

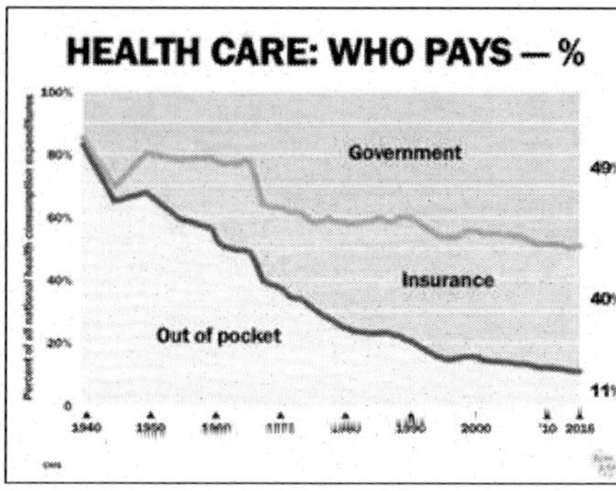

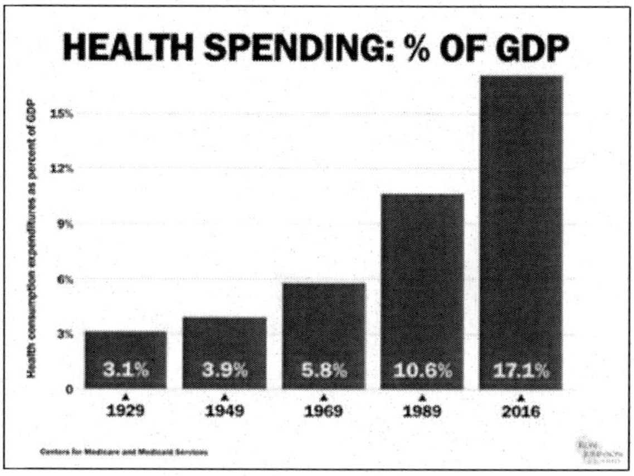

Central to this unsustainable growth is Medicaid. Medicaid began in 1965 as essentially an afterthought, a program so negligible that President Lyndon Johnson did not even mention it when it when he signed it into law alongside Medicare.[75] Envisioned as "a small program to cover poor people's medical bills,"[76] Medicaid enrolled just four million people in its first year, at a per-enrollee cost of only $222.

Today, Medicaid has grown to be the nation's largest health insurer, covering about 70 million people, at a cost to taxpayers of $554 billion per year.[77] Per-enrollee costs are now $7,973—a 3,491 percent increase since 1966.[78] This growth is especially dramatic when current Medicaid spending is compared to the $165 billion that Medicaid would have cost in 2015 if it had grown only at the rate of inflation and growth in population

---

75 Lyndon B. Johnson, Remarks with President Truman at the Signing in Independence of the Medicare Bill (July 30, 1965), *available at* http://www.presidency.ucsb.edu/ws/?pid=27123.

76 Kate Zernike, Abby Goodbough & Pam Belluck, *In Health Bill's Defeat, Medicaid Comes of Age*, N.Y. TIMES (Mar. 27, 2017), *available at* https://www.nytimes.com/2017/03/27/health/medicaid-obamacare.html?_r=0.

77 U.S. Dep't of Health & Human Servs., *2016 Actuarial Report on the Financial Outlook for Medicaid* (2016), *available at* https://www.medicaid.gov/medicaid/finance/downloads/medicaid-actuarial-report-2016.pdf.

78 Medicaid & CHIP Payment & Access Comm'n, *Medicaid Enrollment and Total Spending Levels and Annual Growth, in* MACStats: Medicaid & CHIP Data Book (Dec. 2017), *available at* https://www.macpac.gov/wp-content/uploads/2015/11/EXHIBIT-10.-Medicaid-Enrollment-and-Total-Spending-Levels-and-Annual-Growth-FYs-1966%E2%80%932016.pdf.

since 1990.[79] Federal government projections expect this growth to accelerate in the coming years, primarily due to the Affordable Care Act's (ACA) Medicaid expansion.[80]

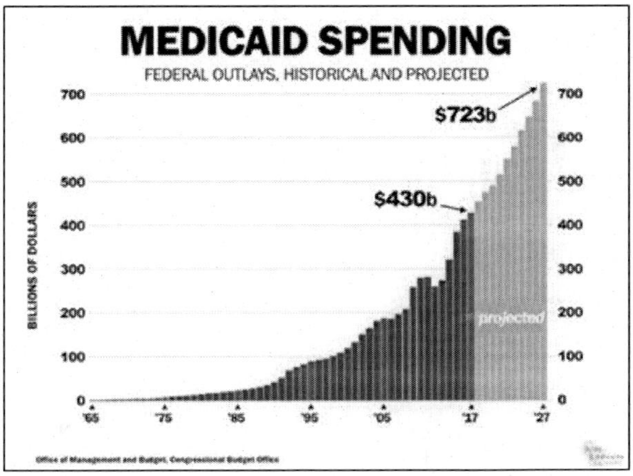

As Medicaid spending consumes even more of the federal budget, it is important that Medicaid dollars are spent properly—*so that the funds flow only to those Americans in need.* However, independent government watchdogs and ongoing oversight by the Committee on Homeland Security and Governmental Affairs show that the Medicaid program is plagued by waste, fraud, and abuse:

- Medicaid overpayments to providers stand at $37 billion per year, a 157 percent increase since 2013.[81]

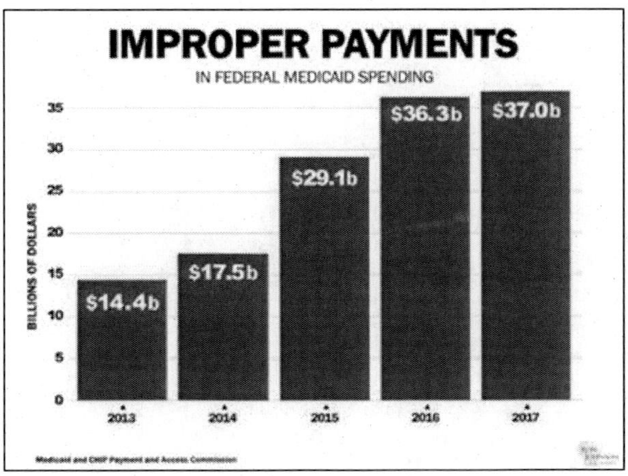

---

[79] Chairman Johnson's staff calculated this number using Consumer Price Index (CPI-U) data and figures from Bureau of Labor Statistics and the U.S. Census Bureau.

[80] Letter from Sen. Ron Johnson, Chairman, S. Comm. on Homeland Sec. & Gov't Affairs, to Seema Verma, Adm'r, Ctrs. for Medicare & Medicaid Servs. (Sept. 27, 2017).

[81] U.S. Gov't Accountability Office, GAO-18-444T, *Medicaid: Opportunities for Improving Program Oversight* (Apr. 2018), *available at* https://www.gao.gov/assets/700/691209.pdf.

- The Department of Health and Human Services Office of Inspector General (HHS OIG) recently estimated that California spent more than $1 billion in federal Medicaid funds for 445,000 ineligible or potentially ineligible beneficiaries.[82]
- The HHS OIG also found that New York made federal Medicaid payments of $26.2 million on behalf of more than 47,000 ineligible people.[83]
- Medicaid fraud convictions by state Medicaid Fraud Control Units nationwide have increased 17 percent since 2013, while criminal recoveries nearly doubled in 2017 compared to the year before.[84] At the end of 2017, state Medicaid Fraud Control Units had nearly 20,000 open fraud investigations.[85]
- The U.S. Government Accountability Office (GAO) has discovered Medicaid benefits for dead people and prisoners; hundreds of thousands of beneficiaries who provided apparently false social security numbers;[86] and an ACA data hub granting coverage to fictitious applicants.[87]
- Private insurers have made "spectacular profits"[88] from Medicaid expansion in California, with one insurer's margins increasing 578 percent in the expansion's first two years, from $71 million to $484 million.[89]
- The Centers for Medicare & Medicaid Services (CMS) has vast authority granted by a 2005 law to police Medicaid fraud,[90] but it has largely failed to do so. GAO and other watchdogs have warned CMS for the past 15 years that Medicaid is uniquely vulnerable to fraud and overpayments.
- CMS has not even attempted to recoup for federal taxpayers the more than one billion in potentially fraudulent Medicaid payments in California, New York and

[82] U.S. Dep't of Health & Human Servs. Off. of Inspector Gen., A-09-16-02023, *California Made Medicaid Payments on Behalf of Newly Eligible Beneficiaries Who Did Not Meet Federal and State Requirements* (Feb. 2018), *available at* https://oig.hhs.gov/oas/reports/region9/91602023.pdf.

[83] U.S. Dep't of Health & Human Servs. Off. of Inspector Gen., A-02-15-01015, *New York Did Not Correctly Determine Medicaid Eligibility for Some Newly Enrolled Beneficiaries* (Jan. 2018), *available at* https://oig.hhs.gov/oas/reports/region2/21501015.pdf.

[84] U.S. Dep't of Health & Human Servs. Off. of Inspector Gen., Medicaid Fraud Control Units Fiscal Year 2017 Annual Report (March 2018), https://oig.hhs.gov/oei/reports/oei-09-18-00180.pdf.

[85] *Id.*

[86] U.S. Gov't Accountability Office, GAO-15-313, *Medicaid: Additional Actions Needed to Help Improve Provider and Beneficiary Fraud Controls* (May 2015), *available at* https://www.gao.gov/products/GAO-15-313.

[87] U.S. Gov't Accountability Office, GAO-16-29, *Patient Protection and Affordable Care Act: CMS Should Act to Strengthen Enrollment Controls and Manage Fraud Risk* (Feb. 2016), *available at* https://www.gao.gov/assets/680/675767.pdf.

[88] Chad Terhune & Anna Gorman, *Insurers make billions off Medicaid in California during Obamacare expansion*, L.A. Times, Nov. 5, 2017.

[89] *Medi-Cal Managed-Care Financial Results, 2012*, KAISER HEALTH NEWS, available at https://kaiserhealthnews.files.wordpress.com/2017/11/medi-cal_financials3.pdf.

[90] Deficit Reduction Act of 2005, Pub. L. No. 109-171, 120 Stat. 4 (2006).

Kentucky,[91] and has not said whether it will go after the excessive payments to insurers in California.

- With the ACA's reimbursement formula giving states an incentive to enroll more beneficiaries to obtain more federal money, CMS has allowed certain states to game the system. California, for example, has received a share of Medicaid expansion dollars vastly disproportionate to other states,[92] even while California officials gave Medicaid money to ineligible people.

Medicaid is a program to assist low-income Americans and others in need. This staff report is not meant to challenge the intentions of such assistance. But for American taxpayers to have confidence that Medicaid funds are only going to those truly in need, CMS must better police waste, fraud, and abuse in the Medicaid program. The depth of Medicaid's fiscal problems shows the need for continued congressional attention on health care reform to slow Medicaid's rate of growth and more equitably fund state Medicaid programs.

Findings

Senator Ron Johnson, Chairman of the Senate Committee on Homeland Security and Governmental Affairs, has been conducting oversight of Medicaid program integrity and escalating costs since February 2017. This oversight has included several letters to CMS and requests for information from eight states. To date, the Chairman's oversight has found:

- Congress substantially expanded CMS's oversight responsibilities in the Deficit Reduction Act of 2005,[93] requiring CMS to root out Medicaid fraud, waste and abuse. Yet CMS has failed to live up to the requirements of this law by conducting only irregular, highly flawed audits of Medicaid providers and failing to meet annual deadlines for program integrity reporting to Congress.
- CMS has not taken basic steps to fight Medicaid fraud, including reviewing federal eligibility determinations for accuracy and even creating an antifraud

---

[91] *"Improper Payments in State-Administered Programs: Medicaid": Hearing before the Subcomm. on Gov't Operations & the Subcomm. on Intergovernmental Affairs of the H. Comm. on Oversight & Gov't Reform*, 115h Cong. (2018).

[92] Letter from Sen. Ron Johnson, Chairman, S. Comm. on Homeland Sec. & Gov't Affairs, to Edmund Brown Jr., Governor of Cal. (Sept. 27, 2017) (California "represents 34 percent of all Medicaid expansion spending, even though California represents only 12 percent of the total U.S. population" (citations omitted)).

[93] Deficit Reduction Act of 2005, Pub. L. No. 109-171, 120 Stat. 4 (2006).

strategy. Since 2015, GAO has made 11 separate anti-fraud recommendations to CMS. CMS has implemented none.[94]

- HHS programs overall are riddled with fraud. New data show that HHS fraud totals nearly $6 billion, by far the highest of any federal agency and 68 percent of the total fraud reported across the government.[95]
- Although there is no specific breakdown for Medicaid in HHS fraud numbers, evidence indicates that Medicaid fraud is rampant.
  - The Committee identified nearly 1,100 people convicted or charged nationwide since 2010 in fraud or related schemes targeting Medicaid to obtain prescription opioids.[96]
  - GAO and other watchdogs have documented potential improper or fraudulent Medicaid payments totaling more than $1 billion in at least eight states—California, New York, Kentucky, Illinois, Arizona, Florida, Michigan, and New Jersey.[97]
- The ACA worsened the problem of Medicaid fraud and overpayments by giving states incentives to declare people newly eligible to receive 100 percent federal reimbursement during the Medicaid expansion's first three years.

The Medicaid Program and CMS's Role in It

Medicaid provides free or low-cost health coverage to low-income people, families and children, pregnant women, the elderly, and people with disabilities.[98] The program is run day-to-day by states and overseen by CMS,[99] which is a component entity of HHS.

Federal taxpayers contribute a specified percentage of Medicaid program expenditures to the states.[100] HHS calculates and annually publishes this federal contribution, known as the Federal Medical Assistance Percentage.[101] There is generally

---

[94] *Improper Payments in State-Administered Programs: Medicaid*, *supra* note 17.

[95] *Resources*, PAYMENTACCURACY.GOV, https://paymentaccuracy.gov/resources/.

[96] Maj. Staff of S. Comm. on Homeland Sec. and Gov't Affairs, *Drugs for Dollars: How Medicaid Helps Fuel the Opioid Epidemic* (2018).

[97] GAO-15-313, *Medicaid: Additional Actions Needed to Help Improve Provider and Beneficiary Fraud Controls*, *supra* note 12.

[98] *Medicaid & CHIP Coverage*, HEALTHCARE.GOV, https://www.healthcare.gov/medicaid-chip/getting-medicaid- chip/.

[99] *Medicaid 101: Administration*, MACPAC, https://www.macpac.gov/medicaid-101/administration/.

[100] *Financial Management*, MEDICAID.GOV, https://www.medicaid.gov/medicaid/finance/.

[101] Office of the Assistant Sec'y for Planning & Evaluation, *Federal Medical Assistance Percentages or Federal Financial Participation in State Assistance Expenditures*, U.S. DEP'T OF HEALTH & HUMAN SERVS. (Mar. 1, 2015), https://aspe.hhs.gov/federal-medical-assistance-percentages-or-federal-financial-participation-state-assistance- expenditures.

no cap on the amount that the federal government contributes to Medicaid in a particular state.[102]

Much of Medicaid's recent growth is due to the ACA, which expanded Medicaid eligibility to include adults under 65 with incomes up to 133 percent of the federal poverty level.[103] CMS significantly understated its projections for per-enrollee spending on adults newly eligible for Medicaid under the ACA.[104] HHS now estimates that federal Medicaid expenditures—which were $299 billion in fiscal year 2014—will rise 96 percent to $588 billion by 2025.[105] CMS recently acknowledged "the heightened potential for waste, fraud and abuse in states that chose to expand their Medicaid program under the [ACA]."[106]

CMS has vast authority to fight this fraud and waste. The ACA provided additional antifraud tools, including allowing "CMS to suspend payments to providers on the basis of a credible allegation of fraud."[107] The Improper Payments Information Act of 2002 also directed CMS and other federal agencies to publicly report overpayments to Medicaid providers.[108] CMS's broadest authorities came in the Deficit Reduction Act of 2005, which provided "a serious restoration of fiscal responsibility . . . closing loopholes and preventing the unscrupulous gaming of the Medicaid system."[109] The legislation expanded CMS's role and responsibilities to combat Medicaid waste, fraud and abuse by creating a Medicaid Integrity Program.[110] Among other provisions, the law required that CMS:

- Review Medicaid providers "to determine whether fraud, waste, or abuse has occurred";
- Audit Medicaid claims to identify "overpayments to individuals or entities receiving Federal funds";
- Hire 100 new employees to focus solely on program integrity;
- Provide anti-fraud education and training
- Prepare anti-fraud plans every five years; and
- Report annually to Congress on the use of anti-Medicaid fraud funds.[111]

---

[102] *See* Alison Mitchell, CONG. RESEARCH SERV., R42865, *Medicaid Disproportionate Share Hospital Payments*, at 1 (June 17, 2016), http://www.crs.gov/reports/pdf/R42865.

[103] *Eligibility*, MEDICAID.GOV, https://www.medicaid.gov/affordable-care-act/eligibility/index.html.

[104] Letter from Sen. Ron Johnson, *supra* note 6.

[105] *Id.*

[106] Email from Emily Felder, CMS, to S. Comm. on Homeland Sec. & Gov't Affairs maj. staff (May 18, 2018).

[107] U.S. Gov't Accountability Office, GAO-12-288T, *Medicaid Program Integrity: Expanded Federal Role Presents Challenges to and Opportunities for Assisting States* (Dec. 2011), *available at* https://www.gao.gov/assets/590/586719.pdf.

[108] Improper Payments Information Act of 2002, Pub. L. No. 107-300, 116 Stat. 2350 (2002).

[109] 151 Cong. Rec. S12, 149-219 (daily ed. Nov. 2, 2005).

[110] 42 U.S.C.A. § 1396u-6.

[111] Deficit Reduction Act of 2005, Pub. L. No. 109-171, 120 Stat. 4 (2006).

CMS'S Lax Oversight of Medicaid Program Integrity

Medicaid program integrity had been considered primarily a state responsibility during the program's first four decades.[112] In the early 2000s, as independent watchdogs shined a light on Medicaid waste, fraud, and abuse, federal policymakers insisted that CMS do more. By 2005—four decades into Medicaid's existence—CMS had only eight full-time employees working to help states fight Medicaid fraud and abuse. That constituted about 0.2 percent of CMS's entire workforce, at a time when federal taxpayers spent more than $168 billion on Medicaid.[113] Each of CMS's eight employees was responsible for monitoring $21 billion in fraud.

In 2006, CMS established a Medicaid Integrity Group. Nearly a decade later, just after the ACA took effect, CMS subsumed that group under a broader Center for Program Integrity also focusing on Medicare—meaning that the Medicaid Integrity Group "no longer exists as a separate unit."[114]

The change highlights what government watchdogs have repeatedly found: that CMS's oversight of Medicaid program integrity—and its compliance with the 2005 law—has been spotty at best. Despite its vast authority to fight Medicaid waste and fraud, CMS struggles with its oversight of Medicaid program integrity.

Medicaid Fraud

Medicaid fraud ranges from billing the government for services not performed to improperly billing for illicit prescriptions such as dangerous opioids. Although health care fraud is difficult to detect and often not prosecuted,[115] evidence indicates that fraud is pervasive in the Medicaid program and that CMS is failing to adequately police Medicaid fraud.

---

[112] U.S. Gov't Accountability Office, GAO-12-627, *National Medicaid Audit Program: CMS Should Improve Reporting and Focus on Audit Collaboration with States* (June 2012), *available at* https://www.gao.gov/assets/600/591601.pdf.

[113] U.S. Gov't Accountability Office, GAO-06-578T, *Medicaid Integrity: Implementation of New Program Provides Opportunities for Federal Leadership to Combat Fraud, Waste, And Abuse* (Mar. 2006), *available at* https://www.gao.gov/assets/120/113123.pdf.

[114] U.S. Gov't Accountability Office, GAO-15-207T, *Medicaid Information Technology: CMS Supports Use of Program Integrity Systems but Should Require States to Determine Effectiveness* (Jan. 2015), *available at* https://www.gao.gov/assets/670/668233.pdf.

[115] Paul Jesilow & Bryan Burton, *Detecting Healthcare Fraud and Abuse in the United States*, OXFORD RESEARCH ENCYCLOPEDIAS: CRIMINOLOGY & CRIMINAL JUSTICE, *available at* http://criminology.oxfordre.com/view/10.1093/acrefore/9780190264079.001.0001/acrefore-9780190264079-e-275; U.S. Gov't Accountability Office, GAO-16-216, *Health Care Fraud: Information on Most Common Schemes and the Likely Effect of Smart Cards* (Jan. 2016), *available at* https://www.gao.gov/assets/680/674771.pdf.

- In 2015, GAO found "thousands of Medicaid beneficiaries and hundreds of providers involved in potential improper or fraudulent payments" in four states—Arizona, Florida, Michigan, and New Jersey.[116]
- The Committee also found evidence of Medicaid fraud in its examination of Medicaid's role in helping to fuel the opioid epidemic.[117] In January 2018, Chairman Johnson released a staff report highlighting nearly 300 criminal cases involving at least 1,072 defendants in which people were convicted or charged with abusing Medicaid to obtain or sell opioids.[118] The criminal schemes identified by the Committee ranged from large drug rings that employ beneficiaries as "runners" to fill oxycodone prescriptions to nurses who steal hydrocodone pills from patients.[119] The Committee held a hearing in conjunction with the report to hear from local law enforcement and a former state Medicaid official about how Medicaid fraud helps to fuel the opioid crisis.[120]
- In a series of undercover operations between 2014 and 2016, GAO submitted applications to the federal ACA marketplace with names of fictitious enrollees and with fake or no documentation.[121] In nearly every instance, the marketplace granted Medicaid coverage to the non-existent enrollees—complete with premium tax credits—including in a number of stings that occurred three years after the ACA took effect.[122] The marketplace verified the fraudulent eligibility through a CMS-created "data hub." GAO warned in 2016 that the hub, which "plays a key role in the eligibility and enrollment process," was vulnerable to fraud.[123]
- In April 2018, GAO testified that CMS had failed to implement 11 separate GAO recommendation to fight Medicaid fraud, including providing regular fraud-awareness training to employees and requiring new hires to undergo such training, conducting Medicaid fraud risk assessments, and creating and implementing "an anti-fraud strategy."[124]

---

[116] GAO-15-313, *Medicaid: Additional Actions Needed to Help Improve Provider and Beneficiary Fraud Controls*, *supra* note 12.
[117] *Drugs for Dollars: How Medicaid Helps Fuel the Opioid Epidemic*, *supra* note 22.
[118] *Id.*
[119] *Id.*
[120] *"Unintended Consequences: Medicaid and the Opioid Epidemic": Hearing before the S. Comm. on Homeland Sec. and Gov't Affairs*, 115th Cong. (2018).
[121] GAO-16-29, *Patient Protection and Affordable Care Act: CMS Should Act to Strengthen Enrollment Controls and Manage Fraud Risk*, *supra* note 13.
[122] *Id.*
[123] *Id.*
[124] *Improper Payments in State-Administered Programs: Medicaid*, *supra* note 17.

Medicaid Overpayments

Federal law defines improper payments as those that should not have been made or were made in incorrect amounts.[125] Although improper payments include overpayments and underpayments, only 0.8 percent of the $36.7 billion in Medicaid improper payments in fiscal year 2017 were underpayments.[126] Although the exact percentage of overpayments that constitute fraud is unclear, there is no doubt that all overpayments waste federal tax dollars. Evidence suggests that CMS could do more to police Medicaid overpayments.

- Federal law required every federal agency to estimate improper payments and report the estimates annually to Congress beginning in FY 2004.[127] HHS, however, did not start reporting improper Medicaid payments until 2007.
- In 2008, the first full year in which HHS disclosed improper Medicaid payments, they were already the highest of any federal program at $18.6 billion.[128] This figure prompted a stern warning from GAO, which linked improper payments to fraud and warned that CMS needed "a culture of accountability over improper payments" to "reduce fraud and address the wasteful spending that results from lapses in controls."[129] GAO added that the magnitude of Medicaid payment errors "indicates that CMS and the states face significant challenges to address the program's vulnerabilities."[130]
- In 2015, GAO reported that while CMS had helped state Medicaid programs implement systems to detect overpayments, it had failed to require states to measure whether those systems worked.[131] With no requirement, most states did not implement metrics to measure success.[132] Around that time, Medicaid improper payments began rising, going from $14.4 billion in 2013[133]—the year before Obamacare took effect—to $37 billion in 2017—a 157 percent increase.[134] During the same period, the Medicaid improper payment rate, the percentage of

---

[125] PAYMENTACCURACY.GOV, https://paymentaccuracy.gov/.

[126] U.S. Dep't of Health & Human Servs., *Agency Financial Report* (2017), *available at* https://www.hhs.gov/sites/default/files/fy-2017-hhs-agency-financial-report.pdf. Because Medicaid improper payments are overwhelmingly overpayments, this chapter is using the term overpayments where appropriate.

[127] Improper Payments Information Act of 2002, Pub. L. No. 107-300, 116 Stat. 2350 (2002).

[128] U.S. Gov't Accountability Office, GAO-09-628T, *Improper Payments: Progress Made but Challenges Remain in Estimating and Reducing Improper Payments* (Apr. 2009), *available at* https://www.gao.gov/products/GAO-09- 628T.

[129] *Id.*

[130] *Id.*

[131] GAO-15-207T, *Medicaid Information Technology: CMS Supports Use of Program Integrity Systems but Should Require States to Determine Effectiveness*, *supra* note 40.

[132] *Id.*

[133] Letter from Beryl Davis, Dir., Fin. Mgmt. & Assurance, U.S. Gov't Accountability Office, to Sen. Thomas Carper, Chairman, S. Comm. on Homeland Sec. & Gov't Affairs, et al. (Dec. 9, 2014), *available at* https://www.gao.gov/assets/670/667332.pdf.

[134] GAO-18-444T, *Medicaid: Opportunities for Improving Program Oversight*, *supra* note 7.

total federal Medicaid expenditures estimated to be improper, rose 74 percent.[135] Medicaid alone now constitutes 26 percent of improper payments across the entire federal government.[136]

- As recently as 2017, GAO warned in its most recent High Risk report that "CMS's improper payment rate estimates may be inaccurate."[137] According to GAO, 13 years after Congress required CMS to better police Medicaid fraud, CMS must still "take appropriate measures to reduce improper payments, as dollars wasted detract from our ability to ensure that the individuals who rely on the Medicaid program— including children, and individuals who are elderly or disabled—are provided adequate care."[138]

Medicaid Audits and Eligibility

CMS's lax oversight has extended into the most vital area of Medicaid program integrity: ensuring only those eligible for Medicaid receive the program's benefits.

- In 2011, CMS was forced to redesign its required audits of Medicaid providers, which were then the largest part of the CMS Medicaid integrity program.[139] Due to poor CMS data that were missing basic provider information, the audits identified less than $20 million in potential overpayments, at a cost of at least $102 million for contractors to conduct the audits.[140]
- Upon the ACA's implementation in 2014, evidence emerged that CMS was not paying enough attention to its fraud-related responsibilities for the fastest-growing part of Medicaid: managed care. GAO found that CMS and other federal entities had "taken few steps to address Medicaid managed care program integrity" and that CMS had failed to update its managed care program integrity guidance to states since 2000.[141] Unless CMS took "a larger role in holding states accountable," GAO warned, "a growing portion of federal Medicaid dollars [would be] vulnerable to improper payments."[142] Although HHS concurred with several GAO recommendations, it contended that a key anti-fraud

---

[135] U.S. Dep't of Health & Human Servs., *Agency Financial Report* (2016), *available at* https://www.hhs.gov/sites/default/files/fy-2016-hhs-agency-financial-report.pdf.

[136] GAO-18-444T, *Medicaid: Opportunities for Improving Program Oversight*, *supra* note 7.

[137] U.S. Gov't Accountability Office, GAO-17-317, *High-Risk Series: Progress on Many High-Risk Areas, While Substantial Efforts Needed on Others* (Feb. 2017), *available at* https://www.gao.gov/products/GAO-17-317.

[138] GAO-18-444T, *Medicaid: Opportunities for Improving Program Oversight*, *supra* note 7.

[139] U.S. Gov't Accountability Office, GAO-12-674T, *Medicaid: Federal Oversight of Payments and Program Integrity Needs Improvement* (Apr. 2012), *available at* https://www.gao.gov/assets/600/590392.pdf.

[140] *Id.*; GAO-12-288T, *Medicaid Program Integrity: Expanded Federal Role Presents Challenges to and Opportunities for Assisting States*, *supra* note 33.

[141] U.S. Gov't Accountability Office, GAO-14-341, *Medicaid Program Integrity: Increased Oversight Needed to Ensure Integrity of Growing Managed Care Expenditures* (May 2014), *available at* https://www.gao.gov/assets/670/663306.pdf.

[142] *Id.*

recommendation—that CMS hold states accountable by requiring them to audit payments to Medicaid managed care providers—was "unclear."[143]

- By 2015, CMS had started interim reviews of Medicaid expansion eligibility determinations. However, CMS officials excluded from review Medicaid eligibility determinations in states where the federal government made such determinations, meaning that 67 percent of the country escaped such scrutiny.[144] In the 17 states that then had their own exchanges, CMS suspended until fiscal year 2018—the first four years of the ACA—its requirement that states review their own eligibility determination.[145] Citing ACA-related changes to Medicaid eligibility standards and state eligibility systems, CMS required states that operate their own exchanges to conduct temporary "pilot eligibility reviews."[146] Those reviews did find Medicaid expansion eligibility errors in eight of nine states—including enrollment of people whose incomes were too high to be eligible.[147]
- CMS is still not reviewing eligibility determinations in states using the ACA's federally-facilitated exchanges as GAO has been recommending since 2015,[148] or filing annual reports on its Medicaid integrity program to Congress as required by the 2005 law.[149] According to GAO's latest High Risk report, CMS filed the 2013 and 2014 reports in 2016—and was more than a year late with the 2015 report. As a result, CMS is still unable to discharge its most fundamental duty to American taxpayers: "to ensure the fiscal integrity of the [Medicaid] program."[150]

CMS's Lax Attention to State Medicaid Programs

As a joint federal-state program, Medicaid varies state-to-state. CMS claims it "works closely with [its] state partners to provide them with the tools and knowledge to effectively operate their programs."[151] While CMS has taken some steps to improve state-based integrity programs—including the establishment of the Medicaid Integrity Institute with the Justice Department in 2007—evidence suggests that CMS can do much more to root out waste, fraud, and abuse in state Medicaid programs.

---

[143] *Id.*

[144] U.S. Gov't Accountability Office, GAO-16-53, *Medicaid: Additional Efforts Needed to Ensure that State Spending is Appropriately Matched with Federal Funds* (Oct. 2015), *available at* https://www.gao.gov/assets/680/673159.pdf.

[145] *Id.*

[146] *Id.*

[147] *Id.*

[148] GAO-18-444T, *Medicaid: Opportunities for Improving Program Oversight*, *supra* note 7.

[149] GAO-17-317, *High-Risk Series: Progress on Many High-Risk Areas, While Substantial Efforts Needed on Others*, *supra* note 63.

[150] *Id.*

[151] Email from Emily Felder, *supra* note 32.

GAO has identified several problems with CMS's oversight of and communication with state Medicaid programs.

- As late as 2014, CMS program integrity guidance issued in 2000 to states for Medicaid managed care was still not available on the CMS website, and state officials reported they did not use the guidance to fight fraud or overpayments. CMS told GAO at the time that the 14-year-old guidance was being "updated" but could not provide "a timeline for its completion."[152]
- CMS has still not provided guidance to states on the availability of automated information through Medicare's enrollment database, which would help states screen Medicaid providers. GAO has been urging this step since 2015.[153]
- CMS has not sought "to identify opportunities to address barriers that limit states' participation in collaborative audits," as GAO has also recommended.[154] Federal officials say CMS has sometimes allowed state officials to refuse to participate in these audits, which limited CMS's oversight of fraud and other program integrity issues.[155]

Fraud in State Medicaid Programs

CMS's lax oversight of states is leading, in part, to Medicaid fraud and wasted taxpayer money.

- In March 2018, the Illinois auditor revealed that the state paid $71 million for Medicaid services for more than 8,000 people without checking whether they were still eligible within the 12-month period required by federal law.[156] Auditors also determined that Illinois paid Medicaid costs for people who were never Medicaid eligible because their immigration status was not verified or they lacked a valid social security number, and that Illinois failed to recoup $76 million in overpayments to private Medicaid-program insurers.[157]
- In New York, the HHS OIG reported in January 2018 that state officials calculated Medicaid eligibility incorrectly for more than 30 percent of

---

[152] GAO-14-341, *Medicaid Program Integrity: Increased Oversight Needed to Ensure Integrity of Growing Managed Care Expenditures*, *supra* note 67.

[153] GAO-18-444T, *Medicaid: Opportunities for Improving Program Oversight*, *supra* note 7.

[154] *Id.*

[155] Interview with Gov't Accountability Office officials and S. Comm. on Homeland Sec. & Gov't Affairs maj. staff (Apr. 23, 2018).

[156] Financial Audit for the Year Ended June 30, 2017, STATE OF ILLINOIS DEP'T OF HEALTHCARE & FAMILY SERVS. (Mar. 6, 2018), *available at* https://www.auditor.illinois.gov/Audit-Reports/Compliance-Agency-List/DHFS/FY17-DHFS-Fin-Full.pdf.

[157] John O'Connor, *Illinois Fails to Recoup $76 Million in Medicaid Overpayment*, U.S. NEWS (March 24, 2018), https://www.usnews.com/news/best-states/illinois/articles/2018-03-24/illinois-fails-to-recoup-76-million-in-medicaid-overpayment.

beneficiaries sampled by auditors.[158] The errors resulted in federal Medicaid payments of an estimated $26.2 million for more than 47,000 ineligible people.[159]

- In August 2017, HHS OIG identified an estimated $73 million in federal Medicaid payments for nearly 70,000 potentially ineligible beneficiaries in Kentucky.[160]

California: More Than $1 Billion in Potentially Fraudulent Medicaid Payments

In California, the HHS OIG identified an estimated than $1 billion in federal Medicaid payments on behalf of 445,000 ineligible or potentially ineligible people.[161] Of that total, the OIG found $629 million in federal taxpayer funds to have been paid for 366,000 ineligible people.[162]

- CMS appears unwilling to recoup taxpayer dollars wrongly paid out from California's Medicaid program. During a hearing of the House Committee on Oversight and Government Reform in April 2018, CMS's deputy director for Medicaid, Timothy Hill, testified that CMS did not intend to collect the more than $1 billion in fraudulent payments from California.[163] Hill testified:

Rep. Meadows: So, Mr. Hill, are you going after the $1.2 billion?

Mr. Hill: The $1.2 [billion] is identified as potential overpayment. There was not a recommendation to collect it because . . .

Rep. Meadows: Well, let me give you a recommendation. Collect it. I mean, it is the American taxpayers' dollars. Is it your sworn testimony here today...because you did not get a recommendation to collect $1.2 billion in improper payments, you are not going after it?

Mr. Hill: No, the recommendations were to fix the systems in California. . .

Rep. Meadows: So are you going after it or not?

Mr. Hill: We are not issuing a disallowance to California ... [164]

- CMS's reluctance to police California is all the more glaring in light of the size of California's Medicaid program. California received $20.3 billion for Medicaid expansion from the federal government in 2015—34 percent of all Medicaid expansion spending, even though California represented only 12 percent of the

---

[158] U.S. Dep't of Health & Human Servs., A-02-15-01015, *supra* note 9.

[159] *Id.*

[160] U.S. Dep't of Health & Human Servs., A-04-16-08047, *Kentucky Did Not Always Perform Medicaid Eligibility Determinations for Non-Newly Eligible Beneficiaries in Accordance with Federal and State Requirements* (Aug. 2017), *available at* https://oig.hhs.gov/oas/reports/region4/41608047.pdf.

[161] U.S. Dep't of Health & Human Servs. Off. of Inspector Gen., A-09-16-02023, *supra* note 8.

[162] *Id.*

[163] *Improper Payments in State-Administered Programs: Medicaid*, *supra* note 17.

[164] *Id.*

U.S. population.[165] As Chairman Johnson wrote to CMS administrator Verma in September 2017, enrollment under Medicaid expansion has substantially exceeded projections in California and many other expansion states.[166]

- California exemplifies how the ACA's Medicaid expansion reimbursement formula has allowed some states to game the system. Although the traditional federal matching rate ranges from 50 percent to as high as 73 percent, there is a far higher matching rate for people made newly eligible for Medicaid under the ACA—100 percent through 2016, before phasing down to 90 percent in 2020 and beyond.[167] This higher matching rate provides states a tremendous financial incentive to categorize more people as newly eligible to obtain more federal money.
- CMS's lax oversight extends to its review of California's state Medicaid plan. Because CMS allowed California to pay higher Medicaid rates to managed care companies during the ACA's first few years, insurance companies profited handsomely.[168] According to managed care financial results from California's Medicaid program, Health Net, the largest Medicaid insurer nationwide, reported a profit of $71 million in California in 2013.[169] In 2014, the first year of the ACA's Medicaid expansion, Health Net's profits rose to $170 million, and reached $484 million in 2015[170]—a 578 percent increase during the ACA's first two years. CMS has not stated publicly whether it will seek to recoup any of this funding from California.

Medicaid Maximization Schemes

Because the federal contribution to Medicaid is generally unlimited, some states choose funding sources for their share of Medicaid's cost in a manner designed to maximize the federal government's contribution.[171] Under these so-called "Medicaid maximization schemes," the states artificially inflate what the federal government contributes while reducing the state contribution.[172] Both GAO and the HHS OIG have

---

[165] Letter from Sen. Ron Johnson, *supra* note 6.

[166] *Id.*

[167] Robin Rudowitz, *Understanding How States Access the ACA Enhanced Medicaid Match Rates*, KAISER FAMILY FOUNDATION (Sept. 29, 2014), https://www.kff.org/medicaid/issue-brief/understanding-how-states-access-the-aca- enhanced-medicaid-match-rates/.

[168] Terhune & Gorman, *supra* note14.

[169] *Medi-Cal Managed-Care Financial Results, 2012*, *supra* note 15.

[170] *Id.*

[171] *See generally Non-Federal Financing*, MACPAC, https://www.macpac.gov/subtopic/non-federal-financing/ (detailing various sources of funding) (last visited May 22, 2018).

[172] *See* U.S. Gov't Accountability Office, GAO-14-627, *Medicaid Financing: States' Increased Reliance on Funds from Health Care Providers and Local Governments Warrants Improved CMS Data Collection*, at 2-3 (July 2014), *available at* https://www.gao.gov/assets/670/665077.pdf.

repeatedly warned that these Medicaid maximization schemes undermine the federal-state Medicaid partnership.[173]

- Intergovernmental transfers (IGTs) include "transfers of . . . funds between State and/or local public Medicaid providers and the State Medicaid agency."[174] IGTs "often do not represent a true expenditure for health care services," which means "states are not fully financing their share of Medicaid costs as was intended."[175] In one instance, Michigan "paid" $122 million of its own funds to county health facilities, along with a federal match—and the same day, the county facilities transferred all but $6 million of the state funds, and the federal match, back to the state.[176] States have used federal matching funds received "for a range of purposes with no direct link to improving quality of care or increasing Medicaid services."[177] According to GAO, CMS "generally does not require (or otherwise collect) information from states on the funds they use to finance Medicaid, nor ensure that the data that it does collect are accurate and complete."[178]
- States tax healthcare providers, then return the funds to the providers and trigger a federal match.[179] This shell game artificially inflates what the federal government contributes.[180] These taxes are "increasingly popular and [have] resulted in billions of dollars in additional Medicaid spending."[181] An Oregon official described the state's provider tax as a "dream tax," where "we [Oregon] collect the tax from hospitals, we put it up as a match for federal money, and then

---

[173] U.S. Gov't Accountability Office, GAO-16-195T, *Medicaid: Improving Transparency and Accountability of Supplemental Payments and State Financing Methods,* at 6 (Nov. 2015), *available at* https://www.gao.gov/assets/680/673493.pdf; *Spotlight on Medicaid: State Policies That Result in Inflated Federal Costs*, U.S. DEP'T OF HEALTH AND HUMAN SERVS., OFFICE OF INSPECTOR GEN., https://oig.hhs.gov/newsroom/spotlight/2014/inflated-federal-costs.asp (last visited May 22, 2018).

[174] *"Examining Medicaid and CHIP's Federal Medical Assistance Percentage": Hearing before the Subcomm. On Health of the House Comm. on Energy and Commerce*, 114th Cong. (2016) (statement of John Hagg, Dir. of Medicaid Audits, Off. of Inspector Gen., Dep't of Health and Human Servs.).

[175] Teresa Coughlin & Stephen Zuckerman, *States' Use of Medicaid Maximization Strategies to Tap Federal Revenues: Program Implications and Consequences*, URBAN INSTITUTE, at 11 (June 1, 2002), https://www.urban.org/sites/default/files/publication/60176/310525-States-Use-of-Medicaid-Maximization-Strategies-to-Tap-Federal-Revenues.PDF.

[176] U.S. Gov't Accountability Office, GAO-04-574T, *Medicaid: Intergovernmental Transfers Have Facilitated State Financing Schemes*, at 5-6 (Mar. 2004), *available at* https://www.gao.gov/assets/120/110702.pdf.

[177] *Spotlight on Medicaid: State Policies That Result in Inflated Federal Costs*, U.S. DEP'T OF HEALTH AND HUMAN SERVS., OFFICE OF INSPECTOR GEN., https://oig.hhs.gov/newsroom/spotlight/2014/inflated-federal-costs.asp (last visited May 22, 2018).

[178] GAO-16-195T, *Medicaid: Improving Transparency and Accountability of Supplemental Payments and State Financing Methods, supra* note 99, at 13; *see also* GAO-14-627, *Medicaid Financing: States' Increased Reliance on Funds from Health Care Providers and Local Governments Warrants Improved CMS Data Collection, supra* note 98, at 39 ("CMS does not collect accurate and complete data from all states on the various sources of funds to finance the nonfederal share …").

[179] *See* GAO-14-627, *Medicaid Financing: States' Increased Reliance on Funds from Health Care Providers and Local Governments Warrants Improved CMS Data Collection*, *supra* note 98, at 2.

[180] *Id.*

[181] Alex Brill, *Medicaid Provider Taxes: Closing a Loophole*, TAX NOTES, at 5 (June 29, 2015), *available at* http://www.aei.org/wp-content/uploads/2015/06/Brill-Medicaid-Provider-Taxes.pdf.

we give it back to the hospitals."[182] Connecticut has a similar scheme that, if approved by CMS, would enable it to pocket funds from federal taxpayers to bolster the state's bottom line.[183]

- Supplemental payments are "payments that are separate from the regular payments states make based on claims submitted for services rendered."[184] One type of supplemental payments, disproportionate share hospital (DSH) payments, helps offset costs that hospitals accrue when serving Medicaid beneficiaries and other low-income patients.[185] Such payments are "capped at a facility-specific level and state level."[186] But states also make non-DSH supplemental payments to hospitals and other providers that "are not subject to firm dollar limits at the facility or state level."[187] In fact, these payments "are not necessarily made on the basis of claims for specific services to particular patients and can amount to tens or hundreds of millions of dollars to a single provider, annually."[188] They can also exceed the costs of services provided.[189] According to GAO, "CMS lacks data at the federal level on [these] non-DSH supplemental payments," and "the payments are not subject to audit."[190] Similarly, according to GAO, CMS should require more "reliable[] and timely information" concerning supplemental payments states make to providers.[191]

The Committee's Oversight of CMS and Medicaid

As the Chairman of the Senate's chief oversight committee, Senator Johnson has a duty to conduct oversight of federal agencies, including CMS, to ensure the government spends federal tax dollars efficiently and effectively.

---

[182] Peter Wong, *Oregon House Extends Hospital Tax*, PORTLAND TRIBUNE, Mar. 11, 2015, *available at* http://portlandtribune.com/pt/9-news/253422-123198-oregon-house-extends-hospital-tax.

[183] Red Jahncke, *Why Tax Hospitals? It's a Medicaid Shell Game*, WALL ST. J., Dec. 29, 2017, *available at* https://www.wsj.com/articles/why-tax-hospitals-its-a-medicaid-shell-game-1514586150.

[184] GAO-14-627, *Medicaid Financing: States' Increased Reliance on Funds from Health Care Providers and Local Governments Warrants Improved CMS Data Collection*, *supra* note 98, at 2.

[185] GAO-16-195T, *Medicaid: Improving Transparency and Accountability of Supplemental Payments and State Financing Methods*, *supra* note 99, at 5.

[186] *Id.*; *see also* Alison Mitchell, CONG. RESEARCH SERV., R42865, *Medicaid Disproportionate Share Hospital Payments*, at 1 (June 17, 2016), http://www.crs.gov/reports/pdf/R42865.

[187] GAO-16-195T, *Medicaid: Improving Transparency and Accountability of Supplemental Payments and State Financing Methods*, *supra* note 99, at 5.

[188] *Id.*

[189] In 2012, GAO reported that "39 states made non-DSH supplemental payments" that exceeded "total costs of providing Medicaid care by about $2.7 billion." *Id.* at 7.

[190] *Id.* at 8.

[191] *See id.* at 6-7; *see also id.* at 8-9 (describing need for "complete and reliable provider-specific data" on non-DSH supplemental payments because such data is needed to identify payments that may be "excessive" and inappropriate).

Medicaid's Escalating Costs and Enrollment Figures

In the early days of the Trump Administration, Chairman Johnson became concerned about growing evidence that Medicaid expansion costs and enrollment were spiraling far beyond initial projections. Committee majority staff sought CMS's help in exploring this problem and understanding CMS's actions to address it.[192]

- On September 27, 2017, Chairman Johnson sent a letter to Administrator Verma formally requesting information about the escalating costs of Medicaid expansion and CMS's efforts to address the rising costs.[193] Chairman Johnson raised concerns that the cost surge could stem "from the Medicaid expansion's reimbursement formula, which gives states a financial incentive to categorize people as newly eligible to obtain more federal money."[194] Chairman Johnson also sent letters to eight states with particularly alarming rates of growth in Medicaid costs or enrollment.[195]
- In October 2017, Administrator Verma responded. She wrote that CMS "takes very seriously [its] responsibility to see that only eligible individuals are enrolled in entitlement programs."[196]
    - Administrator Verma wrote that CMS had provided enhanced funding for modernized or new state Medicaid eligibility systems and taken other steps, such as holding "multiple all-state calls and in-person trainings," to provide guidance to states on how to "implement the federal [Medicaid] match rate methodology appropriately."[197]
    - Administrator Verma's response did not address the repeated warnings from government watchdogs that CMS's actions to police Medicaid program integrity have been insufficient.[198] She wrote that CMS conducts quarterly reviews of state Medicaid expenditure reports and had disallowed only "over $15 million" in claims for services for newly eligible beneficiaries.[199] In comparison to the estimated $37 billion in annual Medicaid overpayments,[200] CMS's disallowance data shows that it could be doing more to police Medicaid program integrity.

---

[192] *See* e.g., meeting with Cntrs. for Medicare & Medicaid Servs. and S. Comm. on Homeland Sec. & Gov't Affairs maj. staff (May 4, 2017); meeting with Brian Neale, Cntrs. for Medicare & Medicaid Servs. and S. Comm. on Homeland Sec. & Gov't Affairs maj. staff (Mar. 31, 2017).

[193] Letter from Sen. Ron Johnson, *supra* note 6.

[194] *Id.*

[195] E.g., Letter from Sen. Ron Johnson, *supra* note 18.

[196] Letter from Seema Verma, Adm'r, Ctrs. For Medicare & Medicaid Servs., to Sen. Ron Johnson, Chairman, S. Comm. on Homeland Sec. & Gov't Affairs (Oct. 27, 2017).

[197] *Id.*

[198] *Id.*

[199] *Id.*

[200] GAO-18-444T, *Medicaid: Opportunities for Improving Program Oversight*, *supra* note 7.

Medicaid Fraud and the Opioid Crisis

Chairman Johnson also uncovered evidence suggesting a correlation between the Medicaid program and the nation's opioid crisis.

- On January 17, 2018, Chairman Johnson convened a hearing of the Committee and released a staff report detailing how the structure of the Medicaid program creates a series of incentives for opioid abuse.[201] The report detailed hundreds of examples of opioid-related fraud in the Medicaid program and explained how Medicaid is serving as a funding source for obtaining and illicitly distributing opioids.[202] Chairman Johnson sent a copy of the report to Administrator Verma, along with specific questions about CMS's efforts to eliminate Medicaid's role in the opioid epidemic.[203]
- Administrator Verma responded on February 9, focusing instead on Medicaid's role in ensuring beneficiaries have treatment for substance abuse disorders.[204] While treatment is certainly an important element of Medicaid, Administrator Verma's response failed to address the key questions Chairman Johnson asked, specifically his request that she explain CMS's "work to improve the structure of the Medicaid program to limit the perverse incentives that lead to opioid abuse."[205] The Committee sought supplementary materials from CMS, which has provided only limited information to date about its work to address Medicaid's role in the opioid crisis.

Union Dues Skimming from Medicaid Funds

On April 30, 2018, Chairman Johnson wrote to Administrator Verma urging CMS to review the practice of "dues skimming," in which states allow unions to classify home health care workers as government employees for purposes of collecting union dues from Medicaid payments.[206] Dues skimming allows states to take an estimated $200 million each year in union dues—money that would otherwise help for the care of Medicaid beneficiaries.[207]

---

[201] *Unintended Consequences: Medicaid and the Opioid Epidemic*, *supra* note 17; *Drugs for Dollars: How Medicaid Helps Fuel the Opioid Epidemic*, *supra* note 22.

[202] *Drugs for Dollars: How Medicaid Helps Fuel the Opioid Epidemic*, *supra* note 22.

[203] Letter from Sen. Ron Johnson, Chairman, S. Comm. on Homeland Sec. & Gov't Affairs, to Seema Verma, Adm'r, Ctrs. For Medicare & Medicaid Servs., & Eric D. Hargan, Acting Secretary, Dep't of Health & Human Servs. (Jan. 17, 2018).

[204] Letter from Seema Verma, Adm'r, Ctrs. For Medicare & Medicaid Servs., to Sen. Ron Johnson, Chairman, S. Comm. on Homeland Sec. & Gov't Affairs (Feb. 9, 2018).

[205] Letter from Sen. Ron Johnson, Chairman, *supra* note 6.

[206] Letter from Sen. Ron Johnson, Chairman, S. Comm. on Homeland Sec. & Gov't Affairs, to Seema Verma, Adm'r, Ctrs. For Medicare & Medicaid Servs. (Apr. 30, 2018).

[207] *Id.*

Administrator Verma responded on June 13, 2018.[208] She informed the Chairman that CMS "does not possess" information about the amount of Medicaid funds diverted for union dues, but that CMS was reviewing whether to implement changes to "ensure Medicaid fund are legally spent."[209] The response enclosed correspondence with the Illinois Governor about Medicaid dues skimming, but otherwise provided no responsive documents.[210]

Steps toward Reform

Medicaid is an important program that helps millions of Americans in need. But as the program has grown over the past half-century, it has expanded at a pace that is now threatening to overwhelm federal and state budgets.[211] The ACA is putting new strains on CMS and Medicaid,[212] making it vitally important that the federal government ensure that no tax dollars go to waste.[213]

Yet as this staff report shows, CMS is failing to safeguard the hundreds of billions of dollars that fund Medicaid each year.[214] A series of government watchdog reports, dating back more than a decade, show that CMS is not effectively policing Medicaid fraud. A succession of CMS administrators have not provided the effective oversight that Congress required in 2005.[215] The Committee's oversight of soaring expansion costs,[216] the pernicious role of opioids,[217] and the plague of Medicaid fraud[218] further demonstrates that CMS has not proven an effective steward of Medicaid taxpayer dollars. This unfortunate trend has continued, despite the Trump Administration's stated goal to reign in Medicaid fraud.[219]

The time is ripe for CMS to take proactive steps to reduce Medicaid fraud and improve program integrity. It must make a more serious commitment to Medicaid

---

[208] Letter from Seema Verma, Adm'r, Ctrs. For Medicare & Medicaid Servs., to Sen. Ron Johnson, Chairman, S. Comm. on Homeland Sec. & Gov't Affairs (June 13, 2018).

[209] *Id.*

[210] *Id.*

[211] Letter from Sen. Ron Johnson, *supra* note 6.

[212] *Id.*

[213] *"Nomination of Seema Verma to be Administrator of the Centers for Medicare and Medicaid Services": Hearing before the S. Comm. on Finance*, 115th Cong. (2017).

[214] Robin Rudowitz & Allison Valentine, *Medicaid Enrollment & Spending Growth: FY 2017 & 2018*, KAISER FAMILY FOUNDATION (Oct. 19, 2014), https://www.kff.org/medicaid/issue-brief/medicaid-enrollment-spending- growth-fy-2017-2018/.

[215] Deficit Reduction Act of 2005, Pub. L. No. 109-171, 120 Stat. 4 (2006).

[216] Letter from Sen. Ron Johnson, *supra* note 6.

[217] *Drugs for Dollars: How Medicaid Helps Fuel the Opioid Epidemic*, *supra* note 22.

[218] Letter from Sen. Ron Johnson, Chairman, S. Comm. on Homeland Sec. & Gov't Affairs, & Claire McCaskill, Ranking Member, S. Comm. on Homeland Sec. & Gov't Affairs, to Seema Verma, Adm'r, Ctrs. for Medicare & Medicaid Servs. (May 15, 2018).

[219] James Swann, *Trump Budget Would Boost Spending to Fight Medicare, Medicaid Fraud*, BLOOMBERG (Mar. 20, 2017), https://www.bna.com/trump-budget-boost-n57982085442/.

program integrity and sustain that effort through smart and effective oversight of state Medicaid programs. That commitment must extend through every part of the agency.

There are several steps that CMS could take toward improving Medicaid's program integrity.

- CMS should enact the 11 open GAO anti-fraud recommendations dating to 2015, especially those urging CMS to review federal Medicaid eligibility determinations for accuracy and to provide fraud-awareness training for all CMS employees.[220]
- CMS should take perhaps the most basic step of all: create, document and implement a Medicaid anti-fraud strategy.[221]
- CMS ought to crack down on states that allow fraud or otherwise abuse Medicaid funding, starting with recouping the more than $1 billion California spent on behalf of ineligible or potentially ineligible beneficiaries.[222]
- CMS should make a sustained effort to slow and then eliminate the $37 billion in overpayments plaguing the Medicaid program each year.[223]
- CMS should take seriously Medicaid's role in the opioid epidemic and make structural changes to the program that eliminate incentives leading to opioid abuse and illicit fraud.[224]
- CMS must work with government watchdogs, especially the non-partisan GAO and HHS OIG, to better police Medicaid fraud.
- CMS must become more responsive to and cooperative with Congressional oversight seeking to identify and eliminate Medicaid fraud.

In addition, Congress could take steps to address fundamental incentives that currently present challenges to Medicaid program integrity.

- Congress should reduce the "safe harbor" for states' taxes on health care providers to limit Medicaid maximization schemes that have inflated federal payments to states.[225]

---

[220] GAO-18-444T, *Medicaid: Opportunities for Improving Program Oversight*, *supra* note 7.

[221] *Id.*

[222] U.S. Dep't of Health & Human Servs. Off. of Inspector Gen., A-09-16-02023, *supra* note 8.

[223] GAO-18-444T, *Medicaid: Opportunities for Improving Program Oversight*, *supra* note 7.

[224] *Drugs for Dollars: How Medicaid Helps Fuel the Opioid Epidemic*, *supra* note 22.

[225] *Limit States' Taxes on Health Care Providers*, CONG. BUDGET OFFICE (Dec. 8, 2016), https://www.cbo.gov/budget-options/2016/52230.

- Congress should transition Medicaid to a block grant funding mechanism for existing Medicaid expansion populations,[226] instead of the current open-ended federal entitlement. This mechanism would help reduce incentives for states that seek to maximize federal funds and potentially enroll ineligible people. A block grant system would also provide a more equitable distribution of federal funding to states that have been good stewards of taxpayer dollars.[227]

MEMORANDUM

January 17, 2018

To: Members of the Senate Committee on Homeland Security & Governmental Affairs (HSGAC)

Fr: HSGAC Minority Staff

Re: Additional Information on the Relationship between Medicaid Expansion and the Opioid Epidemic

Medicaid is a federal program jointly funded by states and the federal government that provides health care coverage to low-income adults, children, pregnant women, people with disabilities, and elderly individuals.[228] When enacted, the Affordable Care Act (ACA) required states to offer Medicaid coverage to adults between the ages of 18 and 65 with incomes up to 133% of the federal poverty level.[229] States were required to provide Medicaid to those individuals regardless of health or family status by 2014.[230] The U.S. Supreme Court subsequently held that the ACA's Medicaid expansion was unconstitutionally coercive, making expansion optional for states.[231] As a result, to date 32 states and the District of Columbia have expanded Medicaid and 18 states have not expanded Medicaid.[232]

---

[226] *Graham-Cassidy-Heller-Johnson Plan to Replace ACA Funding With a New Block Grant and Cap Medicaid Would Decrease Federal Funding for States by $160 Billion from 2020-2026; Then a $240 Billion Loss in 2027 if the Law is Not Reauthorized*, KAISER FAMILY FOUNDATION (Sept. 21, 2017), https://www.kff.org/health-reform/press-release/graham-cassidy-heller-johnson-plan-to-replace-aca-funding-with-a-new-block-grant-and-cap- medicaid-would-decrease-federal-funding-for-states-by-160-billion-from-2020-2026-then-a-240-billion-loss-in/.

[227] *Id.*

[228] U.S. Department of Health and Human Services, Centers for Medicare and Medicaid Services, *Medicaid: Overview* (www.medicaid.gov/medicaid/index.html) (accessed Jan. 16, 2018).

[229] U.S. Department of Health and Human Services, Centers for Medicare and Medicaid Services, *Medicaid & CHIP: Medicaid expansion & what it means for you* (www.healthcare.gov/medicaid-chip/medicaid-expansion-and-you/) (accessed Jan. 17, 2018).

[230] *Id.*

[231] *National Federation of Independent Business v. Sebelius,* 567 U.S. 519 (2012).

[232] Families USA, *A 50-State Look at Medicaid Expansion* (Jan. 2018) (http://familiesusa.org/product/50-state-look-medicaid-expansion).

Critics of the ACA, including Senator Ron Johnson, Chairman of the U.S. Committee on Homeland Security and Governmental Affairs, have recently alleged that Medicaid expansion may be fueling the opioid epidemic in communities across the country.[233] At the request of Ranking Member Claire McCaskill, this memorandum provides information on Medicaid expansion and the opioid epidemic. Key findings include:

- The opioid epidemic predates Medicaid expansion.
- Recent increases in opioid mortality stem from fentanyl and heroin, not prescription opioids.
- Mortality data indicate there is no statistically significant evidence that Medicaid expansion affects drug-related overdoses.
- Empirical research indicates determinants of opioid deaths are demographic characteristics and prescriber behavior.
- States that expand Medicaid under the Affordable Care Act are better equipped to address behavioral health care and substance abuse treatment needs.

Opioid Epidemic Predates Medicaid Expansion

One method to establish causation is to demonstrate that the causes preceded the effects. Historical statistical data indicate that the opioid epidemic predates Medicaid expansion in the ACA. In 1995, Purdue Pharma introduced OxyContin, a controlled-release opioid, and overdoses across the United States increased rapidly. Between 1997 and 2002, OxyContin prescriptions for non-cancer pain grew from 670,000 to 6.2 million.[234] Mortality rates attributed to opioid overdoses doubled between 1999 and 2013.[235]

According to an analysis conducted by Andrew Goodman-Bacon, an assistant professor of economics at Vanderbilt University, a statistical analysis of mortality rates indicate that the upward trend in drug poisoning started in 2010, four years prior to the expansion of Medicaid.[236] He wrote, in conjunction with his co-author Emma Sandoe:

---

[233] *See, e.g.,* Letter from Senator Ron Johnson, Chairman of the U.S. Senate Committee on Homeland Security and Governmental Affairs, to Daniel R. Levinson, Inspector General, U.S. Department of Health and Human Services (Jul. 27, 2017); *Medicaid fueling opioid epidemic? New theory is challenged,* Associated Press (Aug. 31, 2017) (www.apnews.com/a860fb7b0e0c4117b9420b3bcfb928c6).

[234] Andrew Goodman-Bacon and Emma Sandoe, *Did Medicaid Expansion Cause the Opioid Epidemic? There's Little Evidence That It Did,* Health Affairs (blog) (Aug. 23, 2017) (http://healthaffairs.org/blog/2017/08/23/did-medicaid-expansion-cause-the-opioid-epidemic-theres-little-evidence-that-it-did/).

[235] *Id.*

[236] *Id.*

Figure 7 plots age-adjusted drug-related mortality rates among those aged 25-54 in states that did and did not expand Medicaid under the ACA … The figure also plots the difference in mortality between expansion and non-expansion states (relative to the difference in 2009; dashed lines are 95-percent confidence intervals based on standard errors clustered by state). Expansion states did have relatively more drug deaths than non-expansion states in 2015, but the upward trend in deaths in expansion states started in 2010, four years before the Medicaid expansion began. The results are the same if we exclude the six early expansion states. By the simplest criterion for causality, that causes must precede effects, these results cannot be taken as evidence of Medicaid expansion causing these deaths.[237]

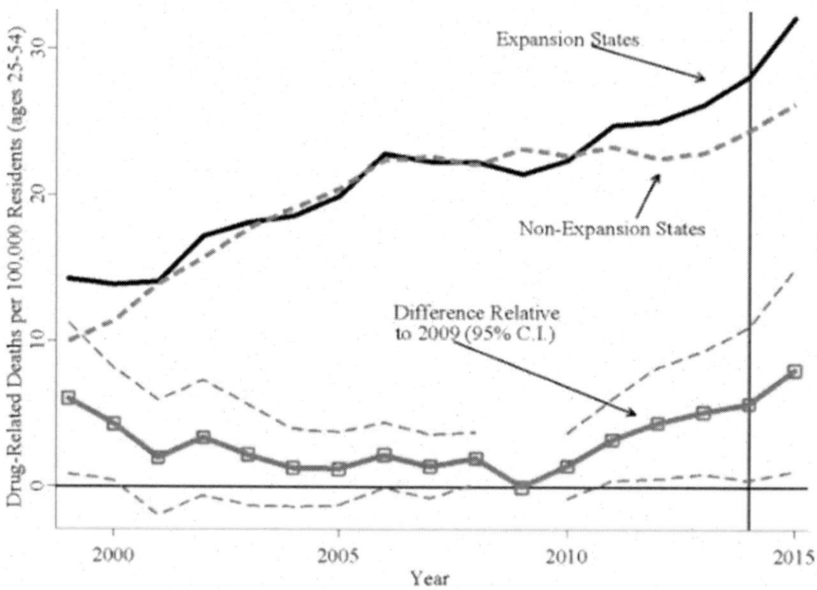

Figure 7. Age-Adjusted Drug-Poisoning Mortality Rate for Ages 25-54 by Medicaid Expansion Status, 1999-2015.[238]

Recent Increases in Opioid Mortality Stem from Fetanyl and Heroin, Not Prescription Opioids

Since 2013, nearly all increases in opioid overdoses are attributable to heroin and heroin substitutes, including fentanyl. Data from the U.S. Centers for Disease Control indicate that although overdose deaths containing any opioid is continuing to increase,

---

[237] *Id.*

[238] *Id.*

recent surges in overdoses result from heroin and other synthetic opioids such as fentanyl, carfentanil, and tramadol.[239]

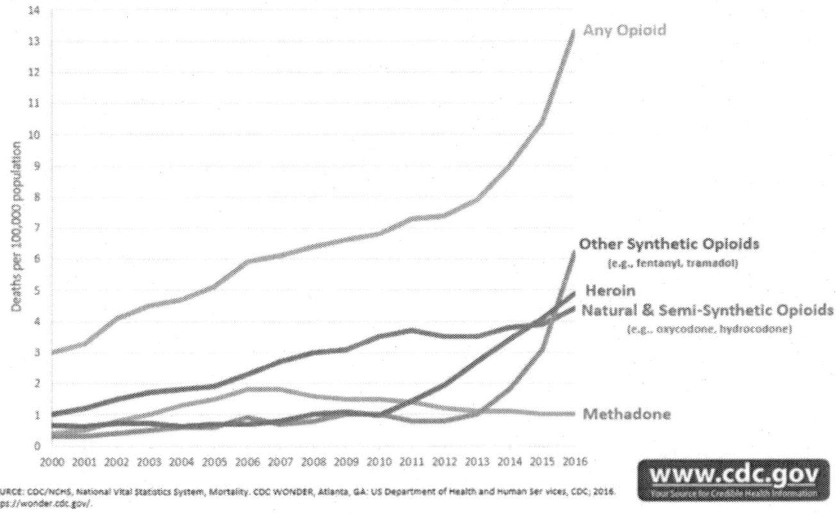

Figure 8. Overdose Deaths Involving Opioids, by Type of Opioid, United States, 2000-2016.[240]

Mortality Data Indicate There Is No Statistically Significant Evidence That Medicaid Expansion Affects Drug-Related Overdoses

In 2017, Brendan Saloner from the Johns Hopkins Bloomberg School of Public Health and Johanna Maclean of Temple University issued a paper on the impact of Medicaid expansion under the Affordable Care Act on substance abuse disorder treatment utilization and financing.[241] In this research, Saloner and Maclean examined data from the National Vital Statistics Mortality Files between 2010 and 2015 and narrowed the data set to deaths classified as alcohol poisonings and drug-related overdoses.[242] They further narrowed the data to poisonings and overdoses among non-elderly adults aged 18 to 64 years and compared deaths within expansion and non-expansion states.[243] The authors found "no statistically significant evidence that Medicaid expansions affected fatal alcohol poisonings or drug-related overdoses."[244]

---

[239] U.S. Centers for Disease Control and Prevention, *Opioid DataAnalysis* (https://www.cdc.gov/drugoverdose/data/analysis.html) (accessed Jan. 16, 2018).

[240] *Id.*

[241] Maclean, J. C., & Saloner, B. (2017), *The Effect of Public Insurance Expansions on Substance Use Disorder Treatment: Evidence from the Affordable Care Act* (No. w23342), National Bureau of Economic Research.

[242] *Id.*

[243] *Id.*

[244] *Id.*

Empirical Research Indicate Determinants of Opioid Deaths Are Demographic Characteristics and Prescriber Behavior

The *American Journal of Public Health* published a literature review of empirical research that found: "Opioid-related mortality trends have been marked by considerable sociodemographic differences."[245] The authors wrote:

> We found 22 studies … that examined the contribution of sociodemographic characteristics, including race/ethnicity, gender, age, socioeconomic status (SES), and rural–urban residence, to increased opioid-related mortality. In general, opioid-related mortality rates have been higher among men, non-Hispanic Whites and American Indian/Alaska Natives, middle-aged individuals, those living in rural areas, and those of lower SES.[246]

The authors also reviewed the empirical data regarding the role of prescriber behavior in increased opioid-related mortality.[247] They found:

- Eight studies providing evidence that increased prescriptions for opioids may have played a role in increased opioid-related mortality;
- Seven studies providing evidence of the contribution of increased dosages to increased opioid-related mortality;
- Seven studies that provided evidence for the contribution of prescription of oxycodone, particularly the long-acting formulation of OxyContin, to increased opioid-related mortality; and
- One study providing evidence that high-volume prescribing may have played a role in increased opioid-related mortality.[248]

States That Expand Medicaid under the Affordable Care Act Are Better Equipped to Address Behavioral Health Care and Substance Abuse Treatment Needs

The Medicaid program plays a critical role in addressing the opioid epidemic. In 2015, Medicaid provided coverage to three in ten people grappling with opioid addiction

---

[245] Nicholas B. King, Ph. D, et al., *Determinants of Increased Opioid-Related Mortality in the United States and Canada, 1990–2013: A Systematic Review,* American Journal of Public Health (Aug. 2014).
[246] *Id.*
[247] *Id.*
[248] *Id.*

in the United States.[249] Medicaid covers services such as intensive outpatient treatment and inpatient detoxification.[250] The ACA broadened Medicaid coverage to include medication assisted treatment, a recovery program that combines medication (methadone, buprenorphine, or naltrexone) with counseling and other therapies.[251] All Medicaid programs cover at least one of the three required medications, and most states cover all three.[252]

The expansion of Medicaid has been critical to confronting substance abuse disorders. Healthcare economists Richard G. Frank, the Margaret T. Morris Professor of Health Economics in the Department of Health Care Policy at Harvard Medical School, and Dr. Sherry A. Glied, Dean of the Wagner School of Public Service at New York University, have estimated that states that expanded Medicaid have helped 1.3 million additional patients access behavioral health care services.[253] Additionally, recent empirical research has shown that states that expanded Medicaid under the ACA were associated with an increase in prescriptions for one of the required medications for medication assisted treatment.[254]

Additionally, the U.S. Department of Health and Human Services found that "evidence is mounting" that Medicaid expansion enables patients to access care to confront opioid addiction.[255] In an issue brief on the role of the ACA in addressing the opioid epidemic, the findings of the Assistant Secretary for Planning and Evaluation are quoted below:

- Among low-income adults, Medicaid expansion was associated with a 7.5 percent reduction in unmet need for mental health treatment and an 18.3 percent reduction in unmet need for substance use disorder treatment services.
- Medicaid expansion in Ohio led to especially large improvements in access to care and financial security for expansion enrollees with opioid use disorder. 75 percent reported improved overall access to care, 83 percent reported improved

---

[249] Kaiser Family Foundation, *Medicaid and the Opioid Epidemic: Enrollment, Spending, and the Implications of Proposed Policy Changes* (Jul. 14, 2017) (www.kff.org/medicaid/issue-brief/medicaid-and-the-opioid-epidemic-enrollment-spending-and-the-implications-of-proposed- policy-changes/).

[250] *Id.*

[251] Kaiser Family Foundation, *Medicaid's Role in Addressing the Opioid Epidemic* (June 2017) (https://kaiserfamilyfoundation.files.wordpress.com/2017/03/medicaid_s-role-in-addressing-the-opioid-epidemic.png).

[252] *Id.*

[253] Richard G. Frank and Sherry A. Glied, *Keep Obamacare to keep progress on treating opioid disorders and mental illnesses (op-ed),* The Hill (Jan. 11, 2017) (http://thehill.com/blogs/pundits-blog/healthcare/313672-keep-obamacare-to-keep-progress-on- treating-opioid-disorders).

[254] Hefei Wen, Ph. D. et al., *Impact of Medicaid Expansion on Medicaid-covered Utilization of Buprenorphine for Opioid Use Disorder Treatment*, Medical Care: Official Journal of the Medical Care Section, American Public Health Association (Apr. 2017).

[255] U.S. Department of Health and Human Services, Assistant Secretary for Planning and Evaluation, *Continuing Progress on the Opioid Epidemic: The Role of the Affordable Care Act* (Jan. 11, 2017) (https://aspe.hhs.gov/system/files/pdf/255456/ACAOpioid.pdf).

access to prescription medications, and 59 percent reported improved access to mental health care.

- Medicaid expansion in Kentucky was linked to a large increase in Kentuckians receiving treatment for substance use disorder.[256]

CMS Announces Initiatives to Strengthen Medicaid Program Integrity

Agency Actions Will Help Ensure the Sustainability of Vital Safety Net Program for All Beneficiaries

Today, the Centers for Medicare and Medicaid Services (CMS) announced new and enhanced initiatives designed to improve Medicaid program integrity through greater transparency and accountability, strengthened data, and innovative and robust analytic tools.

"The initiatives released today are essential to help strengthen and preserve the foundation of the program for the millions of Americans who depend on Medicaid's safety net. With historic growth in Medicaid comes an urgent federal responsibility to ensure sound fiscal stewardship and oversight of the program," said CMS Administrator Seema Verma. "These initiatives are the vital steps necessary to respond to Medicaid's evolving landscape and fulfill our responsibility to beneficiaries and taxpayers."

Recent years have seen a rapid increase in Medicaid spending driven by several factors, including Medicaid expansion, from $456 billion in 2013 to an estimated $576 billion in 2016. Much of this growth came from the program's federal share that grew from $263 billion to an estimated $363 billion during that period. While the responsibility for proper payments in Medicaid primarily lies with the states, oversight of the Medicaid program requires a partnership. CMS plays a significant role in supporting state efforts to meet high program standards.

Administrator Verma has set forth three pillars to guide CMS' work in the Medicaid program: Flexibility, Accountability, and Integrity. Emphasizing these, she expanded on the role of CMS saying, "As we give states the flexibility they need to make Medicaid work best in their communities, integrity and oversight must be at the forefront of our role. Beneficiaries depend on Medicaid and CMS is accountable for the program's long-term viability. As today's initiatives show, we will use the tools we have to hold states accountable as we work with them to keep Medicaid sound and safeguarded for beneficiaries."

---

[256] *Id.*

The initiatives announced today include stronger audit functions, enhanced oversight of state contracts with private insurance companies, increased beneficiary eligibility oversight, and stricter enforcement of state compliance with federal rules.

Important New Initiatives

1) Emphasize program integrity in audits of state claims for federal match funds and medical loss ratios (MLRs). Audits are central to CMS' partnership with states—not only encouraging compliance but also revealing how to improve integrity at all levels. Under this initiative, CMS will begin auditing some states based on the amount spent on clinical services and quality improvement versus administration and profit. The MLR audits will include reviewing states' rate setting. Overall, audits will address issues identified by the Government Accountability Office (GAO) and Office of Inspector General (OIG), as well as other behavior previously found harmful to the Medicaid program.
2) Conduct new audits of state beneficiary eligibility determinations. CMS will audit states that have been previously found to be high risk by the OIG to examine how they determine which groups are eligible for Medicaid benefits. These audits will include assessing the effect of Medicaid expansion and its enhanced federal match rate on state eligibility policy. Current regulations will allow CMS to begin to issue potential disallowances to states based on Payment Error Rate Measurement (PERM) program findings in 2022. The PERM program measures improper payments in the Medicaid program and the Children's Health Insurance Program (CHIP) on a rolling three year cycle and produces national and state-specific improper payment rates.
3) Optimize state-provided claims and provider data: CMS will utilize advanced analytics and other innovative solutions to both improve Medicaid eligibility and payment data and maximize the potential for program integrity purposes. The Trump Administration has made partnering with states a priority. CMS is committed to work closely with states to ensure that the agency and oversight bodies have access to the best, most complete and accurate Medicaid data. For the first time, every state plus Washington, D.C. and Puerto Rico are now submitting enhanced data to CMS. Over the course of the coming months, we will be validating the quality and completeness of the data.

Ongoing Integrity Work

Working with states to ensure Medicaid provides high-quality care for our most vulnerable people is a central part of CMS' mission. To learn about noteworthy efforts in place to protect Medicaid's integrity—including provider screening and education, streamlined access to data, and an enhanced Medicaid Scorecard—see https://www.medicaid.gov/state-resource-center/downloads/program-integrity-strategy-factsheet.pdf.

CMS Medicaid Program Integrity Strategy

Enhanced Medicaid Program Integrity Strategy

The last several years have seen a rapid increase in Medicaid spending driven by several factors, including Medicaid expansion, from $456 billion in 2013 to an estimated $576 billion in 2016. Much of this growth came from the federal share that grew from $263 billion to an estimated $363 billion during the same period. With this historic growth comes an equally growing and urgent responsibility to ensure sound stewardship and oversight of our program resources. As part of CMS's plan to reform Medicaid using the three pillars of flexibility, accountability and integrity, we are announcing a new strategy to ensure we are keeping the Medicaid program sustainable for our future.

While the responsibility for proper payments in Medicaid primarily lies with the states, oversight of the Medicaid program requires a partnership, and CMS plays a significant role in supporting state efforts and increasing state oversight, accountability, and transparency. Because of this responsibility, CMS is announcing new and enhanced initiatives that will create greater transparency in and accountability for Medicaid program integrity performance, enable increased data sharing and robust analytic tools, and seek to reduce Medicaid improper payments across states. The initiatives include stronger audit functions, increased beneficiary eligibility oversight, and enhanced enforcement of state compliance with federal rules.

CMS's Robust Plan for New or Enhanced Medicaid Program Integrity Initiatives

- Strengthen the Program Integrity Focus of Audits of State Claiming for Federal Match Funds and Rate Setting – CMS will begin targeted audits of some states' managed care organization (MCO) financial reporting. Plans have implemented risk mitigation strategies like Medical Loss Ratio; CMS will be checking to make sure claims experience actually matches what plans have been reporting. Audit activities will include review of high-risk vulnerabilities identified by the Government Accountability Office and Office of Inspector General (OIG), as well as other behavior previously found detrimental to the Medicaid program.

- Conduct New Audits of State Beneficiary Eligibility Determinations – CMS will initiate audits of state beneficiary eligibility determinations in states previously reviewed by OIG. These audits will include assessment of the impact of changes to state eligibility policy as a result of Medicaid expansion; for example, we will review whether beneficiaries were found eligible for the correct Medicaid eligibility category.
- Optimize state-provided claims and provider data: It is an administration priority for CMS to work closely with states to ensure that CMS and oversight bodies have access to the best, most complete and accurate Medicaid data. For the first time, all 50 states, D.C. and Puerto Rico are now submitting data on their programs to the Transformed Medicaid Statistical Information System (TMSIS), and over the course of the coming months CMS will be validating the quality and completeness of the data. CMS's ongoing goal is to use advanced analytics and other innovative solutions to both improve TMSIS data and maximize the potential for program integrity purposes. This will allow CMS to identify instances like a beneficiary receiving more hours of treatment than hours in a day or other flags that necessitate further investigation.
- Use Data Innovation to Empower States and Conduct Data Analytics Pilots – CMS will share its extensive knowledge, gained from processing and analyzing large, complex Medicare data sets, to help states apply algorithms and insights to analyze Medicaid state claim data and identify potential areas to target for investigation.
- Offer Provider Screening for States on an Opt-In Basis – CMS will pilot a process to screen Medicaid providers on behalf of states. Centralizing this process will improve efficiency and coordination across Medicare and Medicaid, reduce state and provider burden, and address one of the biggest sources of error as measured by the Payment Error Rate Measurement (PERM) program today.
- Enhanced Data Sharing and Collaboration between CMS and the States. CMS will work with States to enhance data sharing and collaboration to tackle program integrity efforts in both the Medicare and Medicaid programs. For example, CMS is making the Social Security Administration's Death Master File available for States to support provider enrollment activities.
- Publicly Report State Performance on the Medicaid Scorecard – CMS has released a Medicaid scorecard that presents state performance measures related to their Medicaid programs. Future versions of the scorecard will include state

program integrity performance measures like PERM, the Medicaid improper payment error rate.

- Provide Medicaid Provider Education to Reduce Improper Payments – CMS will strengthen efforts to provide effective Medicaid provider education to reduce aberrant billing, including education focused on comparative billing reports. CMS also will work with states on other provider facing tools and investments we are currently making.

CMS's Existing Initiatives Protect Medicaid

- Managed Care Rate Reviews - Beginning in 2014, CMS implemented enhanced review of state capitation rates for coverage of the new expansion population to ensure that capitation rates are consistent with federal requirements and appropriately contain costs. CMS has since expanded that review to all managed care capitation rates and adopted a regulation providing more detailed requirements related to rate setting. All managed care rates are reviewed to ensure that the rates are actuarially sound and based on commonly accepted actuarial principles. Our rate review includes monitoring strategies implemented by states to mitigate rate setting risk, such as MLRs and risk corridors. Based on our review of these strategies states will be paying back an estimated $3.2 billion from the risk-mitigation strategies in 2014 and an estimated $5.5 billion return from those arrangements in 2015. This represents about nine percent of capitation payments for newly eligible adults in 2014 and 2015.
- Ensure State Compliance with the Medicaid Managed Care Final Rule – CMS will monitor state implementation of, and enforce compliance with, program integrity safeguards such as (1) reporting overpayments and fraud, and (2) screening and enrolling Medicaid managed care providers.
- Financial Oversight. CMS engages in robust financial oversight to ensure that when states ultimately claim for federal match on their expenditures, that federal Medicaid funds are spent lawfully and appropriately. We use specialized accountants and financial management specialists to review state claims each quarter, using trend analyses, environmental scanning and the results of external audits to find anomalies, and request additional documentation or justifications when necessary. We also engage in state specific reviews, going on-site to review state Medicaid programs to ensure that state expenditures and corresponding claims for federal matching funds are allowable. In Fiscal Year 2017, these efforts resulted in questioning $2.7 billion in Medicaid costs and averting nearly $500 million in questionable reimbursements.

- Payment Error Rate Measurement (PERM) Reviews – The PERM program measures improper payments in the Medicaid program and the Children's Health Insurance Program (CHIP) where each state is audited on a rolling three year basis and annually produces national and state-specific improper payment rates for each state Medicaid program. The improper payment rates are based on federal reviews of the fee-for-service (FFS), managed care, and eligibility components of Medicaid and CHIP in the fiscal year under review. Through the PERM program each state is reviewed once every three years.
- Medicaid Eligibility Quality Control (MEQC) Program – The MEQC program uses state-directed reviews in the two off-cycle PERM years to address Medicaid beneficiary eligibility vulnerabilities. MEQC focuses on areas not addressed through PERM reviews and on areas identified as error-prone through the PERM program.
- Medicaid Provider Screening and Enrollment – CMS uses multiple tools to assist states with provider screening and enrollment compliance, and allow them to leverage Medicare data and activities. These include the Provider Enrollment, Chain and Ownership System (PECOS), state site visits for technical assistance and education, Medicare data compare services, and the Medicaid Provider Enrollment Compendium (MPEC).
- State Program Integrity Reviews – CMS conducts reviews to determine if state policies and practices comply with federal regulations, identify program vulnerabilities that may not rise to the level of regulatory compliance issues, identify states' program integrity best practices, and monitor state corrective action plans.
- Medicaid Integrity Institute (MII) – CMS's MII provides training and education to more than one thousand state Medicaid PI staff annually. Course topics include provider screening and enrollment, managed care, personal care services, opioids, beneficiary fraud, data analytics, and investigatory techniques.
- Healthcare Fraud Prevention Partnership (HFPP) – The HFPP is a voluntary public-private partnership between the federal government, state agencies, law enforcement, private health insurance plans, and healthcare anti-fraud associations that aims to detect and prevent healthcare fraud through data and information sharing.
- CMS's Unified Program Integrity Contractors (UPICs) - CMS's UPICs are contracted entities that perform activities that identify and reduce fraud, waste, and abuse by individuals and entities furnishing items and services under Medicare and Medicaid. The UPICs work closely with states to perform numerous functions to detect, prevent, and deter specific risks and broader vulnerabilities to the integrity of the Medicaid program, including conducting provider investigations and audits.

AGENT ELIGIBILITY AND UNDERWRITING GUIDE: HUMANA*ONE* HEALTH AND LIFE PRODUCTS

Humana*One*® Eligibility and Underwriting Guide

Humana Is Proud to Offer Humanaone Health, Life and Dental Insurance for Individuals and Families

The Humana*One* brand of individual products are insured by subsidiaries of Humana, Inc.

This is your guide to assessing your client's eligibility for Humana*One* health and life products. Applications are subject to approval. For information on Humana*One* products and processes, please see the Humana*One* Product and Process Guide.

Use the phone numbers and addresses below to get the information you need quickly. You can also contact your sales representative; we're committed to serving you quickly and efficiently. After all, your success is our success. We value your partnership, and we thank you for your support.

IMPORTANT: Please advise your client not to cancel any current health or life insurance coverage until receipt of written approval from our Underwriting department.

This guide is subject to change without notice. Contractual information supersedes information in this guide. This guide does not provide state-specific information.

This guide is for agent use only.

ELIGIBILITY AND UNDERWRITING GUIDE

e-Query Service (Ask an Underwriter)

e-Query is a service which allows you to assess your client's insurance eligibility more accurately with the assistance of a Humana underwriter. It directly links you to a dedicated team of underwriters by means of an electronic form hosted on Humana*One* agent workbench.

e-Query does not replace the Underwriting Guidelines herein, but rather compliments it. To access the e-Query form you will need to log onto the HumanaOne Agent Workbench from the Agent Portal on www.humana.com, and click on the "e-Query/Ask an Underwriter" link under the questions section. e-Query is not currently available in the state of Wisconsin.

Eligibility Requirements

For Health Coverage

- Issue ages: 2 weeks – 64 ½ years
  Newborns on family and child only applications will be eligible for coverage when they have had a two week well baby exam with normal results.
  Please Note: This applies to full term babies. If they are born premature or with complications, we will underwrite as necessary.
- Maximum issue age of a dependent child varies by state.
- Dependents may include stepchildren, and/or legally adopted children. (Dependent definitions vary by state.)

Children-Only Health Coverage

Children can be insured alone. The custodial parent or legal guardian who can attest to child's health history must complete the application. If an underwriting interview is required, the person that completed the application will be interviewed. The youngest child will be the primary applicant, and any others will be listed as dependents.

Newborns applying for coverage require a two week well baby exam with normal results. Medical records are required for any child that is 2 weeks to 2 months of age. A child only health policy is ineligible, if any family member of the applicant(s) is pregnant or currently an expectant parent. See the terms indicated under Current/ Pregnancy/Expectant parent.

Application Scenarios

1) Parent A has custody and resides in a state in which Humana offers coverage. Parent B will be paying for the health insurance. Parent A must complete and sign the application to verify the health history. Parent B must sign the payer portion of the application.
2) Parent A has custody and resides in a state in which Humana does NOT offer coverage. Parent B will be paying for the health insurance. Because benefits are based on the applicant's primary resident, Humana will not be able to accept an application for the child(ren).
3) Both parents share custody and reside in a state in which Humana offers coverage. Either parent can complete and sign the application.

4) Both parents share custody and reside in a state in which Humana offers coverage, however, their dependent student attends school in a state where Humana does not offer coverage. Coverage may be extended to the parents and their dependent college student(s).

Current Pregnancy/Expectant Parent

For family applications, before applying for coverage, the mother must be two weeks postpartum, with no adverse findings, and the newborn must be two weeks old and have had a normal two week baby exam.

For child-only health policies, if any family member of the child is currently an expectant parent, the application is ineligible. Before applying for coverage, the mother must be two weeks postpartum, with no adverse findings, and the newborn must be 2 weeks of age, and have had a normal two week well baby exam with normal results.

Other Coverage

A person who is currently covered by another plan must replace that coverage with Humana. However, it is important that he or she does not cancel existing coverage until written notification is received from Humana that coverage will be issued. Some states may require a replacement form.

U.S. Citizenship

The applicant's primary residence must be in a state where the product is approved for sale. If the applicant is not a U.S. citizen, he or she must have lived in the U.S. for a minimum of one year, plans to remain in the U.S. for over three years, has had a normal physical exam with blood work from a U.S. physician, and has no plans of foreign travel of greater than three months continuously. An immigration physical does not meet the criteria for an acceptable physical exam.

Foreign Travel

An applicant who lives in a foreign country is not eligible for coverage, nor is an applicant who has plans for extended foreign travel of three consecutive months at a time or longer. (May vary by state.)

Exceptions

An applicant who, for the purpose of Missionary Work, has plans for extended foreign travel for 0-2 years from the time of the application is eligible for coverage. An applicant with foreign travel plans exceeding 2 years for Missionary Work would not be eligible.

An applicant who, for the purpose of studying abroad or occupational/business travel has plans for extended foreign travel for 0-2 years from the time of the application is eligible for coverage. An applicant with foreign travel plans exceeding 2 years for studying abroad or occupational/business travel would not be eligible.

Tobacco Usage - Health

Humana has two tobacco classes:

1) Non-user: Does not use ANY form of tobacco currently or has not used ANY tobacco cessation products in the last 12 months.
2) Tobacco user

People who do not smoke or use any form of tobacco have their premium discounted. Humana conducts random nicotine testing during underwriting review.

Health Underwriting Guidelines

The following circumstances may result in a person not being eligible for health coverage:

1) Currently pregnant, an expectant parent (including fathers and/or other family members)—entire application is ineligible;
2) Health history that includes one of the ineligible health conditions;
3) Height/weight that exceeds the limits identified in the health build chart; or
4) Employment in an ineligible occupation. Not applicable in Florida.
5) Non-U.S. citizen who has not consulted a physician in the U.S.
6) Health history that includes 3 or more risk factors (build/overweight, elevated cholesterol/elevated triglycerides, hypertension, tobacco use).
7) Hypertension with 50% rateable build.
8) Hypertension with current treatment for Sleep Apnea.

A "yes" answer to any one of these circumstances may result in a declination of coverage. However, this information only provides their potential eligibility; it is not a final determination. All final coverage decisions are made by our Underwriting department upon receipt of an application. This assessment is not an offer of coverage or a notice of declination for your client.

Ineligible Occupations (Not Applicable in Florida)

- Air traffic controllers
- Asbestos and toxic chemical workers
- Commercial fishermen who do not return to port every day
- Divers (professional scuba or skin)
- Explosive workers
- High-risk aviation (experimental and test pilots, crop dusters)
- Oil and natural gas workers, including offshore operations
- Professional auto racers
- Professional rodeo participants
- Professional and semi-professional athletes (**Note:** Golfers are acceptable)
- Structural steel workers, iron workers and steeplejacks
- Underground miners

Health Build Charts

Use this table as a guide to determine if an applicant is rateable because of his or her build. Humana may request a paramedical exam (at our expense) to confirm an applicant's height and weight. An applicant must have maintained an acceptable build within the 12 months prior to applying to be considered eligible. If an individual's weight exceeds our "Standard" class but less than our "Decline" limit, they will be subject to a premium increase of 25-50%.

To qualify for the lower build rating, an applicant must lose the weight to reach the lower range and maintain the weight loss for 12 months.

Applicants who have applied for individual insurance and who have been offered a rating due to build may also have an obesity rider added to his or her offer. Any diagnostic procedure, treatment, or surgery for obesity including any complications thereof, will be excluded from coverage. In states where riders are not offered, coverage may be declined.

If an applicant is applying for both a Humana*One* health plan as well as for Humana*One* Term Life Insurance, the Health Build Chart will be followed during the underwriting process. (May vary by state.)

Female		
	standard	decline
4’11”	88-151 lbs	175 lbs
5’0”	90-155 lbs	180 lbs
5’1”	93-160 lbs	187 lbs
5’2”	97-167 lbs	193 lbs
5’3”	100-172 lbs	199 lbs
5’4”	102-178 lbs	206 lbs
5’5”	106-183 lbs	212 lbs
5’6”	110-189 lbs	219 lbs
5’7”	113-195 lbs	225 lbs
5’8”	116-200 lbs	232 lbs
5’9”	119-206 lbs	239 lbs
5’10”	123-212 lbs	246 lbs
5’11”	127-219 lbs	253 lbs
6’0”	130-224 lbs	260 lbs
6’1”	134-232 lbs	266 lbs
Male		
	standard	decline
5’2”	97-177 lbs	198 lbs
5’3”	100-182 lbs	205 lbs
5’4”	102-189 lbs	211 lbs
5’5”	106-194 lbs	218 lbs
5’6”	110-200 lbs	224 lbs
5’7”	113-206 lbs	232 lbs
5’8”	116-212 lbs	238 lbs
5’9”	119-219 lbs	245 lbs
5’10”	123-225 lbs	252 lbs
5’11”	127-232 lbs	260 lbs
6’0”	130-238 lbs	267 lbs
6’1”	134-246 lbs	274 lbs
6’2”	138-252 lbs	282 lbs
6’3”	141-259 lbs	289 lbs
6’4”	145-266 lbs	298 lbs

Ineligible Health Conditions

A series of medical questions will be asked of each of the proposed insured. Any applicant age 18 and older must review and attest to the questions individually, (age requirements vary by state). Below is a partial listing of conditions that may cause Humana to decline coverage. The list is not all-inclusive.

Please note that if your client is applying for both a health plan and a life policy at the same time, and they are denied a health plan based on their health status, the process will discontinue as well for the life policy.

Below conditions are permanent declines, unless otherwise indicated. Handling of the below conditions may vary by state.

A

- Achalasia, cardio spasm
- Achondroplasia
- Acromegaly
- Addison's disease
- Adrenal disorders AIDS, ARC, or HIV
- Alcohol dependence or abuse—individual consideration, after 5 years of recovery
- Alport syndrome
- Alzheimer's disease
- Amyloidosis
- Amyotrophic lateral sclerosis (ALS or Lou Gehrig's disease)
- Anemia—aplastic Cooley's, B-12 deficiency, hemolytic, Mediterranean, pernicious, sickle cell or Thalassemia Major
- Anencephaly
- Aneurysm—if present or within 5 years
- Angina
- Angioplasty
- Ankylosing spondylitis
- Anorexia nervosa—individual consideration, after 8 years of recovery
- Anticoagulant therapy
- Antiphospholipid syndrome
- Anticardiolipin antibody syndrome
- Aortic arch arteritis
- Aortic insufficiency/stenosis/regurgitation—moderate or severe
- Aortitis
- Arnold-Chiari malformation
- Arterial embolism (clot)
- Arterial occlusion
- Arteriosclerosis, atherosclerosis
- Arteriosclerosis obliterans (ASO)

- Arteriovenous malformation (A-V malformation)
- Arteritis
- Artificial heart valve
- Asperger's syndrome—except in Indiana
- Ascites
- Ataxia telangiectasia
- Atherosclerosis obliterans
- Atherosclerosis thrombotic disease
- Atrial fibrillation—one event less than 2 years ago or multiple events or chronic or with Pacemaker or Cardiverter
- Atrial septal defect—present or if surgically corrected with complications
- Autism—varies by state

B

- Banti's syndrome
- Basal cell carcinoma—if present
- Berger's disease
- Biliary cirrhosis
- Bipolar disorders
- Bladder entropy—symptomatic
- Blastomycosis
- Brachial plexus disorder
- Brain attack
- Brain tumors
- Bright's disease
- Bronchiectasis—if lung resection, no residuals, no tobacco – individual consideration
- Bronchiolectasis
- Bruit
- Buerger's disease (thromboangiitis obliterans)
- Bulimia—individual considration, after 8 years of recovery
- Burkitt's lymphoma (malignant lymphoma)
- Bypass surgery

C

- Cachexia
- Cancer with lymph node involvement or metastasis
- Cardiac decompensation
- Cardiac defibrillator (implantable)
- Cardiac or comorbidity risk factors—3 or more (build/overweight, elevated cholesterol/ triglyercerides, hypertension, tobacco use)
- Cardiomegaly
- Cardiomyopathy
- Cardiospasm
- Celiac Disease
- Central serous retinopathy
- Cerebral palsy
- Cerebrovascular accident
- Cerebrovascular disease
- Charcot-Marie-Tooth disease
- Chediak Kigaski syndrome
- Chondrocalcinosis
- Christmas disease
- Chromosomal abnormalities
- Chronic granulomatous disease
- Chronic glomerulonephritis
- Chronic hepatitis
- Chronic obstructive pulmonary disease (COPD)
- Chronic progressive external opthalmoplegia (CPEO)
- Cirrhosis of the liver
- Coarctation of the aorta
- Cocaine abuse
- Colitis (ulcerative)
- Collagen diseases
- Congenital heart anomalies
- Congenital lymphedema
- Congestive heart failure (CHF)
- Connective tissue disorder
- Cor pulmonale
- Coronary artery bypass surgery (CABS)
- Coronary artery disease (CAD)

- Coronary Fistula
- Coronary heart disease (CHD)
- CREST syndrome
- Creutzfeldt-Jakob disease
- Crigleer-Najaar syndrome
- Crohn disease
- Curvature of the spine with pulmonary, cardiac or spinal cord involvement
- Cushing syndrome/disease
- Cystic fibrosis
- Cystic kidney diseases
- Cystic medial necrosis

D

- Dejerine type sclerosis
- Delirium
- Delusions
- Dementia
- Demyelinating diseases
- Depressant addiction—current history of addiction with current usage
- Dermatitis herpetiformis—with evidence of significant immunologic compromise
- Dermatomyositis
- Depression—major, if hospitalization required or with suicidal attempt or ideation
- DiGeorge syndrome
- Diabetes insipidus
- Diabetes mellitus (type 1 and type 2)
- Down syndrome
- Drug dependence or abuse (illicit, illegal, over the counter or prescription)
- Drug psychosis
- Dwarfism

E

- Eaton-Lambert syndrome
- Ebstein's malformation (Ebstein's anomaly)
- Edward's syndrome

- Ehlers-Danlos syndrome
- Eisenmenger's complex (Eisenmenger's syndrome)
- Ejection Fraction-less than 50% or more than 75%
- Embolism—arterial is permanent decline; pulmonary depends on frequency, treatment, etc.
- Emphysema
- Encephalocele
- Encephalocystocele
- Encephalopathy
- Eosinophilic granuloma
- Epidermolysis bullosa
- Erythema Multiforme (Stevens Johnson syndrome)—if present or less than one year since complete recovery or residuals
- Esophageal varices

F

- Fabry disease
- Factor V deficiency
- Factor VIII or IX deficiency
- Familial Aadenomatous polyposis
- Fanconi syndrome-fanconi anemia
- Fibromyalgia
- Flexure-hepatic or splenic
- Fragile X syndrome
- Fragilitas ossium

G

- Galactorrhea—if present
- Galactosemia
- Gargoylism (mucopolysaccharidosis)
- Gastrectomy—total removal
- Gastric bypass/stapling
- Gastroparesis
- Gaucher's disease
- Gender identity disorder
- General paresis

- Glycogen storage disease
- Guillain-Barre Syndrome/Polyneuritis—if present or less than 3 years since recovered or if residual disability/permanent impairment

H

- Hallucinations
- Hand-Schueller-Christian disease
- Heart attack or disease
- Heart enlargement/hypertrophy
- Heart-lung transplants
- Heavy chain disease
- Hemiplegia
- Hemochromatosis
- Hemophilia A or B
- Hemophilia vascular
- Henoch-Schoenlein purpura
- Hepatic flexure
- Hepatomegaly
- Hepatitis (autoimmune)
- Hepatitis A—if less than 6 months after complete recovery
- Hepatitis B carrier
- Hepatitis C
- Hepatitis D (HDC or delta virus)
- Hepatitis E (HEV)
- Hepatitis G (HGV)
- Hepatomegaly
- Hereditary angioedema
- Hereditary spherocytosis—if present
- Hirschsprung's disease—if unoperated or symptomatic
- Histocytosis X
- Histoplasmosis—if present or disseminated and less than 3 years since complete recovery
- HIV positive
- Hodgkin's disease
- Hughes syndrome
- Human T-cell leukemia virus
- Human T-cell lymphotropic virus

- Hunner's ulcer
- Huntington's chorea
- Hydrocephalus
- Hydronephrosis—if present or bilateral
- Hyperhydrosis—if present or if surgically corrected with residual symptoms or any complications
- Hyperparathyroidism—if unoperated
- Hypersplenism
- Hypogonadism (primary)
- Hypoparathyroidism
- Hypoplastic anemia
- Hysteria

I

- Idiopathic thrombocytopenic purpura (child form)—if present
- IgA nephropathy/Berger's Disease IgG subclass deficiency
- Immune deficiency
- Infectious neuritis—if present or multiple episodes Insulin resistance
- Intermittent claudication
- Interstitial cystitis (chronic)/Hunner's Ulcer
- Intestinal infarction/Intestinal ischemia—unless acute with complete recovery more than 6 weeks ago
- Intestinal obstruction—if present
- Iritis—if one episode, less than 6 months ago or multiple episodes
- Ischemic heart disease
- Ischemic/ulcerative colitis IV drug use

J

- Jaundice (adult)—present or less than 6 months since complete recovery
- Juvenile dermatomyositis—if present or less than 2 years since complete recovery

K

- Kahler's disease
- Karposi's sarcoma

- Kartagener's syndrome
- Keratoconus—present and surgery recommended
- Kidney injury—major injury with history of dialysis
- Kidney failure—if chronic or acute less than 2 months since recovery
- Kidney stone—if present or if more than 4 episodes
- Kidney transplant
- Klinefelter's syndrome
- Korsakoff's psychosis

L

- Left bundle branch block
- Left ventricular hypertrophy
- Legionella pneumophilia (Legionnaire's disease)
- Letterer-Siwe disease
- Leukemia
- Leukoencephalopathy
- Lipidosis (Niemann Pick disease)
- Liver abscess with residuals
- Liver cancer
- Liver transplant
- Lobstein's disease
- Lou Gehrig's disease (ALS)
- Lung cancer
- Lung transplant
- Lyme's disease—if present
- Lymphoblastoma
- Lymphoma
- Lymphoma, Hodgkins
- Lymphomatoid papulosis

M

- Malaria—more than one occurrence with complications or frequent disabling attacks
- Manic disorders
- Marchiafava-Micheli syndrome
- Marfan's syndrome

- Medullary cystic kidney
- Medullary sponge kidney—if present or less than 18 years of age or if more than 18 years of age—bilateral
- Mental retardation—severe, emotionally unstable, seizures or psychiatric impairments
- Mesenteric vascular disease
- Metabolic syndrome
- Microcephaly
- Milroy's disease
- Mitral insufficiency
- Mitral stenosis
- Mixed connective tissue disease
- Moebius syndrome/Mobius syndrome
- Mucopolysaccharidosis
- Multicystic kidney
- Multiple myeloma
- Multiple personality disorder
- Multiple sclerosis
- Muscular dystrophy
- Myasthenia gravis
- Myelitis—if present or less than 6 months since complete recovery
- Myocardial infarction (MI)
- Myocardial ischemia
- Myotonic dystrophy
- Myxedema—if present

N

- Nail-Patella syndrome
- Narcotic use/addiction
- Nephritis (chronic)
- Nephrocalcinosis
- Nephrosclerosis
- Nephrotic syndrome
- Neuritis—if present
- Neurofibromatosis
- Neurogenic bladder—if present
-

- Neuromuscular disorders
- Niemann-Pick disease (Lipidosis)

O

- Occlusion
- Organic brain disorder/syndrome
- Organ transplant recipient
- Osteitis fibrosa cystica
- Osteitis fibrosa cystica disseminata
- Osteitis fibrosa cystica generalisata
- Osteogenesis imperfecta/Lobstein's Disease
- Ovarian cancer

P

- Pacemaker
- Paget's disease
- Pancreatic cyst or pseudocyst
- Pancytopenia
- Paralysis
- Paranoid disorder
- Paraplegia
- Parkinson's disease
- Paroxysmal nocturnal hemoglobinuria
- Pathological fractures
- Pemphigus
- Percutaneous transluminal coronary angioplasty
- Periarteritis nodosa
- Peripheral occlusive arterial disease (POAD)
- Peripheral vascular disease or intermittent claudication
- Pernicious anemia
- Pick's disease
- Pierre Robin's syndrome
- Pituitary Adenoma—if present
- Pituitary dwarfism/Achondroplasia
- Plasmacytoma
- Pneumocystis carinii pneumonia (PCP)

- Pneumonitis
- Poliomyelitis—if present or more than one limb involved
- Polyarteritis
- Polycystic kidney
- Polycystic ovarian syndrome (PCOS)
- Polycythemia vera
- Polyglandular autoimmune disease
- Polyneuritis (Guillain-Barre syndrome)—if present or less than 3 years since recovered or residual disability/permanent impairment
- Porphyria—diagnosed less than 5 years prior to application
- Portal hypertension
- Post-Polio syndrome
- Pregnant, an expectant parent (including fathers and/or other family members)—the entire application is ineligible
- Primary biliary cirrhosis
- Primary pulmonary hypertension
- Primary sclerosing cholangitis
- Prinzmental's angina
- Pseudocyst—if present
- Pseudotumor cerebri
- Psittacosis—with extensive respiratory involvement
- Psoriasis—if severe or use of UV light
- Psychiatric disorder—severe including childhood and adolescence
- Psychosis
- Pulmonary embolism/thrombosis—if present, on anticoagulants or if less than 1 year
- Pulmonary fibrosis
- Pulmonary heart disease
- Pulmonic insufficiency—if moderate to severe
- Pulmonic stenosis
- Pulseless disease
- Pyloric Stenosis—if present
- Pyogenic arthritis

Q

- Quadriplegia

R

- Reflex sympathetic dystrophy
- Renal failure—chronic, uremia
- Renal hypertension
- Renal Insufficiency—chronic or renal failure
- Respiratory failure
- Retinal detachment—if present
- Retinopathy—central serous and diabetic
- Rhabdomyosarcoma
- Rheumatic heart disease
- Rheumatoid arthritis
- Russel-Silver syndrome—if less than 24 years of age

S

- Sarcoidosis
- Schizo-affective disorders
- Schizophrenia
- Scleroderma—generalized
- Senility
- Severe combined immunodeficiency
- Sexual deviation or disorder
- Shunt
- Sialadenitis
- Sialdenosis
- Sick sinus syndrome
- Sickle cell anemia
- Silent myocardial ischemia
- Sjogren's disease
- Sleep apnea—central or mixed sleep apnea, or current tobacco user, or with ratable build, or with hypertension or if surgery suggested
- Spherocytosis/Hereditary
- Spherocytosis—if present
- Spina bifida (Manifesta)
- Splenic flexure
- Spondylitis
- Sprue disease

- Spurway's disease
- Status Asthmaticus
- Stents—artery or blood vessel
- Stevens Johnson syndrome/Erythema Multiforme—if present or less than one year since complete recovery or history of with residuals
- Still's disease
- Stimulant usage
- Stokes-Adams syndrome
- Stroke
- Sturge-Weber syndrome
- Suicide attempt/ideation
- Syndrome
- Syphilis—if present or less than one year since complete recovery or more than 1 year since complete recovery without two normal lab results
- Syringomyelia
- Systemic fibrosclerosing syndrome
- Systemic lupus erythematosis (SLE or lupus)
- Systemic sclerosis

T

- Takayasu's arteritis
- Tetrology of fallot
- Thalassemia major
- Thrombocythemia
- Total anomalous pulmonary venous connection
- Transient ischemic attack (TIA)
- Transplant (except corneal)
- Transposition of the great vessels
- Transsexualism
- Tricuspid atresia
- Tricuspid insufficiency/regurgitation—moderate or severe
- Tricuspid stenosis
- Trisomy 21 syndrome (Down syndrome)
- Truncus arteriosus
- Tuberous sclerosis
- Turner's syndrome

U

- Ulcerative colitis/proctitis
- Underdeveloped left ventricle syndrome
- Urachal remnant—if present
- Uveitis—if chronic or less than 6 months since recovery

V

- Valve disorder
- Valve replacement
- Varicose veins of the esophagus
- Vascular hemophilia
- Ventricular arrhythmias
- Ventricular septal defect—present or less than 1 year since repaired or if surgically corrected with complications
- Von Hypple-Lindau syndrome
- Von Willebrand's disease/Pseudohemophilia

W

- Waldenstrom's macroglobulinemia
- Warnick's disease
- Wegener's granulomatosis (Wegener's syndrome)
- Weight reduction surgery—other than gastric banding
- Williams syndrome
- Wilson's disease
- Wiskott-Aldrich syndrome

X

- XYY syndrome

Z

- Zollinger-Ellison syndrome

Actions for Common Medical Conditions-Rider States

These guidelines may vary due to state-specific laws and regulations but can be followed as a general outline. This is not all inclusive. Final decision is based on underwriting review. Underwriting assessments in the below grid are based on customary and usual treatment seen for the conditions noted. Below are examples only; Humana will be solely responsible for the final underwriting decision, which is based on the completed application and the applicant's health history. Guidelines are subject to change without prior notice.

NOTE: If an applicant on an application requires more than three exclusion riders (two in Indiana), the applicant will be declined.

Condition *We reserve the right to rate for the condition and/or medication use when appropriate. A modified rating is determined based on the severity of the condition and treatment and/or prescription medication cost, dosage, and premium amount.*	\$1500 or lower deductible plus Rx	\$2500 - \$5000 deductible plus Rx	\$2000 - \$5200 deductible no Rx	\$6000 or higher deductible plus Rx
Acid Reflux/ GERD/ Heartburn				
Present, no hiatal hernia, non prescription medication (OTC only), no recommended consultations or testing	Standard	Standard	Standard	Standard
Present, prescription medication, no hiatal hernia present	Rider	Standard or Rate Up KY & OH: Standard or Rider	Standard	Standard or Rate Up KY & OH: Standard or Rider
Prescription Medication use currently, hiatal hernia present	Rider	Rider	Rider	Rider
Acne/Rosacea				
Present, no treatment or OTC medication	Standard	Standard	Standard	Standard
Prescription meds, or < 6 months since med use, no Accutane or equivalent	Rider	Standard or Rating KY & OH: Standard or Rider	Standard	Standard or Rating KY & OH: Standard or Rider
Prescription meds, completed ≥ 6 months ago, complete recovery, no Accutane or equivalent	Standard	Standard	Standard	Standard
Accutane treatment of equivalent, or ≤ 1 year since treatment completed	Rider	Rider	Rider	Rider
Accutane treatment of equivalent, or > 1 year ago since treatment, complete recovery	Standard	Standard	Standard	Standard

Condition *We reserve the right to rate for the condition and/or medication use when appropriate. A modified rating is determined based on the severity of the condition and treatment and/or prescription medication cost, dosage, and premium amount.*	$1500 or lower deductible plus Rx	$2500 - $5000 deductible plus Rx	$2000 - $5200 deductible no Rx	$6000 or higher deductible plus Rx
Allergies				
Recommended, pending or scheduled testing	Rate 50% NV: Decline if tobacco user	Rate 50% NV: Decline if tobacco use	Rate 50% NV: Decline if tobacco use	Standard
Seasonal prescription meds (3 refills or less per year, or OTC, no immunotherapy treatment	Standard	Standard	Standard	Standard
Prescription meds, more than 3 refills per year, no immunotherapy treatment	Standard or Rating KY & OH: Standard or Rider	Standard or Rating KY & OH: Standard or Rider	Standard	Standard or Rating KY & OH: Standard or Rider
With or without prescribed medications, current or recent immunotherapy	Rider	Rider	Standard - for prescribed medications Rider - immunotherapy	Rider
Amputation/Prosthesis				
Finger or toes, with or without prosthesis	Standard	Standard	Standard	Standard
Eye	Standard	Standard	Standard	Standard
All other amputations, with or without prosthesis	Rider KY: Decline	Rider KY: Decline	Rider KY: Decline	Rider KY: Decline
Caused by diabetes, severe artery disease or other disease	Decline	Decline	Decline	Decline
Anemia - other than anemia listed in the ineligible health conditions list				
Present	Standard	Standard	Standard	Standard
Aneurysm				
Present	Decline	Decline	Decline	Decline
History of, more than 5 years after repaired	Individual consideration	Individual consideration	Individual consideration	Individual consideration
Anxiety				
Well controlled with prescription medication, no counseling, no more than 2 ER visits in the last 12 months	Standard or Rating KY & OH: Standard or Rider	Standard or Rating KY & OH: Standard or Rider	Standard	Standard or Rating KY & OH: Standard or Rider
Counseling only, no medication	Rate 10-20%	Rate 10-20%	Standard	Rate 10-20%
Asthma				
Exercise induced, no regular medication required	Standard	Standard	Standard	Standard
Medication use only	Rider	Standard or Rating KY & OH: Standard or Rider	Standard	Standard or Rating KY & OH: Standard or Rider
Medication use, steroid treatment (not including Albuterol inhaler) less than 3 times and/or no emergency room visits in the past 12 months	Rider	Rider	Rider	Standard or Rating KY & OH: Standard or Rider

(Continued)

Condition *We reserve the right to rate for the condition and/or medication use when appropriate. A modified rating is determined based on the severity of the condition and treatment and/or prescription medication cost, dosage, and premium amount.*	$1500 or lower deductible plus Rx	$2500 - $5000 deductible plus Rx	$2000 - $5200 deductible no Rx	$6000 or higher deductible plus Rx
Oral steriods required ≥ 3 times or more than 2 ER visits in the past 12 months	Decline	Decline	Decline	Decline
Attention Deficit Disorder/ADD/ADHD				
No medication or counseling, more than 2 years	Standard	Standard	Standard	Standard
One medication	Rider IN: Rate only KY & OH: Standard or Rider	Rider or Rating IN: Rate only KY & OH: Standard or Rider	Standard	Rating IN: Rate only KY & OH: Standard or Rider
More than one medication	Rider IN: Rate only KY & OH: Standard or Rider	Rider or Rating IN: Rate only KY & OH: Standard or Rider	Standard	Rating IN: Rate only KY & OH: Standard or Rider
Atrial Fibrillation				
Single event, more than 2 years ago	Standard	Standard	Standard	Standard
Chronic or ongoing treatment	Decline	Decline	Decline	Decline
Single event less than 2 years ago or multiple events or pacemaker/defibrillator	Decline	Decline	Decline	Decline
Back Sprain/Strain/Whiplash				
≥ 1 year ago - complete recovery	Standard	Standard	Standard	Standard
Less than 1 year ago or not recovered	Rider	Rider	Rider	Standard
Baker's Cyst				
History of no recurrence	Standard	Standard	Standard	Standard
Present, asymptomatic	Rider	Standard	Standard	Standard
Present, symptomatic	Rider	Rider	Rider	Standard
Basal Cell Carcinoma				
Present	Decline	Decline	Decline	Decline
Single occurrence, complete recovery	Standard	Standard	Standard	Standard
Multiple occurences, or recurrent, removed (regardless of timeframe)	Rider - permanent	Rider - permanent	Rider - permanent	Standard
Benign Prostatic Hypertrophy/BPH				
Incidental finding, no symptoms, no treatment or medication use	Standard	Standard	Standard	Standard
Well controlled on one medication	Standard or Rate up	Standard or Rate up	Standard or Rate up	Standard or Rate up

Condition *We reserve the right to rate for the condition and/or medication use when appropriate. A modified rating is determined based on the severity of the condition and treatment and/or prescription medication cost, dosage, and premium amount.*	$1500 or lower deductible plus Rx	$2500 - $5000 deductible plus Rx	$2000 - $5200 deductible no Rx	$6000 or higher deductible plus Rx
More than one medication	Permanent Rider plus Rating for meds UT - Decline	Permanent Rider plus Rating for meds UT - Decline	Permanent Rider UT - Decline	Permanent Rider plus Rating for meds UT - Decline
Prostatectomy, TURP, TUNA, TUIP, TUMT, or Lazer surgery completed, no follow up needed, complete recovery, no residual complications or medication use	Standard	Standard	Standard	Standard
Bladder Infections (Cystitis)				
Less than 4 per year	Standard	Standard	Standard	Standard
4 - 6 or more per year	Decline	Standard	Standard	Standard
More than 6	Decline	Decline	Decline	Decline
Breast Cyst, Nodule or Mass				
Present & benign	Rider VA: Rate 25%	Rider VA: Rate 25%	Rider VA: Rate 25%	Standard
Removed & benign	Standard	Standard	Standard	Standard
Present, pathology unknown	Decline	Decline	Decline	Decline
Breast Implants				
Present, no complications, placed for cosmetic purposes	Standard	Standard	Standard	Standard
Breast Reduction/Macromastia				
Condition present, no surgery completed	Rider	Rider	Rider	Rider
Surgery completed < 1 year ago, with complete recovery	Standard	Standard	Standard	Standard
Surgery completed < 1 year ago, with residuals	Rider	Rider	Rider	Rider
Surgery completed > 1 year ago, no residuals	Standard	Standard	Standard	Standard
Bronchitis				
1 - 3 episodes in the past year, non tobacco user, complete recovery	Standard	Standard	Standard	Standard
1 - 2 episodes in the past year, Tobacco user, complete recovery	Standard	Standard	Standard	Standard
3 episodes a year, Tobacco user, complete recovery	Individual consideration	Individual consideration	Individual consideration	Individual consideration
3 episodes a year or Chronic Bronchitis	Decline	Decline	Decline	Decline
Bundle Branch Block (right)				
Complete, no tobacco use for the last 12 months, symptoms & treatment free for last 12 months, build not ratable	Standard	Standard	Standard	Standard

(Continued)

Condition *We reserve the right to rate for the condition and/or medication use when appropriate. A modified rating is determined based on the severity of the condition and treatment and/or prescription medication cost, dosage, and premium amount.*	$1500 or lower deductible plus Rx	$2500 - $5000 deductible plus Rx	$2000 - $5200 deductible no Rx	$6000 or higher deductible plus Rx
Bursitis/Tendonitis/Tenosynovitis				
Single occurrence with complete recovery	Standard	Standard	Standard	Standard
Single occurrence, not recovered	Rider	Standard	Standard	Standard
Multiple occurrences	Rider	Rider	Rider	Rider
Carpal Tunnel				
Present or residuals	Rider	Rider	Rider	Standard
Surgical repair complete recovery	Standard	Standard	Standard	Standard
Cataracts				
Present	Rider KY: Decline	Rider KY: Decline	Rider KY: Decline	Standard
Surgically corrected, fully recovered, no residuals	Standard	Standard	Standard	Standard
Chlamydia				
Present or under treatment, no other STD history	Standard	Standard	Standard	Standard
Complete recovery	Standard	Standard	Standard	Standard
Colon Polyps				
Present	Decline	Decline	Decline	Decline
More than 1 benign polyp removed within the past 5 years during colonoscopy, scheduled f/u is every 10 years	Rider (permanent)	Rider (permanent)	Rider (permanent)	Rider (permanent)
Single benign polyp removed during colonoscopy within the last 5 years, no colon resection, f/u schedue every 5 years	Standard	Standard	Standard	Standard
Single benign polyp removed during colonoscopy, within the past 5 years no colon resection, follow up scheduled every 3 - 5 years	Rider (permanent)	Rider (permanent)	Rider (permanent)	Rider (permanent)
More than 1 polyp removed within the past 5 years. Surgically removed (not during colonoscopy) or part of colon surgically removed or follow up scheduled every 1 - 2 years	Decline	Decline	Decline	Decline

Condition *We reserve the right to rate for the condition and/or medication use when appropriate. A modified rating is determined based on the severity of the condition and treatment and/or prescription medication cost, dosage, and premium amount.*	$1500 or lower deductible plus Rx	$2500 - $5000 deductible plus Rx	$2000 - $5200 deductible no Rx	$6000 or higher deductible plus Rx
1 - 2 polyps removed within the past 5 years during colonoscopy, only 1 colonoscopy completed within the past 5 years. Follow up scheduled every 3 - 5 years	Rider (permanent) UT: Decline tobacco user or Max rating applies	Rider (permanent) UT: Decline tobacco user or max rating applies	Rider (permanent) UT: Decline tobacco user or max rating applies	Rider (permanent) UT: Decline tobacco user or max rating applies
More than 2 polyps removed within the past 5 years, follow up scheduled every 3 - 5 years	Decline	Decline	Decline	Decline
Condyloma				
Present or history of - no HPV	Rider UT: 85% rating, non tobacco users UT: Decline tobacco users	Standard	Standard	Standard
Present of history of - with HPV	Rider UT: 85% rating, non tobacco users UT: Decline tobacco users HPV underwritten separately	Rider UT: 85% rating, non tobacco users UT: Decline tobacco users HPV underwritten separately	Rider UT: 85% rating, non tobacco users UT: Decline tobacco users HPV underwritten separately	Rider UT: 85% rating, non tobacco users UT: Decline tobacco users HPV underwritten separately
Deep Vein Thrombosis (DVT)				
On anticoagulants or one episode less than 3 months ago	Decline	Decline	Decline	Decline
One episode—3 mos - 2 years with complete recovery	Rider	Rider	Rider	Standard
Recurrent	Decline	Decline	Decline	Decline
Depression				
Well controlled with prescription medication, no counseling	Standard or Rating KY & OH: Standard or Rider	Standard or Rating KY & OH: Standard or Rider	Standard	Standard or Rating KY & OH: Standard or Rider
Counseling only, no medication	Rate 10-20%	Rate 10-20%	Rate 10-20%	Rate 10-20%
Deviated Septum (nasal)				
Present, asymptomatic or surgically repaired	Standard	Standard	Standard	Standard
Symptomatic	Rider	Rider	Rider	Rider
Disc Disorder (herniated, bulging, ruptured)				
Present, surgically repaired less than 1 year ago or with residuals	Rider	Rider	Rider	Rider
Asymptomatic, surgically repaired more than 1 year ago with full recovery	Standard	Standard	Standard	Standard
Diverticulitis				
Present, No Surgery	Rider	Rider	Rider	Rider
Surgery within 0-2 years	Rider	Rider	Rider	Rider

(Continued)

Condition *We reserve the right to rate for the condition and/or medication use when appropriate. A modified rating is determined based on the severity of the condition and treatment and/or prescription medication cost, dosage, and premium amount.*	$1500 or lower deductible plus Rx	$2500 - $5000 deductible plus Rx	$2000 - $5200 deductible no Rx	$6000 or higher deductible plus Rx
Surgically corrected > 2 years ago	Standard	Standard	Standard	Standard
Diverticulosis				
Present or with history of diverticulitis, No Surgery	Decline	Decline	Decline	Decline
Surgery within 0-2 years	Decline	Decline	Decline	Decline
Surgically corrected > 2 years ago	Standard	Standard	Standard	Standard
DUI - Paramed exam is required				
Single occurrence, within 5 years	Rate 30%-Decline	Rate 30%-Decline	Rate 30%-Decline	Rate 30%-Decline
Single occurrence, more than 5 years	Standard	Standard	Standard	Standard
Multiple occurrences, within 5 years	Decline	Decline	Decline	Decline
Multiple occurrences, more than 5 years	Individual consideration	Individual consideration	Individual consideration	Individual consideration
Ear Infection (Otitis Media)				
< 3 in the past 12 months	Standard	Standard	Standard	Standard
3 in the past 12 months	Rider	Rider	Rider	Standard
Tubes Present	Rider	Standard	Standard	Standard
Tubes no longer present, no recurrence	Standard	Standard	Standard	Standard
Eczema				
Present or less than 2 years since symptomatic	Rider	Standard or Rating KY & OH: Standard or Rider	Standard	Standard or Rating KY & OH: Standard or Rider
2 years since treatment or symptoms	Standard	Standard	Standard	Standard
Endometriosis				
Present or within 5 years of treatment	Rider KY: Decline	Rider KY: Decline	Rider KY: Decline	Rider KY: Decline
5 years since symptoms or treatment	Standard	Standard	Standard	Standard
Surgery < 3 years ago	Rider KY: Decline	Rider KY: Decline	Rider KY: Decline	Standard KY: Decline
Surgery > 3 years ago	Standard	Standard	Standard	Standard
Enlarged Prostate - See Benign Prostatic Hypertrophy				
Epilepsy, Grand Mal (Generalized)				
Seizure within past 2 years	Decline	Decline	Decline	Decline
Last seizure > 2 years ago	Standard or Rate up	Standard or Rate up	Standard	Standard or Rate up
Epilepsy, Petit Mal (Generalized)				
Seizure within past 2 years	Decline	Decline	Decline	Decline

Condition *We reserve the right to rate for the condition and/or medication use when appropriate. A modified rating is determined based on the severity of the condition and treatment and/or prescription medication cost, dosage, and premium amount.*	$1500 or lower deductible plus Rx	$2500 - $5000 deductible plus Rx	$2000 - $5200 deductible no Rx	$6000 or higher deductible plus Rx
Last seizure > 2 years ago	Standard or Rate up	Standard or Rate up	Standard	Standard or Rate up
Epilepsy, Temporal Lobe (Partial)				
Seizure < 1 year ago	Decline	Decline	Decline	Decline
Seizure > 1 year ago	Standard or Rate up	Standard or Rate up	Standard	Standard or Rate up
Fractures				
Present - No fixation device	Rider	Standard	Standard	Standard
Present - with permanent fixation device	Standard	Standard	Standard	Standard
Present - with temporary fixation device	Rider	Standard	Standard	Standard
Recovered & released from care with no fixation device or permanent fixation device	Standard	Standard	Standard	Standard
Recovered, released from care with temporary fixation device	Rider	Rider	Rider	Standard
Pathological	Decline	Decline	Decline	Decline
Ganglion Cyst				
Present & symptomatic	Rider	Standard	Standard	Standard
Surgically removed or history of and resolved	Standard	Standard	Standard	Standard
Gastric banding - weight loss surgery				
Lap band removed, no rateable build, weight maintained for one year	Standard	Standard	Standard	Standard
Lap Band removed, rateable build, or weight loss not maintained for one year	Decline	Decline	Decline	Decline
Lap Band present	Decline	Decline	Decline	Decline
Gastric Bypass / Gastric Stapling	Decline	Decline	Decline	Decline
GERD (reflux) - see Acid Reflux/GERD				
Gestational Diabetes				
< 5 yrs ago, diet controlled during pregnancy, no recurrence	Rate 25%	Rate 25%	Rate 25%	Rate 25%
5 yrs ago, diet controlled during pregnancy, no recurrence	Standard	Standard	Standard	Standard
< 5 yrs ago, controlled with insulin during pregnancy, no recurrence<	Rate 50%	Rate 50%	Rate 50%	Rate 50%
5 yrs ago, controlled with insulin during pregnancy, no recurrence	Rate 25%	Rate 25%	Rate 25%	Rate 25%
History of, no glucose test following pregnancy or glucose levels did not return to normal	Decline	Decline	Decline	Decline

(Continued)

Condition *We reserve the right to rate for the condition and/or medication use when appropriate. A modified rating is determined based on the severity of the condition and treatment and/or prescription medication cost, dosage, and premium amount.*	$1500 or lower deductible plus Rx	$2500 - $5000 deductible plus Rx	$2000 - $5200 deductible no Rx	$6000 or higher deductible plus Rx
Glaucoma				
Symptomatic, but not diagnosed	Rider and rating for medications	Rider and rating for medications	Rider for condition, no action for medications	Rider and rating for medications
Present, well controlled	Rating OH & KY: Rider	Rating OH & KY: Rider	Standard	Rating OH & KY: Rider
Present, not controlled: with or without medications	Rider	Rider	Rider	Rider
Surgically corrected both eyes, with or without medications	If no medications: Standard Medication use: Rating OH & KY: Rider	If no medications: Standard Medication use: Rating OH & KY: Rider	Standard	If no medications: Standard Medication use: Rating OH & KY: Rider
Surgically corrected in one eye: with or without medication use	Rider	Rider	Rider	Rider
Gout				
Present or within 2 years of symptoms or treatment	Rider	Rider	Rider	Standard
Recovered and time from last symptoms or treatment > 2 years	Standard	Standard	Standard	Standard
Grave's Disease - See Hyperthyroidism				
Guillain-Barre Syndrome				
Present or < 3 years since recovered or Residual disability/permanent impairment	Decline	Decline	Decline	Decline
3 years since recovered, no disability, minimal weakness, no relapse	Rate 25%	Standard	Standard	Standard
Gynecomastia				
Present	Rider	Rider	Rider	Rider
Surgical correction > 6 months ago	Standard	Standard	Standard	Standard
Hashimoto's Thyroiditis - See Hypothyroidism				
Heartburn - see Acid Reflux				
Heart Murmur				
Functional/Innocent, Grade I or II - Systolic	Standard	Standard	Standard	Standard
Organic, Grade III or greater, continuous - Diastolic	Decline	Decline	Decline	Decline
Hemorrhoids				
Present, asymptomatic	Standard	Standard	Standard	Standard

Condition *We reserve the right to rate for the condition and/or medication use when appropriate. A modified rating is determined based on the severity of the condition and treatment and/or prescription medication cost, dosage, and premium amount.*	$1500 or lower deductible plus Rx	$2500 - $5000 deductible plus Rx	$2000 - $5200 deductible no Rx	$6000 or higher deductible plus Rx
Present, symptomatic	Rider	Standard or Rate up	Standard	Standard
1 year since symptoms or surgery	Standard	Standard	Standard	Standard
Hepatitis A				
6 months since treatment with normal liver tests	Standard	Standard	Standard	Standard
Hepatitis B				
Carrier	Decline	Decline	Decline	Decline
Present or < 6 months since treatment	Decline	Decline	Decline	Decline
Others	Individual consideration	Individual consideration	Individual consideration	Individual consideration
Hernia				
Present, all types other than Hiatal Hernia	Rider	Rider	Rider	Rider
Surgically repaired	Standard	Standard	Standard	Standard
Herpes				
OTC medication	Standard	Standard	Standard	Standard
Prescription medication	Rating or Rider KY & OH: Standard or Rider	Rating or Rider KY & OH: Standard or Rider	Standard	Rating or Rider KY & OH: Standard or Rider
Herpes Zoster (shingles)				
Present	Standard or Rate up	Standard or Rate up	Standard	Standard
Complete recovery, no medication	Standard	Standard	Standard	Standard
Hiatal Hernia - see Acid Reflux/GERD				
High Blood Pressure/Hypertension				
Underwritten based on age of onset, stability and comorbidity				
Stable, average readings 150/90 or less, no other cardiac risk factors, controlled with medication	Standard or Rate up	Standard or Rate up	Standard	Standard or Rate up
High Blood Pressure + 50% Ratable Build				
	Decline	Decline	Decline	Decline
High Blood Pressure + Ratable Build + Tobacco User				
	Decline	Decline	Decline	Decline
High Blood Pressure + High Cholesterol controlled with medication				
	Standard or Rating KY & OH: Hypertenstion: Standard or Rating Cholesterol: Standard or Rider	Standard or Rating KY & OH: Hypertension: Standard or Rating Cholesterol: Standard or Rider	Standard	Standard or Rating KY & OH: Hypertension: Standard or Rating Cholesterol: Standard or Rider

(Continued)

Condition *We reserve the right to rate for the condition and/or medication use when appropriate. A modified rating is determined based on the severity of the condition and treatment and/or prescription medication cost, dosage, and premium amount.*	$1500 or lower deductible plus Rx	$2500 - $5000 deductible plus Rx	$2000 - $5200 deductible no Rx	$6000 or higher deductible plus Rx
High Blood Pressure + Sleep Apnea				
	Decline	Decline	Decline	Decline
High Blood Pressure + High Cholesterol + Ratable Build				
	Decline	Decline	Decline	Decline
High Blood Pressure + High Cholesterol + Tobacco User				
	Decline	Decline	Decline	Decline
High Cholesterol				
Lipid panel results within normal limits, compliant with follow up, controlled with medication	Standard or Rating KY & OH: Standard or Rider	Standard or Rating KY & OH: Standard or Rider	Standard	Standard or Rating KY & OH: Standard or Rider
High Cholesterol + Ratable Build + Tobacco User				
	Decline	Decline	Decline	Decline
High Cholesterol + Ratable Build + Hypertension				
	Decline	Decline	Decline	Decline
Human Papilloma Virus (HPV)				
Low risk - no condyloma	Standard	Standard	Standard	Standard
High risk	Rider CO & KY: Decline UT: Rate 85%-non tobacco user, Decline-tobacco user	Rider CO & KY: Decline UT: Rate 85%-non tobacco user, Decline-tobacco user	Rider CO & KY: Decline UT: Rate 85%-non tobacco user, Decline-tobacco user	Rider CO & KY: Decline UT: Rate 85%-non tobacco user, Decline-tobacco user
Hyperthyroidism				
Present - untreated	Decline	Decline	Decline	Decline
Present - treated with medication	Rider	Standard	Standard	Standard
Hypoglycemia				
Present, follow up recommended	Decline	Decline	Decline	Decline
Present, or history of, diet controlled, no follow-up recommended	Standard	Standard	Standard	Standard
Present, treated with medication	Decline	Decline	Decline	Decline
Hypothyroid				
Present or history of	Standard	Standard	Standard	Standard
Infertility Treatment - male and female				
Current infertility drug treatment	Decline - entire family	Decline - entire family	Decline - entire family	Decline - entire family
Last treatment with infertility drugs ≤ a year without a live birth	Decline - entire family	Decline - entire family	Decline - entire family	Decline - entire family
Last treatment with infertility drugs with a live birth, family planning complete	Standard	Standard	Standard	Standard

Condition *We reserve the right to rate for the condition and/or medication use when appropriate. A modified rating is determined based on the severity of the condition and treatment and/or prescription medication cost, dosage, and premium amount.*	$1500 or lower deductible plus Rx	$2500 - $5000 deductible plus Rx	$2000 - $5200 deductible no Rx	$6000 or higher deductible plus Rx
Last treatment with infertility drugs with a live birth, family planning is not complete	Decline - entire family	Decline - entire family	Decline - entire family	Decline - entire family
Last treatment with IVF, ZIFT, GIFT or others, family planning complete	Standard	Standard	Standard	Standard
Last treatment with IVF, ZIFT, GIFT or others, family planning is not complete	Decline - entire family	Decline - entire family	Decline - entire family	Decline - entire family
Insomnia				
Treated with medication	Standard or Rating KY & OH: Standard or Rider	Standard or Rating KY & OH: Standard or Rider	Standard	Standard or Rating KY & OH: Standard or Rider
Irritable Bowel Syndrome				
Treated with OTC medication	Standard	Standard	Standard	Standard
Controlled w/prescription GI medication	Rider	Standard or Rating KY & OH: Standard or Rider	Standard	Standard or Rating KY & OH: Standard or Rider
Treated w/non-GI prescription medication	Rider and Rating for non-GI meds	Standard or Rating	Standard	Standard or Rating
ITP (blood disorder)				
Child form, complete recovery, platelet count returned to normal	Standard	Standard	Standard	Standard
Child form, present	Decline	Decline	Decline	Decline
Adult form or chronic, less than 40 years of age, more than 3 years since treatment and a complete recovery	Rate 25%	Rate 25%	Rate 25%	Rate 25%
Adult form or chronic, more than 6 years since treatment and a complete recovery, no current treatment, normal platelet count	Standard	Standard	Standard	Standard
Joint replacement				
Hip replaced	Permanent Rider KY: Decline	Permanent Rider KY: Decline	Permanent rider KY: Decline	Permanent Rider KY: Decline
Knee replaced	Permanent Rider KY: Decline	Permanent Rider KY: Decline	Permanent Rider KY: Decline	Permanent Rider KY: Decline
Shoulder replaced	Permanent Rider KY: Rate 100% - Decline tobacco user	Permanent Rider KY: Rate 100% - Decline tobacco user	Permanent Rider KY: Rate 100% - Decline tobacco user	Standard
Kidney Infection/Pyelonephritis/Pyelitis				
1 episode, within 0-3 years	Rider	Standard	Standard	Standard
1 episode > 3 years ago	Standard	Standard	Standard	Standard
2 episodes, < 2 years ago	Decline	Decline	Decline	Standard

(Continued)

Condition *We reserve the right to rate for the condition and/or medication use when appropriate. A modified rating is determined based on the severity of the condition and treatment and/or prescription medication cost, dosage, and premium amount.*	$1500 or lower deductible plus Rx	$2500 - $5000 deductible plus Rx	$2000 - $5200 deductible no Rx	$6000 or higher deductible plus Rx
2 episodes, 2-5 years ago	Rider	Standard	Standard	Standard
2 episodes, > 5 years ago	Standard	Standard	Standard	Standard
3 or more episodes, regardless of time frame	Decline	Decline	Decline	Decline
Kidney Stones				
Present	Decline	Decline	Decline	Rider
Passed or surgically removed < 2 years ago	Rider	Rider	Rider	Standard
Passed or surgically removed > 2 years	Standard	Standard	Standard	Standard
5 or more episodes	Decline	Decline	Decline	Decline
Lichen Planus				
Mild infrequent attacks	Standard	Standard	Standard	Standard
Frequent or severe attacks	Rider plus Rate	Standard or Rate up	Rider	Standard or Rate up
Lipoma				
Present, asymptomatic, no surgery anticipated	Standard	Standard	Standard	Standard
Present and symptomatic	Rider	Standard	Standard	Standard
Lyme Disease				
Present or treatment completed less than 6 months ago	Decline	Decline	Decline	Decline
6 months since recovery, no residuals	Standard	Standard	Standard	Standard
Macular Degeneration				
Dry or wet	Rider	Rider	Rider	Rider
Meniere's Disease				
Present, confirmed diagnosis, stable, current or history of med use, no ongoing follow-up or treatment	Standard or Rating KY & OH: Standard or Rider (permanent)	Standard or Rating KY & OH: Standard or Rider (permanent)	Standard	Standard
Present, confirmed diagnosis, stable, current or history of med use, ongoing follow-up or treatment	Rider (permanent)	Rider (permanent)	Rider (permanent)	Rider (permanent)
Migraines				
Occasional (□ 3 episodes yearly) treated with OTC medication	Standard	Standard	Standard	Standard
≥ 4 episodes in the last 12 months, or severe. Workup completed, symptoms controlled with current treatment	Rider	Standard or Rating KY & OH: Standard or Rider	Standard	Standard or Rating KY & OH: Standard or Rider

Condition *We reserve the right to rate for the condition and/or medication use when appropriate. A modified rating is determined based on the severity of the condition and treatment and/or prescription medication cost, dosage, and premium amount.*	\$1500 or lower deductible plus Rx	\$2500 - \$5000 deductible plus Rx	\$2000 - \$5200 deductible no Rx	\$6000 or higher deductible plus Rx
≥ 4 episodes in the last 12 months, No workup completed	Decline	Decline	Decline	Decline
Miscarriage				
1 - 2, no underlying cause	Standard	Standard	Standard	Standard
2, no full term deliveries	Rider	Rider	Rider	Rider
History of with full term delivery	Standard	Standard	Standard	Standard
Mitral Valve Prolapse				
No symptoms or treatment	Standard	Standard	Standard	Standard
Mild symptoms controlled with one med, no other heart disorder	Standard or Rate up	Standard or Rate up	Standard	Standard or Rate up
Molluscum Contagiosum				
Present or complete recovery < 1 year	Rider	Standard	Standard	Standard
Complete recovery > 1 year	Standard	Standard	Standard	Standard
MRSA - Methicillin-Resistant Staphylococcus Aureus				
Present, currently under treatment	Decline	Decline	Decline	Decline
Completed treatment, follow-up pending	Decline	Decline	Decline	Decline
Treated, full recovery of over 60 days	Standard	Standard	Standard	Standard
Nephritis/Glomerulonephritis				
1 episodes > 3 years ago	Standard	Standard	Standard	Standard
1 episode < 2 years ago	Decline	Decline	Decline	Decline
Osteoarthritis				
Present, only OTC meds, no PT or OT, no shoulder, hip, pelvis, back or spine, knee or ankle involvement	Standard	Standard	Standard	Standard
Present, all treatment except OTC meds, no shoulder, hip, pelvis, back or spine, knee or ankle involvement	Rider	Rider	Rider	Standard or Rating
Present, regardless of treatment, with shoulder, hip, pelvis, back or spine, knee or ankle involvement and no joint replacement	Rider	Rider	Rider	Rider
Joint replacement (see joint replacements)				
Osteoporosis/Osteopenia				
Current use of Prophylactic medication, due to age/ menopause, no diagnosis of osteoporosis or osteopenia, no fractures or Dexa scans done	Standard or Rate up	Standard or Rate up	Standard	Standard or Rate up

(Continued)

Condition *We reserve the right to rate for the condition and/or medication use when appropriate. A modified rating is determined based on the severity of the condition and treatment and/or prescription medication cost, dosage, and premium amount.*	$1500 or lower deductible plus Rx	$2500 - $5000 deductible plus Rx	$2000 - $5200 deductible no Rx	$6000 or higher deductible plus Rx
Diagnosis of Osteoporosis or Osteopenia with or without medication use, Dexa scans stable or improved	Rider (permanent)	Rider (permanent)	Rider (permanent)	Standard or Rate up
Present, severe, history of pathologic fractures, crippling, Dexa scans worsening	Decline	Decline	Decline	Decline
Ovarian Cyst				
Present, asymptomatic	Standard	Standard	Standard	Standard
Symptomatic	Rider	Rider	Rider	Rider
Removed	Standard	Standard	Standard	Standard
Pancreatitis				
History of attack, no underlying cause, resolved	Individual consideration, medical records required	Individual consideration, medical records required	Individual consideration, medical records required	Individual consideration, medical records required
Chronic or recurrent	Decline	Decline	Decline	Decline
Pap Smear - Abnormal				
ASCUS, no high risk HPV, Class II or Class III followed by one normal pap, Class IV, treated, followed by three normal pap smears	Standard	Standard	Standard	Standard
Phlebitis				
Current use of blood thinners	Decline	Decline	Decline	Decline
One episode, < 3 months, complete recovery, no varicose veins or edema	Rider	Rider	Rider	Standard
One episode, 3 months - 2 years, complete recovery, no varicose veins or edema	Standard	Standard	Standard	Standard
Recurrent episodes within 0 - 2 years	Rider	Rider	Rider	Standard
History of ≥ 2 years ago	Standard	Standard	Standard	Standard
Varicose Veins - (see Varicose Veins)				
Pneumonia				
Present	Decline	Decline	Decline	Decline
Complete recovery	Standard	Standard	Standard	Standard
Prostatitis				
One episode, full recovery	Standard	Standard	Standard	Standard
1 episode or chronic	Rider	Rider	Rider	Rider
Prosthesis/Prosthetics Device See Amputation				

Condition *We reserve the right to rate for the condition and/or medication use when appropriate. A modified rating is determined based on the severity of the condition and treatment and/or prescription medication cost, dosage, and premium amount.*	$1500 or lower deductible plus Rx	$2500 - $5000 deductible plus Rx	$2000 - $5200 deductible no Rx	$6000 or higher deductible plus Rx
Prostate - Enlarged See Benign Prostatic Hypertrophy/BPH				
Psoriasis				
Mild symptoms, OTC medications or no treatment	Standard	Standard	Standard	Standard
Mild to moderate symptoms, conservative treatments, including prescription topical agents	Rider	Standard or Rating KY & OH: Standard or Rider	Standard	Standard or Rating KY & OH: Standard or Rider
Severe symptoms requiring RX medication such as Enbrel, Remicade, Sulfasalazine, gold therapy or Methotrexate	Decline	Decline	Decline	Decline
Psoriatic Arthritis (See Psoriatic Arthritis)				
Use of tanning bed only	Standard	Standard	Standard	Standard
Use of UVA/PUVA light at a medical facility	Decline	Decline	Decline	Decline
Psoriatic Arthritis				
All cases	Decline	Decline	Decline	Decline
Pyloric Stenosis				
Present	Decline	Decline	Decline	Decline
Surgically corrected with complete recovery	Standard	Standard	Standard	Standard
Respiratory Syncytial Virus (RSV)/Bronchiolitis				
Present or history of, < 2 years of age, Synagis/ Palivizumab use	Decline	Decline	Decline	Decline
2 years of age, Last occurrence < 1 year ago and Synagis/Palivizumab use	Decline	Decline	Decline	Decline
2 years of age, Last occurrence > 1 year ago, No medications for > 1 year, Complete recovery, No other respiratory conditions	Standard	Standard	Standard	Standard
Restless Leg Syndrome				
Confirmed diagnosis, no medication, or treatment for 12 months	Standard	Standard	Standard	Standard
Confirmed diagnosis, controlled with medication or treatment or no medication use for 12 months	Standard or Rating KY & OH: Standard or Rider	Standard or Rating KY & OH: Standard or Rider	Standard	Standard or Rating KY & OH: Standard or Rider
Unconfirmed diagnosis or testing pending or recommended	Decline	Decline	Decline	Decline
Retinal Detachment				
Present	Decline	Decline	Decline	Decline
Surgically corrected < 2 years	Rider	Standard	Standard	Standard
Rheumatoid Arthritis				

(Continued)

Condition *We reserve the right to rate for the condition and/or medication use when appropriate. A modified rating is determined based on the severity of the condition and treatment and/or prescription medication cost, dosage, and premium amount.*	$1500 or lower deductible plus Rx	$2500 - $5000 deductible plus Rx	$2000 - $5200 deductible no Rx	$6000 or higher deductible plus Rx
	Decline	Decline	Decline	Decline
Scoliosis				
Present, no surgery, under age of 20	Rider	Rider	Rider	Rider
Present, over age of 20	Standard	Standard	Standard	Standard
Surgery completed, rod in place, full recovery	Standard	Standard	Standard	Standard
Any cardiac, pulmonary or spinal cord involvement	Decline	Decline	Decline	Decline
Sinusitis				
< 3 episodes in the past year	Standard	Standard	Standard	Standard
3 - 6 episodes in the past 12 months	Rider	Standard	Standard	Standard
6 episodes in the past 12 months	Rider	Rider	Rider	Standard
Sleep Apnea				
Controlled with CPAP	Rider	Rider	Rider	Standard
Surgically corrected	Standard	Standard	Standard	Standard
Sleep Apnea + Ratable build	Decline	Decline	Decline	Decline
Sleep Apnea + Tobacco User	Decline	Decline	Decline	Decline
Sleep Apnea + Hypertension	Decline	Decline	Decline	Decline
Central or Mixed	Decline	Decline	Decline	Decline
Spina Bifida				
Occulta, incidental finding, asymptomatic	Standard	Standard	Standard	Standard
Occulta - symptomatic	Decline	Decline	Decline	Decline
Manifesta	Decline	Decline	Decline	Decline
Spinal Manipulations				
0 - 2 visits per year	Standard	Standard	Standard	Standard
3 - 5 visits per year	All states Standard except: NV: Rider Portrait plan only (all other plans standard)	All states Standard except: NV - Rider Portrait plan & Autoshare 80 plus RX only (all other plans standard)	Standard	All states Standard except: NV - Rider Autoshare 80 plus RX only (all other plans standard)
6 - 10 visits per year	All states Ridered except: AZ, CO & WI: Rate 25%	All states Standard except: NV - Rider Portrait plan & Autoshare 80 plus RX only (all other plans standard)	Standard	All states Standard except: NV - Rider Autoshare 80 plus RX only (all other plans standard)

Condition *We reserve the right to rate for the condition and/or medication use when appropriate. A modified rating is determined based on the severity of the condition and treatment and/or prescription medication cost, dosage, and premium amount.*	$1500 or lower deductible plus Rx	$2500 - $5000 deductible plus Rx	$2000 - $5200 deductible no Rx	$6000 or higher deductible plus Rx
11 - 15 visits per year	All states Ridered except: AZ, CO & WI: Rate 50%	All states Standard except: NV - Rider Portrait plan & Autoshare 80 plus RX only (all other plans standard)	Standard	All states Standard except: NV - Rider Autoshare 80 plus RX only (all other plans standard)
16 - 20 visits per year	All states Ridered except: AZ, CO & WI: Rate 75%	All states Ridered except: AZ, CO & WI: Rate 15%	All states Ridered except: AZ, CO & WI: Rate 15%	All states Standard except: NV - Rider Autoshare 80 plus RX only (all other plans standard)
21 - 25 visits per year	All states Ridered except: AZ, CO & WI: Rate 100%	All states Ridered except: AZ, CO & WI: Rate 25%	All states Ridered except: AZ, CO & WI: Rate 25%	All states Standard except: NV - Rider Autoshare 80 plus RX only (all other plans standard)
26 - 30 visits per year	All states Ridered except: AZ, CO & WI: Rate 125%	All states Ridered except: AZ, CO & WI: Rate 40%	All states Ridered except: AZ, CO & WI: Rate 740%	All states Standard except: NV - Rider Autoshare 80 plus RX only (all other plans standard)
31 - 35 visits per year	All states Ridered except: AZ, CO & WI: Rate 150%	All states Ridered except: AZ, CO & WI: Rate 50%	All states Ridered except: AZ, CO & WI: Rate 50%	All states Standard except: NV - Rider Autoshare 80 plus RX only (all other plans standard)
36+ visits per year	All states Ridered except: AZ, CO & WI: Decline	All states Ridered except: AZ, CO & WI: Rate 75%	All states Ridered except: AZ, CO & WI: Rate 75%	All states Ridered except: AZ, CO & WI: Rate 75%
Stents				
Heart	Decline	Decline	Decline	Decline
Other locations	Individual consideration	Individual consideration	Individual consideration	Individual consideration
Tachycardia				
No attacks in past 12 months, maintained and well controlled on medications to control attacks and symptoms, no other cardiovascular disorders	Rider + Rating for meds	Rider + Rating for meds	Rider	Standard or Rate-up

(Continued)

Condition *We reserve the right to rate for the condition and/or medication use when appropriate. A modified rating is determined based on the severity of the condition and treatment and/or prescription medication cost, dosage, and premium amount.*	$1500 or lower deductible plus Rx	$2500 - $5000 deductible plus Rx	$2000 - $5200 deductible no Rx	$6000 or higher deductible plus Rx
≤ 3 attacks per year, < 1 year since last attack	Decline	Decline	Decline	Decline
≤ 3 attacks per year, 1-3 years since last attack, prompt response to treatment, no other cardivascular disorders	Rider	Rider	Rider	Rider
< 3 attacks per year, > 3 years since last attack, prompt response to treatment, no other cardiovascular disorders	Standard	Standard	Standard	Standard
Others	Decline	Decline	Decline	Decline
Surgical ablation □ 6 months ago	Decline	Decline	Decline	Decline
Surgical ablation > 6 months ago, no residuals	Standard	Standard	Standard	Standard
Tendonitis - SEE BURSITIS				
Tenosynovitis - SEE BURSITIS				
Tonsillitis				
< 3 episodes per year	Standard	Standard	Standard	Standard
3 - 5 episodes per year	Rider	Standard	Standard	Standard
5 episodes per year	Rider	Rider	Rider	Standard
Tourettes Syndrome				
Simple tics, no behavioral disorders	Standard	Standard	Standard	Standard
Controlled with medication	Standard or Rate up	Standard or Rate up	Standard	Standard or Rate up
Disabling, behavioral issues, extensive psychotherapy	Decline	Decline	Decline	Decline
Tuberculosis				
TB infection without disease, + skin test, Negative bacteriologic studies, Negative chest x-ray, No evidence of active disease, Prophylactic drug therapy complete > 6 months ago	Standard	Standard	Standard	Standard
TB infection without disease, + skin test, Negative bacteriologic studies, Negative chest x-ray, No evidence of active disease, Current use of < 6 months of prophylactic drugs	Decline	Standard	Standard	Standard
Ulcer (Peptic)				
One episode, complete recovery	Standard	Standard	Standard	Standard

Condition *We reserve the right to rate for the condition and/or medication use when appropriate. A modified rating is determined based on the severity of the condition and treatment and/or prescription medication cost, dosage, and premium amount.*	$1500 or lower deductible plus Rx	$2500 - $5000 deductible plus Rx	$2000 - $5200 deductible no Rx	$6000 or higher deductible plus Rx
1 episode, well controlled with medications	Rider UT - Decline	Rider UT - Decline	Rider UT - Decline	Standard
History of bleeding or perforation, < 2 years after episode, OR multiple occurrences of bleeding or perforation	Decline	Decline	Decline	Decline
History of bleeding or perforation, > 2 years after episode, single occurrence, no known cause OR NSAID's discontinued, Vagotomy performed > 3 years ago, No symptoms	Standard	Standard	Standard	Standard
Uterine Fibroids				
Post-menopausal, no HRT, asymptomatic or myomectomy or hysterectomy completed	Standard	Standard	Standard	Standard
Others	Rider	Rider	Rider	Rider
Vaginitis				
One occurrence, complete recovery	Standard	Standard	Standard	Standard
1 occurrence, < 1 year since last occurrence	Rider	Standard	Standard	Standard
Varicose Veins of the lower extremities - UT only				
Present-asymptomatic, no recommendations for treatment	Standard	Standard	Standard	Standard
Present with ulcer	Decline	Decline	Decline	Decline
Treated with lazer, stripping or sclerotherapy, full recovery no symptoms or treatment < 1yr ago	Rider	Standard	Standard	Standard
Treated with lazer, stripping or sclerotherapy, full recovery no symptoms or treatment > 1yr ago	Standard	Standard	Standard	Standard
Varicose Veins				
Present-asymptomatic, no recommendations for treatment	Standard	Standard	Standard	Standard
Present with ulcer	Decline	Decline	Decline	Decline
Treated with lazer, stripping or sclerotherapy, full recovery no symptoms or treatment < 1yr ago	Rider	Standard	Standard	Standard
Treated with lazer, stripping or sclerotherapy, full recovery no symptoms or treatment >1yr ago	Standard	Standard	Standard	Standard

(Continued)

Condition *We reserve the right to rate for the condition and/or medication use when appropriate. A modified rating is determined based on the severity of the condition and treatment and/or prescription medication cost, dosage, and premium amount.*	$1500 or lower deductible plus Rx	$2500 - $5000 deductible plus Rx	$2000 - $5200 deductible no Rx	$6000 or higher deductible plus Rx
Ventricular Septal Defect - APS REQUIRED				
Repaired > 1 year ago, complete recovery, normal cardiac exam	Standard	Standard	Standard	Standard
Present or repaired with symptoms or abnormal cardiac exam	Decline	Decline	Decline	Decline
Weight loss medication use				
Use of any weight loss medication (other than Xenical) in combination with hypertension or cardiac issues	Individual consideration - medical records required	Individual consideration - medical records required	Individual consideration - medical records required	Individual consideration - medical records required
Continuous use of any weight loss medications for more than one year	Decline	Decline	Decline	Decline
All other scenarios or Xenical use in combination with hypertension or cardiac disease	Standard	Standard	Standard	Standard
Weight loss surgery - Gastric banding				
Lap band removed, no rateable build, weight maintained for one year	Standard	Standard	Standard	Standard
Lap Band removed, rateable build, or weight loss not maintained for one year	Decline	Decline	Decline	Decline
Lap Band present	Decline	Decline	Decline	Decline
Gastric Bypass / Gastric Stapling	Decline	Decline	Decline	Decline

Actions for Common Medical Conditions — Non-Rider States (LA & MI)

Below are underwriting actions for conditions for which Humana does not place exclusion riders.

These guidelines may vary due to state-specific laws and regulations but can be followed as a general outline. This is not all inclusive. Final decision is based on underwriting review. Underwriting assessments in the below grid are based on customary and usual treatment seen for the conditions noted. Below are examples only; Humana will be solely responsible for the final underwriting decision, which is based on the completed application and the applicant's health history. Guidelines are subject to change without prior notice.

Condition *We reserve the right to rate for the condition and/or medication use when appropriate. A modified rating is determined based on the severity of the condition and treatment and/or prescription medication cost, dosage, and premium amount.*	$1500 or lower deductible plus Rx	$2500 - $5000 deductible plus Rx	$2000 - $5200 deductible no Rx	$6000 or higher deductible plus Rx
Acid Reflux/ GERD/ Heartburn				
Present, no hiatal hernia, non prescription medication (OTC only), no recommended consultations or testing	Standard	Standard	Standard	Standard
Present, prescription medication, no hiatal hernia present	Standard or Rating	Standard or Rating	Standard	Standard or Rating
Prescription Medication use currently, hiatal hernia present	Decline	Decline	Decline	Standard or Rating
Acne/Rosacea				
Present, no treatment or OTC medication	Standard	Standard	Standard	Standard
Prescription meds, or < 6 months since med use, no Accutane or equivalent	Standard or Rating	Standard or Rating	Standard	Standard or Rating
Prescription meds, completed ≥ 6 months ago, complete recovery, no Accutane or equivalent	Standard	Standard	Standard	Standard
Accutane treatment of equivalent, or ≤ 1 year since treatment completed	Decline	Decline	Decline	Decline
Accutane treatment of equivalent, or > 1 year ago since treatment, complete recovery	Standard	Standard	Standard	Standard
Allergies				
Recommended, pending or scheduled testing	Rate 50%	Rate 50%	Rate 50%	Standard
Seasonal prescription meds (3 refills or less per year, or OTC, no immunotherapy treatment.	Standard	Standard	Standard	Standard
Prescription meds, more than 3 refills per year, no immunotherapy treatment	Standard or Rating	Standard or Rating	Standard	Standard or Rating
With or without prescribed medications, current or recent immunotherapy	Individual Consideration with Max Rating	Individual Consideration with Max Rating	Individual Consideration with Max Rating	Individual Consideration with Max Rating
Amputation/Prosthesis				
Finger or toes - with or without prosthesis	Standard	Standard	Standard	Standard
Eye	Standard	Standard	Standard	Standard
All other amputations, with or without prosthesis	Decline	Decline	Decline	Decline
Caused by diabetes, severe artery disease or other disease	Decline	Decline	Decline	Decline
Anemia - other than anemia listed in the ineligible health conditions list				
Present	Standard	Standard	Standard	Standard
Aneurysm				
Present	Decline	Decline	Decline	Decline
Surgically repaired > 5 years, no residuals	Individual consideration	Individual consideration	Individual consideration	Individual consideration
Anxiety				

(Continued)

Condition *We reserve the right to rate for the condition and/or medication use when appropriate. A modified rating is determined based on the severity of the condition and treatment and/or prescription medication cost, dosage, and premium amount.*	$1500 or lower deductible plus Rx	$2500 - $5000 deductible plus Rx	$2000 - $5200 deductible no Rx	$6000 or higher deductible plus Rx
Well controlled with prescription medication, no counseling, no more than 2 ER visits in the last 12 months	Standard or Rate up	Standard or Rate up	Standard	Standard or Rate up
Counseling only, no medication	Standard or Rate up	Standard or Rate up	Standard	Standard or Rate up
Asthma				
Exercise induced, no regular medication required	Standard	Standard	Standard	Standard
Medication use only	Standard or Rate up	Standard or Rate up	Standard	Standard or Rate up
Medication use, steroid treatment (not including Albuterol inhaler) less than 3 times and/or no more than 1-2 emergency room visits in the past 12 months	Standard or Rate up	Standard or Rate up	Standard	Standard or Rate up
Oral steriods required ≥ 3 times or more than 2 ER visits in the past 12 months	Decline	Decline	Decline	Decline
Attention Deficit Disorder/ADD/ADHD				
No medication or counseling, more than 2 years	Standard	Standard or Rate up	Standard	Standard
One medication	Standard or Rate up	Standard or Rate up	Standard	Standard or Rate up
More than one medication	Standard or Rate up	Standard or Rate up	Standard	Standard or Rate up
Atrial Fibrillation				
Single event, more than 2 years ago	Standard	Standard	Standard	Standard
Chronic or ongoing treatment	Decline	Decline	Decline	Decline
Single event less than 2 years ago or multiple events or pacemaker/defibrillator	Decline	Decline	Decline	Decline
Back Sprain/Strain/Whiplash				
≥ 1 year ago - complete recovery	Standard	Standard	Standard	Standard
Less than 1 year ago or not recovered	Rate 50%	Rate 50%	Rate 50%	Standard
Baker's Cyst				
Present and symptomatic	Decline	Decline	Decline	Standard
Present and asymptomatic	Decline	Standard	Standard	Standard
History of and no recurrence	Standard	Standard	Standard	Standard
Basal Cell Carcinoma				
Present	Decline	Decline	Decline	Decline
Single occurrence, removed within 2 years	Rate 25%	Rate 25%	Rate 25%	Standard
Single occurrence, complete recovery	Standard	Standard	Standard	Standard
Multiple occurences, or recurrent, removed (regardless of timeframe)	Rate 25% permanent	Rate 25% permanent	Rate 25% permanent	Standard
Benign Prostatic Hypertrophy/BPH				
Incidental finding, no symptoms, no treatment or medication use	Standard	Standard	Standard	Standard

Condition *We reserve the right to rate for the condition and/or medication use when appropriate. A modified rating is determined based on the severity of the condition and treatment and/or prescription medication cost, dosage, and premium amount.*	$1500 or lower deductible plus Rx	$2500 - $5000 deductible plus Rx	$2000 - $5200 deductible no Rx	$6000 or higher deductible plus Rx
Well controlled on one medication	Standard or Rate up	Standard or Rate up	Standard or Rate up	Standard or Rate up
More than one medication	Decline	Decline	Decline	Decline
Prostatectomy, TURP, TUNA, TUIP, TUMT, or Lazer surgery completed, no follow up needed, complete recovery, no residual complications or medication use	Standard	Standard	Standard	Standard
Bladder Infections (Cystitis)				
Less than 4 per year	Standard	Standard	Standard	Standard
4 - 6 per year	Decline	Standard	Standard	Standard
More than 6 per year	Decline	Decline	Decline	Decline
Breast Cyst, Nodule or Mass				
Present & benign	Rate 25%	Rate 25%	Rate 25%	Standard
Removed & benign	Standard	Standard	Standard	Standard
Present, pathology unknown	Decline	Decline	Decline	Decline
Breast Implants				
Present	Standard	Standard	Standard	Standard
Breast Reduction/Macromastia				
Condition present, no surgery completed	Decline	Decline	Decline	Decline
Surgery completed < 1 year ago, with complete recovery	Standard	Standard	Standard	Standard
Surgery completed < 1 year ago, with residuals	Rate 25%	Rate 25%	Rate 25%	Standard
Surgery completed > 1 year ago, no residuals	Standard	Standard	Standard	Standard
Bronchitis				
1 - 3 episodes in the past year, non tobacco user, complete recovery	Standard	Standard	Standard	Standard
1 - 2 episodes in the past year, Tobacco user, complete recovery	Standard	Standard	Standard	Standard
3 episodes a year, Tobacco user, complete recovery	Individual consideration	Individual consideration	Individual consideration	Individual consideration
> 3 episodes a year or Chronic Bronchitis	Decline	Decline	Decline	Decline
Bundle Branch Block (right)				
Complete right, no tobacco use for last 12 months, symptoms and treatment free for last 12 months, build not ratable	Standard	Standard	Standard	Standard
Bursitis/Tendonitis				
Single occurrence with complete recovery	Standard	Standard	Standard	Standard
Single occurrence, not recovered	Rate 25%	Standard	Standard	Standard
Multiple occurrences	Rate 25%	Rate 25%	Rate 25%	Standard
Carpal Tunnel				
Present or residuals	Decline	Decline	Decline	Standard
Surgical repair, full recovery	Standard	Standard	Standard	Standard
Cataracts				
Present	Decline	Decline	Decline	Standard

(Continued)

Condition *We reserve the right to rate for the condition and/or medication use when appropriate. A modified rating is determined based on the severity of the condition and treatment and/or prescription medication cost, dosage, and premium amount.*	$1500 or lower deductible plus Rx	$2500 - $5000 deductible plus Rx	$2000 - $5200 deductible no Rx	$6000 or higher deductible plus Rx
Surgically corrected, fully recovered, no residuals	Standard	Standard	Standard	Standard
Chlamydia				
Present or under treatment, no other STD history	Standard	Standard	Standard	Standard
Complete recovery	Standard	Standard	Standard	Standard
Colon Polyps				
Present	Decline	Decline	Decline	Decline
More than 1 benign polyp removed within the past 5 years during colonoscopy, follow up scheduled every 10 years	Max Rating or Individual Consideration	Max Rating or Individual Consideration	Max Rating or Individual Consideration	Max Rating or Individual Consideration
Single benign polyp removed during colonoscopy within the last 5 years, no colon resection, follow up scheduled every 5 years	Standard	Standard	Standard	Standard
Single benign polyp removed during colonoscopy, within the past 5 years no colon resection, follow up scheduled every 3 - 5 years	Max Rating or Individual Consideration	Max Rating or Individual Consideration	Max Rating or Individual Consideration	Max Rating or Individual Consideration
More than 1 polyp removed within the past 5 years. Surgically removed (not during colonoscopy) or part of colon surgically removed or follow up scheduled every 1 - 2 years	Decline	Decline	Decline	Decline
1 - 2 polyps removed within the past 5 years during colonoscopy, only 1 colonoscopy completed within the past 5 years. Follow up scheduled every 3 - 5 years	Max Rating or Individual Consideration	Max Rating or Individual Consideration	Max Rating or Individual Consideration	Max Rating or Individual Consideration
More than 2 polyps removed within the past 5 years, follow up scheduled every 3 - 5 years	Decline	Decline	Decline	Decline
Condyloma				
Present or history of - No HPV	Rate 100% LA: 84%	Standard	Standard	Standard
Present of history of - with HPV	Rate 100% LA: Rate 84% HPV underwritten separately	Rate 100% LA: Rate 84% HPV underwritten separately	Rate 100% LA: Rate 84% HPV underwritten separately	Rate 100% LA: Rate 84% HPV underwritten separately
Deep Vein Thrombosis (DVT)				
On anticoagulants or 1 episode < 3 months	Decline	Decline	Decline	Decline
1 episode 3 months - 2 years	Rate 25%	Rate 25%	Rate 25%	Standard
Recurrent	Decline	Decline	Decline	Decline
Depression				

Condition *We reserve the right to rate for the condition and/or medication use when appropriate. A modified rating is determined based on the severity of the condition and treatment and/or prescription medication cost, dosage, and premium amount.*	$1500 or lower deductible plus Rx	$2500 - $5000 deductible plus Rx	$2000 - $5200 deductible no Rx	$6000 or higher deductible plus Rx
Well controlled with prescription medication, no counseling	Standard or Rate up	Standard or Rate up	Standard	Standard or Rate up
Counseling only, no medication	Rate 10-20%	Rate 10-20%	Rate 10-20%	Rate 10-20%
Deviated Septum (nasal)				
Present, asymptomatic or surgically repaired	Standard	Standard	Standard	Standard
Symptomatic	Rate 100% LA: Rate 84%	Rate 100% LA: Rate 84%	Rate 100% LA: Rate 84%	Rate 100% LA: Rate 84%
Disc Disorder (herniated, bulging, ruptured)				
Present, surgically repaired less than 1 year ago or with residuals	Decline	Decline	Decline	Decline
Asymptomatic for more than 1 year without surgery or surgically repaired more than 1 year ago with full recovery	Standard	Standard	Standard	Standard
Diverticulitis				
Present, No Surgery	Decline	Decline	Decline	Decline
Surgery within 0-2 years	Decline	Decline	Decline	Decline
Surgically corrected > 2 years ago	Standard	Standard	Standard	Standard
Diverticulosis				
Present or with history of diverticulitis, No Surgery	Decline	Decline	Decline	Decline
Surgery within 0-2 years	Decline	Decline	Decline	Decline
Surgically corrected > 2 years ago	Standard	Standard	Standard	Standard
DUI - Paramed Exam is required				
Single occurrence, within 5 years	Rate 30% - Decline	Rate 30% - Decline	Rate 30% - Decline	Rate 30% - Decline
Single occurrence, more than 5 years	Standard	Standard	Standard	Standard
Multiple occurrences, within 5 years	Decline	Decline	Decline	Decline
Multiple occurrences, more than 5 years	Individual consideration	Individual consideration	Individual consideration	Individual consideration
Ear Infection (Otitis Media)				
< 3 in the past 12 months	Standard	Standard	Standard	Standard
3 or more in the past 12 months	Decline	Decline	Decline	Standard
Tubes Present	Rate 25%	Standard	Standard	Standard
Tubes no longer present, no recurrence	Standard	Standard	Standard	Standard
Eczema				
Present or less than 2 years since symptomatic	Standard or Rate up	Standard or Rate up	Standard	Standard or Rate up
> 2 years since treatment or symptoms	Standard	Standard	Standard	Standard
Endometriosis				
Present or within 5 years of treatment	Decline	Decline	Decline	Decline
> 5 years since symptoms or treatment	Standard	Standard	Standard	Standard
Surgery < 3 years ago	Decline	Decline	Decline	Standard
Surgery > 3 years ago	Standard	Standard	Standard	Standard
Enlarged Prostate - See Benign Prostatic Hypertrophy				

(Continued)

Condition *We reserve the right to rate for the condition and/or medication use when appropriate. A modified rating is determined based on the severity of the condition and treatment and/or prescription medication cost, dosage, and premium amount.*	$1500 or lower deductible plus Rx	$2500 - $5000 deductible plus Rx	$2000 - $5200 deductible no Rx	$6000 or higher deductible plus Rx
Epilepsy, Grand Mal (Generalized)				
Seizure within past 2 years	Decline	Decline	Decline	Decline
Last seizure > 2 years ago	Standard or Rate up	Standard or Rate up	Standard	Standard or Rate up
Epilepsy, Petit Mal (Generalized)				
Seizure within past 2 years	Decline	Decline	Decline	Decline
Last seizure > 2 years ago	Standard or Rate up	Standard or Rate up	Standard	Standard or Rate up
Epilepsy, Temporal Lobe (Partial)				
Seizure < 1 year ago	Decline	Decline	Decline	Decline
Seizure > 1 year ago	Standard or Rate up	Standard or Rate up	Standard	Standard or Rate up
Fibromyalgia				
Present or history of	Decline	Decline	Decline	Decline
Fractures				
Present - No fixation device	Rate 75%	Standard	Standard	Standard
Present - with permanent fixation device	Standard	Standard	Standard	Standard
Present - with temporary fixation device	Decline	Decline	Decline	Decline
Recovered & released from care with no fixation device or permanent fixation device	Standard	Standard	Standard	Standard
Recovered, released from care with temporary fixation device	Decline	Decline	Decline	Decline
Pathological	Decline	Decline	Decline	Decline
Ganglion Cyst				
Present & symptomatic	Rate 25%	Standard	Standard	Standard
Surgically removed, asymptomatic or history of and resolved	Standard	Standard	Standard	Standard
Gastric banding - weight loss surgery				
Lap band removed, no rateable build, weight maintained for one year	Standard	Standard	Standard	Standard
Lap Band removed, rateable build, or weight loss not maintained for one year	Decline	Decline	Decline	Decline
Lap Band present	Decline	Decline	Decline	Decline
Gastric Bypass / Gastric Stapling	Decline	Decline	Decline	Decline
GERD (reflux) - see Acid Reflux/GERD				
Gestational Diabetes				
< 5 yrs ago, diet controlled during pregnancy, no recurrence	Rate 25%	Rate 25%	Rate 25%	Rate 25%
> 5 yrs ago, diet controlled during pregnancy, no recurrence	Standard	Standard	Standard	Standard
< 5 yrs ago, controlled with insulin during pregnancy, no recurrence<	Rate 50%	Rate 50%	Rate 50%	Rate 50%

Condition *We reserve the right to rate for the condition and/or medication use when appropriate. A modified rating is determined based on the severity of the condition and treatment and/or prescription medication cost, dosage, and premium amount.*	$1500 or lower deductible plus Rx	$2500 - $5000 deductible plus Rx	$2000 - $5200 deductible no Rx	$6000 or higher deductible plus Rx
> 5 yrs ago, controlled with insulin during pregnancy, no recurrence	Rate 25%	Rate 25%	Rate 25%	Rate 25%
History of, no glucose test following pregnancy or glucose levels did not return to normal	Decline	Decline	Decline	Decline
Glaucoma				
Symptomatic, but not diagnosed	Rate 25% for condition and additional rating for meds	Rate 25% for condition and additional rating for meds	Rate 25% for condition and additional rating for meds	Rate 25% for condition and additional rating for meds
Present, well controlled	Rating	Rating	Standard	Rating
Present, not controlled: with or without medications	Decline	50-75% rating for condition, and additional rating for medications	Rate 50%, no action for meds	Rate 50% and additional rating for meds
Surgically corrected both eyes, with or without medications	If no medications: Standard: Medication use: Rating	If no medications: Standard: Medication use: Rating	Standard	If no medications: Standard: Medication use: Rating
Surgically corrected in one eye: with or without medication use	Decline	50-75% rating for condition, and additional rating for medications	Rate 50% for condition, no action for meds	Rate 50% and additional rating for meds
Surgically corrected	Std	Std	Std	Std
Gout				
Present or within 2 years of symptoms or treatment	Rate 75%	Rate 75%	Rate 75%	Standard
Recovered and time from last symptoms or treatment > 2 years	Standard	Standard	Standard	Standard
Grave's Disease - See Hyperthyroidism				
Guillain-Barre Syndrome				
Present or < 3 years since recovered OT residual disability/permanent impairment	Decline	Decline	Decline	Decline
> 3 years since recovered, no disability, minimal weakness, no relapse	Rate 25%	Standard	Standard	Standard
Gynecomastia				
Present	Decline	Decline	Decline	Decline
History of, complete recovery	Standard	Standard	Standard	Standard
Hashimoto's Thyroiditis - See Hypothyroidism				
Heartburn - SEE ACID REFLUX				
Heart Murmur Diastolic				
Functional/Innocent, Grade I or II - Systolic	Standard	Standard	Standard	Standard

(Continued)

Condition *We reserve the right to rate for the condition and/or medication use when appropriate. A modified rating is determined based on the severity of the condition and treatment and/or prescription medication cost, dosage, and premium amount.*	$1500 or lower deductible plus Rx	$2500 - $5000 deductible plus Rx	$2000 - $5200 deductible no Rx	$6000 or higher deductible plus Rx
Organic, Grade III or greater, continuous - Diastolic	Decline	Decline	Decline	Decline
Hemorrhoids				
Present, asymptomatic	Standard	Standard	Standard	Standard
Present, symptomatic	Rate 50%	Standard or Rate up	Standard	Standard or Rate up
> 1 year since symptoms or surgery	Standard	Standard	Standard	Standard
Hepatitis A				
> 6 months since treatment with normal liver tests	Standard	Standard	Standard	Standard
Hepatitis B				
Carrier	Decline	Decline	Decline	Decline
Present or < 6 months since treatment	Decline	Decline	Decline	Decline
Others	Individual consideration	Individual consideration	Individual consideration	Individual consideration
Hernia				
Present, all types other than Hiatal Hernia	Decline	Decline	Decline	Decline
Surgically repaired, with complete recovery and no residuals	Standard	Standard	Standard	Standard
Hiatal Hernia - see Acid Reflux/GERD				
Herpes				
OTC medication	Standard	Standard	Standard	Standard
Prescription medication	Standard or Rate up	Standard or Rate up	Standard	Standard or Rate up
Herpes Zoster (shingles)				
Present	Standard or Rate up	Standard or Rate up	Standard	Standard
Complete recovery, no medication	Standard	Standard	Standard	Standard
High Blood Pressure/Hypertension				
Underwritten based on age of onset, stability and comorbidity				
Stable, average readings 150/90 or less, no other cardiac risk factors, controlled with medication	Standard or Rate up	Standard or Rate up	Standard	Standard or Rate up
High Blood Pressure + 50% Ratable Build				
	Decline	Decline	Decline	Decline
High Blood Pressure + Ratable Build + Tobacco User				
	Decline	Decline	Decline	Decline
High Blood Pressure + High Cholesterol controlled with medication				
	Standard or Rate up	Standard or Rate up	Standard	Standard or Rate up
High Blood Pressure + High Cholesterol + Ratable Build				
	Decline	Decline	Decline	Decline
High Blood Pressure + High Cholesterol + Tobacco User				

Condition *We reserve the right to rate for the condition and/or medication use when appropriate. A modified rating is determined based on the severity of the condition and treatment and/or prescription medication cost, dosage, and premium amount.*	\$1500 or lower deductible plus Rx	\$2500 - \$5000 deductible plus Rx	\$2000 - \$5200 deductible no Rx	\$6000 or higher deductible plus Rx
	Decline	Decline	Decline	Decline
High Blood Pressure + Ratable Build + Tobacco User				
	Decline	Decline	Decline	Decline
High Blood Pressure + Sleep Apnea				
	Decline	Decline	Decline	Decline
High Cholesterol				
Lipid panel results within normal limits, compliant with follow up	Standard or Rate up	Standard or Rate up	Standard	Standard or Rate up
High Cholesterol + Rateable Build + Tobacco User				
	Decline	Decline	Decline	Decline
High Cholesterol + Rateable Build + Hypertension				
	Decline	Decline	Decline	Decline
Human Papilloma Virus (HPV)				
Low risk - no condyloma	Standard	Standard	Standard	Standard
High risk	Decline	Decline	Decline	Decline
Hyperthyroidism				
Present - untreated	Decline	Decline	Decline	Decline
Present - treated with medication	Rate 25% or higher	Standard	Standard	Standard
Hypoglycemia				
Present, follow up recommended	Decline	Decline	Decline	Decline
Present, or history of, diet controlled, no follow-up recommended	Standard	Standard	Standard	Standard
Present, treated with medication	Decline	Decline	Decline	Decline
Hypothyroid				
Present or history of	Standard	Standard	Standard	Standard
Infertility Treatment - male and female				
Current infertility drug treatment	Decline - entire family	Decline - entire family	Decline - entire family	Decline - entire family
Last treatment with infertility drugs □ a year without a live birth	Decline - entire family	Decline - entire family	Decline - entire family	Decline - entire family
Last treatment with infertility drugs with a live birth, family planning complete	Standard	Standard	Standard	Standard
Last treatment with infertility drugs with a live birth, family planning is not complete	Decline - entire family	Decline - entire family	Decline - entire family	Decline - entire family
Last treatment with IVF, ZIFT, GIFT or others, family planning complete	Standard	Standard	Standard	Standard
Last treatment with IVF, ZIFT, GIFT or others, family planning is not complete	Decline - entire family	Decline - entire family	Decline - entire family	Decline - entire family
Insomnia				
Treated with medication	Standard or Rate up	Standard or Rate up	Standard	Standard or Rate up
Irritable Bowel Syndrome				
Treated with OTC medication	Standard	Standard	Standard	Standard

(Continued)

Condition *We reserve the right to rate for the condition and/or medication use when appropriate. A modified rating is determined based on the severity of the condition and treatment and/or prescription medication cost, dosage, and premium amount.*	$1500 or lower deductible plus Rx	$2500 - $5000 deductible plus Rx	$2000 - $5200 deductible no Rx	$6000 or higher deductible plus Rx
Treated with medication	Standard or Rate up	Standard or Rate up	Standard	Standard or Rate up
Treated with non-GI prescription medication	Standard or Rate up	Standard or Rate up	Standard	Standard or Rate up
ITP (blood disorder)				
Child form, complete recovery, platelet count returned to normal	Standard	Standard	Standard	Standard
Child form, present	Decline	Decline	Decline	Decline
Adult form or chronic, less than 40 years of age, more than 3 years since treatment and a complete recovery	Rate 25%	Rate 25%	Rate 25%	Rate 25%
Adult form or chronic, more than 6 years since treatment and a complete recovery, no current treatment, normal platelet count	Standard	Standard	Standard	Standard
Joint replacement				
Hip replaced	Decline	Decline	Decline	Decline
Knee Replaced	Decline	Decline	Decline	Decline
Shoulder replaced	Rate 100% LA: Rate 84%	Rate 100% LA: Rate 84%	Rate 100% LA: Rate 84%	Standard
Kidney Infection/Pyelonephritis/Pyelitis				
1 episode, within 0 - 3 years	Rate 25%	Standard	Standard	Standard
1 episode > 3 years ago	Standard	Standard	Standard	Standard
2 episodes, < 2 years ago	Decline	Decline	Decline	Standard
2 episodes, 2-5 years ago	Rate 25%	Standard	Standard	Standard
2 episodes, > 5 years ago	Standard	Standard	Standard	Standard
3 or more episodes, regardless of time frame	Decline	Decline	Decline	Decline
Kidney Stones				
Present	Decline	Decline	Decline	Decline
Passed - on its own or surgically > 2 years	Standard	Standard	Standard	Standard
> 5 episodes	Decline	Decline	Decline	Decline
Lichen Planus				
Mild infrequent attacks	Standard	Standard	Standard	Standard
Frequent or severe attacks	Rate 25% or higher	Rate	Rate 25%	Rate
Lipoma				
Present, asymptomatic, no surgery anticipated	Standard	Standard	Standard	Standard
Present and symptomatic	Rate 25%	Standard	Standard	Standard
Lyme Disease				
Present or treatment completed less than 6 months ago	Decline	Decline	Decline	Decline
> 6 months since recovery	Standard	Standard	Standard	Standard

Condition *We reserve the right to rate for the condition and/or medication use when appropriate. A modified rating is determined based on the severity of the condition and treatment and/or prescription medication cost, dosage, and premium amount.*	$1500 or lower deductible plus Rx	$2500 - $5000 deductible plus Rx	$2000 - $5200 deductible no Rx	$6000 or higher deductible plus Rx
Macular Degeneration				
Dry or wet	Decline	Decline	Decline	Decline
Meniere's Disease				
Present, confirmed diagnosis, stable, current or history of med use, no ongoing follow-up or treatment	Standard or Rating	Standard or Rating	Standard	Standard
Present, confirmed diagnosis, stable, current or history of med use, ongoing follow-up or treatment	Decline	Decline	Decline	Standard
Migraines				
Occasional (□ 3 episodes yearly) treated with OTC medication	Standard	Standard	Standard	Standard
≥ 4 episodes in the last 12 months, or severe. Workup completed, symptoms controlled with current treatment	Rating	Rating	Standard	Rating
≥ 4 episodes in the last 12 months, No workup completed	Decline	Decline	Decline	Decline
Prescription medication	Standard or Rate up	Standard or Rate up	Standard	Standard or Rate up
Miscarriage				
1-2, no underlying cause	Standard	Standard	Standard	Standard
> 2, no full term deliveries	Rate 50%	Rate 50%	Rate 50%	Rate 50%
History of with full term delivery	Standard	Standard	Standard	Standard
Mitral Valve Prolapse				
No symptoms or treatment	Standard	Standard	Standard	Standard
Mild symptoms controlled with one med, no other heart disorder	Standard or Rate up	Standard or Rate up	Standard	Standard or Rate up
Molluscum Contagiosum				
Present of complete recovery < 1 year	Rate 50%	Standard	Standard	Standard
Complete recovery > 1 year	Standard	Standard	Standard	Standard
Nephritis/Glomerulonephritis				
One episodes > 3 years ago	Standard	Standard	Standard	Standard
One episode < 3 years ago	Decline	Decline	Decline	Decline
Osteoarthritis				
Present, only OTC meds, no PT or OT, no shoulder, hip, pelvis, back or spine, knee or ankle involvement	Standard	Standard	Standard	Standard
Present, all treatment except OTC meds, no shoulder, hip, pelvis, back or spine, knee or ankle involvement	Rating	Rating	Rating	Rating
Present, regardless of treatment, with shoulder, hip, pelvis, back or spine, knee or ankle involvement and no joint replacement	Decline	Decline	Decline	Decline

(Continued)

Condition *We reserve the right to rate for the condition and/or medication use when appropriate. A modified rating is determined based on the severity of the condition and treatment and/or prescription medication cost, dosage, and premium amount.*	$1500 or lower deductible plus Rx	$2500 - $5000 deductible plus Rx	$2000 - $5200 deductible no Rx	$6000 or higher deductible plus Rx
Joint replacement (see joint replacements)				
Osteoporosis/Osteopenia				
Current use of Prophylactic medication, due to age/ menopause, no diagnosis of osteoporosis or osteopenia, no fractures or Dexa scans done	Standard or Rate up	Standard or Rate up	Standard	Standard or Rate up
Diagnosis of Osteoporosis or Osteopenia with or without medication use, Dexa scans stable or improved	Minimum rate of 25% + pharmacy rating if on meds, or 50% Rate if not on meds	Minimum rate of 25% + pharmacy rating if on meds, or 50% Rate if not on meds	Rate 25%	Standard or Rate up
Present, severe, history of pathologic fractures, crippling, Dexa scans worsening	Decline	Decline	Decline	Decline
Ovarian Cyst				
Present, asymptomatic	Standard	Standard	Standard	Standard
Symptomatic	Decline	Rate 50%	Rate 50%	Standard
Removed	Standard	Standard	Standard	Standard
Pancreatitis				
History of attack, no underlying cause, resolved	Individual consideration, medical records required	Individual consideration, medical records required	Individual consideration, medical records required	Individual consideration, medical records required
Chronic or recurrent	Decline	Decline	Decline	Decline
Pap Smear - Abnormal				
ASCUS, no high risk HPV, Class II or Class III followed by one normal pap, Class IV, treated, followed by three normal pap smears	Standard	Standard	Standard	Standard
Phlebitis				
Current use of blood thinners	Decline	Decline	Decline	Decline
One episode, <3 months, complete recovery, no varicose veins or edema	Rate 25%	Rate 25%	Rate 25%	Standard
One episode, 3 months - 2 years, complete recovery, no varicose veins or edema	Standard	Standard	Standard	Standard
Recurrent episodes within 0-2 years	Rate 25%	Rate 25%	Rate 25%	Standard
History of - ≥ 2 years ago	Standard	Standard	Standard	Standard
Varicose Veins - (see Varicose Veins)				
Pneumonia				
Present	Decline	Decline	Decline	Decline
Complete recovery	Standard	Standard	Standard	Standard
Prostatitis				
One episode, full recovery	Standard	Standard	Standard	Standard

Condition *We reserve the right to rate for the condition and/or medication use when appropriate. A modified rating is determined based on the severity of the condition and treatment and/or prescription medication cost, dosage, and premium amount.*	$1500 or lower deductible plus Rx	$2500 - $5000 deductible plus Rx	$2000 - $5200 deductible no Rx	$6000 or higher deductible plus Rx
> One episode or chronic	Rate 25%	Rate 25%	Rate 25%	Rate 25%
Prosthesis/Prosthetics Device See Amputation				
Prostate - Enlarged See Benign Prostatic Hypertrophy/BPH				
Psoriasis				
Mild symptoms, OTC medications or no treatment	Standard	Standard	Standard	Standard
Mild to moderate symptoms, conservative treatments, including prescription topical agents	Standard or Rate up	Standard or Rate up	Standard	Standard or Rate up
Severe symptoms requiring RX medication such as Enbrel, Remicade, Sulfasalazine, gold therapy or Methotrexate	Decline	Decline	Decline	Decline
Use of tanning bed only	Standard	Standard	Standard	Standard
Use of UVA/PUVA light at a medical facility	Standard	Standard	Standard	Standard
Psoriatic Arthritis				
All cases	Decline	Decline	Decline	Decline
Pyloric Stenosis				
Present	Decline	Decline	Decline	Decline
Surgically corrected with complete recovery	Standard	Standard	Standard	Standard
Respiratory Syncytial Virus (RSV)/Bronchiolitis				
Present or history of, < 2 years of age, Synagis/ Palivizumab use	Decline	Decline	Decline	Decline
> 2 years of age, Last occurrence < 1 year ago and Synagis/Palivizumab use	Decline	Decline	Decline	Decline
> 2 years of age, Last occurrence > 1 year ago, no medications for > 1 year, Complete recovery, no other respiratory conditions	Standard	Standard	Standard	Standard
Restless Leg Syndrome				
No medication, no treatment for 2+ years	Standard	Standard	Standard	Standard
Controlled with medication	Standard or Rate up	Standard or Rate up	Standard	Standard or Rate up
Diagnosis not confirmed, secondary condition not ruled out	Decline	Decline	Decline	Decline
Retinal Detachment				
Present	Decline	Decline	Decline	Decline
Surgically correct < 2 years	Rate 50%	Standard	Standard	Standard
Rheumatoid Arthritis				
	Decline	Decline	Decline	Decline
Scoliosis				
Present, no surgery, under age of 20	Decline	Decline	Decline	Decline
Present, over age of 20	Standard	Standard	Standard	Standard

(Continued)

Condition *We reserve the right to rate for the condition and/or medication use when appropriate. A modified rating is determined based on the severity of the condition and treatment and/or prescription medication cost, dosage, and premium amount.*	$1500 or lower deductible plus Rx	$2500 - $5000 deductible plus Rx	$2000 - $5200 deductible no Rx	$6000 or higher deductible plus Rx
Surgery completed, rod in place, full recovery	Standard	Standard	Standard	Standard
Condition *We reserve the right to rate for the condition and/or medication use when appropriate. A modified rating is determined based on the severity of the condition and treatment and/or prescription medication cost, dosage, and premium amount.*	$1500 or lower deductible plus Rx	$2500 - $5000 deductible plus Rx	$2000 - $5200 deductible no Rx	$6000 or higher deductible plus Rx
Any cardiac, pulmonary or spinal cord involvement	Decline	Decline	Decline	Decline
Sinusitis				
< 3 episodes in the past year or chronic	Standard	Standard	Standard	Standard
3 - 6 episodes in the past 12 months	Rate 25%	Standard	Standard	Standard
> 6 episodes on the past 12 months	Rate 25%	Rate 25%	Rate 25%	Standard
Sleep Apnea				
Controlled with CPAP	Rate 150% LA: Decline	Rate 150% LA: Decline	Rate 150% LA: Decline	Standard
Surgically Corrected	Standard	Standard	Standard	Standard
Sleep Apnea + Ratable Build	Decline	Decline	Decline	Decline
Sleep Apnea + Tobacco User	Decline	Decline	Decline	Decline
Sleep Apnea + Hypertension	Decline	Decline	Decline	Decline
Central or Mixed	Decline	Decline	Decline	Decline
Spina Bifida				
Occulta, incidental finding, asymptomatic	Standard	Standard	Standard	Standard
Occulta - symptomatic	Decline	Decline	Decline	Decline
Manifesta	Decline	Decline	Decline	Decline
Spinal Manipulations				
0 - 5 visits per year	Standard	Standard	Standard	Standard
6 - 10 visits per year	Standard	Standard	Standard	Standard
11 - 15 visits per year	Rate 50%	Standard	Standard	Standard
16 - 20 visits per year	Rate 75%	Rate 15%	Rate 15%	Standard
21 - 25 visits per year	Rate 75% Except: LA: Rate 84%	Rate 15% Except: LA: Rate 25%	Rate 15% Except: LA: Rate 25%	Standard
26 - 30 visits per year	Rate 75% Except: LA: Rate 84%	Rate 15% Except: LA: Rate 40%	Rate 15% Except: LA: Rate 40%	Standard
31 - 35 visits per year	Rate 75% Except: LA: Rate 84%	Rate 15% Except: LA: Rate 50%	Rate 15% Except: LA: Rate 50%	Standard
36+ visits per year	Rate 75% Except: LA: Decline	Rate 75% Except: LA: Decline	Rate 15% Except: LA: Rate 75%	Rate 15%

Condition *We reserve the right to rate for the condition and/or medication use when appropriate. A modified rating is determined based on the severity of the condition and treatment and/or prescription medication cost, dosage, and premium amount.*	$1500 or lower deductible plus Rx	$2500 - $5000 deductible plus Rx	$2000 - $5200 deductible no Rx	$6000 or higher deductible plus Rx
Stents				
Heart	Decline	Decline	Decline	Decline
Other locations	Individual consideration	Individual consideration	Individual consideration	Individual consideration
Tachycardia				
No attacks in past 12 months, maintained and well controlled on medications to control attacks and symptoms, no other cardiovascular disorders	Rate 25% or higher	Rate 25% or higher	Rate 25%	Std-Rate
≤ 3 attacks per year, < 1 year since last attack	Decline	Decline	Decline	Decline
≤ 3 attacks per year, 1-3 years since last attack, prompt response to treatment, no other cardivascular disorders	Rate 75%	Rate 75%	Rate 75%	Rate 75%
< 3 attacks per year, > 3 years since last attack, prompt response to treatment, no other cardiovascular disorders	Standard	Standard	Standard	Standard
Others	Decline	Decline	Decline	Decline
Surgical ablation □ 6 months ago	Decline	Decline	Decline	Decline
Surgical ablation > 6 months ago, no residuals	Standard	Standard	Standard	Standard
Tendonitis - SEE BURSITIS				
Tonsillitis				
Less than 3 per year	Standard	Standard	Standard	Standard
3 - 5 per year	Decline	Standard	Standard	Standard
> 5 per year	Decline	Decline	Decline	Standard
Tourettes Syndrome				
Simple tics, no behavioral disorders	Standard	Standard	Standard	Standard
Controlled with medication	Standard or Rate up	Standard or Rate up	Standard	Standard or Rate up
Disabling, behavioral issues, extensive psychotherapy	Decline	Decline	Decline	Decline
Tuberculosis				
TB infection without disease: + skin test, negative bacteriologic studies, negative chest x-ray, no clinical evidence of active TB disease, Prophylactic drug therapy completed > 6 months ago	Standard	Standard	Standard	Standard
TB infection without disease: + skin test, negative bacteriologic studies, negative chest x-ray, no clinical evidence of active TB disease, current use of < 6 months of prophylactic drugs	Decline	Standard	Standard	Standard
Ulcer (Peptic)				
One episodes, complete recovery	Standard	Standard	Standard	Standard

(Continued)

Condition *We reserve the right to rate for the condition and/or medication use when appropriate. A modified rating is determined based on the severity of the condition and treatment and/or prescription medication cost, dosage, and premium amount.*	$1500 or lower deductible plus Rx	$2500 - $5000 deductible plus Rx	$2000 - $5200 deductible no Rx	$6000 or higher deductible plus Rx
History of bleeding or perforation less than 2 years ago or multiple episodes of bleeding or perforation	Decline	Decline	Decline	Decline
One episode of bleeding or perforation > 2 years ago, no symptoms or vagotomy completed > 3 years ago	Standard	Standard	Standard	Standard
Uterine Fibroids				
Post-menopausal, no HRT, asymptomatic or myomectomy or hysterectomy completed	Standard	Standard	Standard	Standard
Others	Decline	Decline	Decline	Decline
Vaginitis				
One occurrence - complete recovery	Standard	Standard	Standard	Standard
> 1 occurrence, < 1 year since last occurrence	Rate 25%	Standard	Standard	Standard
Varicose Veins				
Present-asymptomatic, no recommendations for treatment	Standard	Standard	Standard	Standard
Present with ulcer	Decline	Decline	Decline	Decline
Treated with lazer, stripping or sclerotherapy, full recovery no symptoms or treatment <1yr ago	Rate 25%	Standard	Standard	Standard
Treated with lazer, stripping or sclerotherapy, full recovery no symptoms or treatment >1yr ago	Standard	Standard	Standard	Standard
Ventricular Septal Defect - APS REQUIRED				
Repaired > 1 year ago, complete recovery, normal cardiac exam	Standard	Standard	Standard	Standard
Present or repaired with symptoms or abnormal cardiac exam	Decline	Decline	Decline	Decline
Weight loss medication use				
Use of any weight loss medication (other than Xenical) in combination with hypertension or cardiac issues	Individual consideration medical records required	Individual consideration medical records required	Individual consideration medical records required	Individual consideration medical records required
Continuous use of any weight loss medications for more than one year	Decline	Decline	Decline	Decline
All other scenarios or Xenical use in combination with hypertension or cardiac disease	Standard	Standard	Standard	Standard
Weight loss surgery - Gastric banding				

Condition *We reserve the right to rate for the condition and/or medication use when appropriate. A modified rating is determined based on the severity of the condition and treatment and/or prescription medication cost, dosage, and premium amount.*	$1500 or lower deductible plus Rx	$2500 - $5000 deductible plus Rx	$2000 - $5200 deductible no Rx	$6000 or higher deductible plus Rx
Lap band removed, no rateable build, weight maintained for one year	Standard	Standard	Standard	Standard
Lap Band removed, rateable build, or weight loss not maintained for one year	Decline	Decline	Decline	Decline
Lap Band present	Decline	Decline	Decline	Decline

Actions for Cancer

The following grid includes possible underwriting actions for applicants with cancer history. This is not an all-inclusive list. Medical records are required for all cancer history, regardless of the original diagnosis date.

Eligibility is determined based on the underwriter assessment of complete medical records, confirmation of compliance with all physician recommended follow-up, a current physician assessment of the condition, supporting stability and no recurrence of the condition. Treatment for cancer may be defined as: office visits, preventive maintenance medication, screenings, monitoring, diagnostics, and lab work.

Condition *We reserve the right to rate for the condition and/or medication use when appropriate. A modified rating is determined based on the severity of the condition and treatment and/or prescription medication cost, dosage, and premium amount.*	$1500 or lower deductible plus Rx	$2500 - $5000 deductible plus Rx	$2000 - $5200 deductible no Rx	$6000 or higher deductible plus Rx
Basal Cell Carcinoma				
Present	Decline	Decline	Decline	Decline
Single occurrence, complete recovery	Standard	Standard	Standard	Standard
Multiple occurences, or recurrent, removed (regardless of timeframe)	Rate 25% - permanent	Rate 25% - permanent	Rate 25% - permanent	Standard
Breast				
Stage 0, > 4 yrs from treatment	All states: Rate 25%	All states: Rate 25%	All states: Rate 25%	All states: Rate 25%
Stage 0, ≥ 2 yrs from treatment	FL only: Rating if cancer free for ≥ 2 years	FL only: Rating if cancer free for ≥ 2 years	FL only: Rating if cancer free for ≥ 2 years	FL only: Rating if cancer free for ≥ 2 years
Stage 1, > 11 yrs from treatment	All states: Rate 25-50%	All states: Rate 25-50%	All states: Rate 25-50%	All states: Rate 25-50%
Stage 1, ≥ 2 yrs from treatment	FL only: Rating if cancer free for ≥ 2 years	FL only: Rating if cancer free for ≥ 2 years	FL only: Rating if cancer free for ≥ 2 years	FL only: Rating if cancer free for ≥ 2 years

(Continued)

Condition *We reserve the right to rate for the condition and/or medication use when appropriate. A modified rating is determined based on the severity of the condition and treatment and/or prescription medication cost, dosage, and premium amount.*	$1500 or lower deductible plus Rx	$2500 - $5000 deductible plus Rx	$2000 - $5200 deductible no Rx	$6000 or higher deductible plus Rx
Stage II, III, IV,	Decline FL only: Exception ≥ 2 years cancer free, 150% rating applies	Decline FL only: Exception ≥2 years cancer free, 150% rating applies	Decline FL only: Exception ≥ 2 years cancer free, 150% rating applies	Decline FL only: Exception ≥ 2 years cancer free, 150% rating applies
Bladder				
Stage 0, 10+ years from treatment	Rate 25 - 50%	Rate 25 - 50%	Rate 25 - 50%	Rate 25 - 50%
Stage I, > 10 years from treatment	Individual consideration	Individual consideration	Individual consideration	Individual consideration
Cervical				
Stage 0 (carcinoma in situ), > 3 years from treatment	Rate 25%	Rate 25%	Rate 25%	Rate 25%
Stage I, IA1, IA2, IB1, IB2 (lymph node removed), > 10 years from treatment	Rate 25 - 50%	Rate 25 - 50%	Rate 25 - 50%	Rate 25 - 50%
Stage IA, IIA, IIIA, IBA & IVB, > 10 years ago	Individual consideration	Individual consideration	Individual consideration	Individual consideration
Colon				
Stage 0 or Carcinoma in situ, 3+ years from treatment	Rate 25 - 50%	Rate 25 - 50%	Rate 25%	Rate 25%
Stage I or Duke's A, > 5 years from treatment	Rate 25 - 50%	Rate 25 - 50%	Rate 25 - 50%	Rate 25 - 50%
Stage II or Duke's B, > 12 years from treatment	Rate 25 - 50%	Rate 25 - 50%	Rate 25 - 50%	Rate 25 - 50%
Stage III or IV, Duke's C or D, > 10 years from treatment	Individual consideration	Individual consideration	Individual consideration	Individual consideration
Kidney				
Stage I & II, normal kidney function, > 10 years from treatment:	Rate 25 - 50%	Rate 25 - 50%	Rate 25 - 50%	Rate 25 - 50%
Stage 1 & II, abnormal kidney function, 10 years from treatment	Individual consideration	Individual consideration	Individual consideration	Individual consideration
Stage III & IV, > 10 years from treatment	Individual consideration	Individual consideration	Individual consideration	Individual consideration
Melanoma, localized				
Clark's Level I, II & III - .76 - 1.5 mm thick, > 5 years	Rate 25 - 50%	Rate 25 - 50%	Rate 25 - 50%	Rate 25 - 50%
Clark's Level I, II & III, > 1.5 mm thick, > 10 years	Individual consideration	Individual consideration	Individual consideration	Individual consideration
Clark's Level I, II & III, < .75 mm thick, > 3 years	Rate 25%	Rate 25%	Rate 25%	Rate 25%

(Continued)

Condition *We reserve the right to rate for the condition and/or medication use when appropriate. A modified rating is determined based on the severity of the condition and treatment and/or prescription medication cost, dosage, and premium amount.*	$1500 or lower deductible plus Rx	$2500 - $5000 deductible plus Rx	$2000 - $5200 deductible no Rx	$6000 or higher deductible plus Rx
Clark Level I, II & III, unknown thickness, > 10 years	Individual consideration	Individual consideration	Individual consideration	Individual consideration
Clark level IV or V, > 10 years	Individual consideration	Individual consideration	Individual consideration	Individual consideration
Melanoma In Situ, > 2 years	Rate 25%	Rate 25%	Rate 25%	Rate 25%
Multiple Malignant Melanoma, > 10 years	Individual consideration	Individual consideration	Individual consideration	Individual consideration
Osteoid Osteoma				
Removed with complete recovery	Standard	Standard	Standard	Standard
Prostate				
Stage I or Gleason score 2 - 4, > 2 years	Rate 25%	Rate 25%	Rate 25%	Rate 25%
Gleason Score 5, > 3 years	Rate 25%	Rate 25%	Rate 25%	Rate 25%
Stage II or Gleason Score 6, > 5 years	Rate 25 - 50%	Rate 25 - 50%	Rate 25 - 50%	Rate 25 - 50%
Gleason score 7, > 5 years	Rate 25 - 50%	Rate 25 - 50%	Rate 25 - 50%	Rate 25 - 50%
Stage III or Gleason Score 8 - 10, > 10 years	Rate 25 - 50%	Rate 25 - 50%	Rate 25 - 50%	Rate 25 - 50%
Stage IV or Recurrent, > 10 years	Individual consideration	Individual consideration	Individual consideration	Individual consideration
Skin, Sarcoma				
Adult				
Stage I, G1 or G2, T1, > 3 years	Rate 25%	Rate 25%	Rate 25%	Rate 25%
Stage I, G1 or G2, T2: > 10 years	Individual consideration	Individual consideration	Individual consideration	Individual consideration
Stage II, III or IV, > 10 years	Individual consideration	Individual consideration	Individual consideration	Individual consideration
Under age 20:				
Group I, > 3 years	Rate 25%	Rate 25%	Rate 25%	Rate 25%
Group II, > 5 years	Rate 25 - 50%	Rate 25 - 50%	Rate 25 - 50%	Rate 25 - 50%
Group II, IV or Recurrent, > 10 years	Individual consideration	Individual consideration	Individual consideration	Individual consideration
Skin, Squamous Cell				
Present	Decline	Decline	Decline	Decline
Single occurrence, complete recovery - margins free of tumor	Standard	Standard	Standard	Standard
Multiple occurrences or recurrent, last removal < 3 years ago	Rider - permanent	Rider - permanent	Rider - permanent	Rider - permanent
Multiple occurrences or recurrent, last removal ≥ 3 years ago	Rider - permanent	Rider - permanent	Rider - permanent	Standard
Deep Tumor: invaded muscle, cartilage or bone, no metastasis	Decline	Decline	Decline	Decline
Metastasis	Decline	Decline	Decline	Decline

(Continued)

Condition *We reserve the right to rate for the condition and/or medication use when appropriate. A modified rating is determined based on the severity of the condition and treatment and/or prescription medication cost, dosage, and premium amount.*	$1500 or lower deductible plus Rx	$2500 - $5000 deductible plus Rx	$2000 - $5200 deductible no Rx	$6000 or higher deductible plus Rx
Stomach				
	Individual consideration	Individual consideration	Individual consideration	Individual consideration
Testicular				
Nonseminoma & Seminoma combination, Stage I, 3 years ago	Rate 25%	Rate 25%	Rate 25%	Rate 25%
Nonseminoma & Seminoma Combination Stage II or Stage III > 10 years	Individual consideration	Individual consideration	Individual consideration	Individual consideration
Nonseminoma Stage I, > 3 years	Rate 25%	Rate 25%	Rate 25%	Rate 25%
Nonseminoma, Stage II or III, > 10 years	Individual consideration	Individual consideration	Individual consideration	Individual consideration
Seminoma State I, > 3 years	Rate 25%	Rate 25%	Rate 25%	Rate 25%
Seminoma Stage II or III, > 10 years	Individual consideration	Individual consideration	Individual consideration	Individual consideration
Throat				
	Individual consideration	Individual consideration	Individual consideration	Individual consideration
Tongue - oropharyngeal				
Stage O, > 5 years	Rate 25 - 50%	Rate 25 - 50%	Rate 25-50%	Rate 25 - 50%
Stage I, no alcohol or tobacco use within the past 2 years, > 5 years from treatment	Rate 25 - 50%	Rate 25 - 50%	Rate 25 - 50%	Rate 25 - 50%
Stage I, current alcohol or tobacco use, 10 years from treatment	Individual consideration	Individual consideration	Individual consideration	Individual consideration
Stage II, no alcohol or tobacco use within the past 2 years, > 10 years from treatment	Rate 25-50%	Rate 25-50%	Rate 25-50%	Rate 25-50%
Stage II, current alcohol or tobacco use, 10 years from treatment	Individual consideration	Individual consideration	Individual consideration	Individual consideration
Stage III, IV or Recurrent, > 10 years from treatment	Individual consideration	Individual consideration	Individual consideration	Individual consideration
Thyroid, Papillary				
5 years from treatment	Rate 25 - 50%	Rate 25-50%	Rate 25 - 50%	Rate 25 - 50%
Uterine				
Stage I, II, > 5 years from treatment	Rate 25 - 50%	Rate 25 - 50%	Rate 25 - 50%	Rate 25 - 50%
Stage III, > 10 years from treatment	Rate 25 - 50%	Rate 25 - 50%	Rate 25 - 50%	Rate 25 - 50%
Stage IV, > 10 years	Individual consideration	Individual consideration	Individual consideration	Individual consideration
Uterine sarcoma, > 10 years	Individual consideration	Individual consideration	Individual consideration	Individual consideration

Humana*One* Short Term Medical Plans

Humana*One*'s Short Term Medical Plans are not subject to complete underwriting like other Humana*One* plans. Instead, applicants will be asked four or five eligibility and health questions to determine their eligibility. The following questions must be answered fully and truthfully; including information related to spouse and/or dependents applying for coverage:

- □ No □ Yes Are you or is any immediate family member (whether or not named in this application) pregnant, an expectant parent, in the process of adopting a child, or undergoing infertility treatment?
- □ No □ Yes Have/Are you, your spouse, or any person applying for coverage resided in the U.S. for less than 6 months?
- □ No □ Yes Are you, your spouse, or any person applying for coverage over 300 pounds if male, or over 250 pounds if female?
- □ No □ Yes For any of the following conditions, has any person to be insured received, in the past 5 years, any abnormal test results; medical or surgical consultation, treatment, or advice; consulted a health care professional; or taken medication for: diabetes, emphysema, cancer or tumor, stroke, heart disorder including but not limited to heart attack or chest pain, AIDS or tested positive for HIV, kidney disorder (excluding kidney stones), alcoholism, chemical dependency, drug or alcohol abuse?

In Colorado, an additional question will be asked of the applicants:

- □ No □ Yes Have you or any other person to be insured been covered under two or more non-renewable short term plans during the past 12 months?

Eligibility

If "no" is answered to all of the following questions, your client will be eligible for coverage. If "yes" is answered to any of the following questions, your client will need to provide the name of the person the answer applies to: The person(s) named will not be covered under the policy. If your client is not eligible for coverage, they may choose to apply for a different Humana*One* plan that is fully underwritten.

If you have any questions about Humana*One*'s Short Term Medical plans, please contact your local sales representative.

We agreed to provide Senator Heitkamp details about whether there is appropriate civil penalties for fraud, waste, and abuse to provide a substantial deterrent (on page 41 (lines 20-24) of transcript).

The authority of federal agencies to assess and collect civil monetary penalties (CMP) can be a powerful method for enforcing regulatory policies and deterring violations. In 2017, federal agencies assessed millions of dollars in CMP for violations of statutory requirements, such as phone calls that violated federal telemarketing law and failure to report suspicious orders for controlled substances. GAO has not examined specifically whether these civil penalties are sufficient to deter fraud, waste, or abuse. However, according to the HHS Office of the Inspector General (OIG) website, "The OIG has the authority to seek CMP, assessments, and exclusion against an individual or entity based on a wide variety of prohibited conduct" OIG lists its CMP authorities on the CMP Authorities page and its exclusion authorities on the Exclusion Authorities page.

We agreed to provide Senator McCaskill details about priority open Medicaid recommendations (on page 65 (lines 21-23) of transcript).

Medicaid Managed Care: Improvements Needed to Better Oversee Payment Risks. GA0-18-528 (Washington, D.C.: July 26, 2018).

Recommendation: The Administrator of CMS should expedite the planned efforts to communicate guidance, such as its compendium on Medicaid managed care program integrity, to state stakeholders related to Medicaid managed care program integrity.

Recommendation: The Administrator of CMS should eliminate impediments to collaborative audits in managed care conducted by audit contractors and states, by ensuring that managed care audits are conducted regardless of which entity-the state or the managed care organization--recoups any identified overpayments.

Recommendation: The Administrator of CMS should require states to report and document the amount of MCO overpayments to providers and how they are accounted for in capitation rate- setting.

Action Needed: HHS agreed with our recommendations. We will continue to monitor the implementation of these recommendations.

Medicaid: CMS Should Take Steps to Mitigate Program Risks in Managed Care, GA0-18-291 (Washington, D.C.: May 7, 2018).

Recommendation: The Administrator of CMS should consider and take steps to mitigate the program risks that are not measured in the Payment Error Rate Measurement (PERM); such an effort could include actions such as revising the PERM methodology or focusing additional audit resources on managed care.

Action Needed: HHS agreed with our recommendation. We will continue to monitor the implementation of this recommendation.

Medicaid Assisted Living Services: Improved Federal Oversight of Beneficiary Health and Welfare Is Needed, GA0-18-179 (Washington, D.C.: January 5, 2018).

Recommendation: The Administrator of CMS should establish standard Medicaid reporting requirements for all states to annually report key information on critical incidents, considering, at a minimum, the type of critical incidents involving Medicaid beneficiaries, and the type of residential facilities, including assisted living facilities, where critical incidents occurred.

Action Needed: As of August 2018, HHS concurs with this recommendation. According to CMS, throughout calendar year 2018, the agency will be releasing a series of three informational bulletins on home and community based service waiver beneficiary health and welfare that are based on feedback solicited from a workgroup consisting of states and state associations. We will continue to monitor the implementation of this recommendation.

Medicaid: Further Action Needed to Expedite Use of National Data for Program Oversight, GA0-18-70 (Washington, D.C.: December 8, 2017).

Recommendation: The Administrator of CMS, in partnership with the states, should take additionai steps to expedite the use ofT-MSIS data for program oversight Such steps should include, but are not limited to, efforts to (1) obtain complete information from all states on unreported T-MSIS data elements and their plans to report applicable data elements; (2) identify and share information across states on known T-MSIS data limitations to improve data comparability; and (3) implement mechanisms, such as the Learning Collaborative, by which states can collaborate on an ongoing basis to improve the completeness, comparability, and 1utility ofT-MSIS data.

Action Needed: HHS concurred with this recommendation. In March 2018, HHS stated that it developed a database on data quality findings, which could be used to identify solutions for common problems across states, and has begun to develop a data quality scorecard forT-MSIS users, which aggregates data quality findings in a user-friendly tooL HHS stated that it will (1) continue to work to obtain complete T-MSIS information from all states; (2) take additional steps to share infonmation across states on T-MSIS data limitations; and (3) implement ways for states to collaborate regarding T-MSIS. We will assess HHS's actions once completed.

Recommendation: The Administrator of CMS should articulate a specific plan and associated time frames for using T-MSIS data for oversight.

Action Needed: HHS concurred with the recommendation, but as of April2018, HHS had not yet informed us of any actions taken.

Medicare and Medicaid: CMS Needs to Fully Align Its Antifraud Efforts with the Fraud Risk Framework. GA0-18-88 (Washington, D.C.: December 5, 2017).

Recommendation: The Administrator of CMS should provide fraud-awareness training relevant to risks facing CMS programs and require new hires to undergo such training and all employees to undergo training on a recurring basis.

Recommendation: The Administrator of CMS should conduct fraud risk assessments for Medicare and Medicaid that include respective fraud risk profiles and plans for regularly updating the assessments and profiles.

Recommendation: The Administrator of CMS should create, document, implement, and communicate an antifraud strategy that is aligned with and responsive to regularly assessed fraud risks. This strategy should include an approach for monitoring and evaluation.

Action Needed: HHS agreed with our recommendations. CMS reported that, as of August 2018, the agency is developing annual fraud, waste, abuse training for all CMS employees. Additionally, CMS is working to apply the fraud risk framework to the Medicaid program more broadly. We will continue to monitor the implementation of these recommendations.

Medicaid Program Integrity: CMS Should Build on Current Oversight Efforts by Further Enhancing Collaboration with States, GA0-17-277 (Washington, D.C.: March 15, 2017).

Recommendation: To build upon CMS's collaborative audit efforts and help enhance future collaboration, CMS should identify opportunities to address barriers that limit states' participation in collaborative audits. Such opportunities could include improving communication with states before, during, and after audits are completed; and ensuring that audits align with states' program integrity needs, including the need for oversight of services provided in managed care delivery systems.

Action Needed: HHS concurred with this recommendation. CMS has taken steps to identify opportunities to improve state participation in collaborative audits. Notably, as of January 2018, CMS is in the process of awarding and implementing contracts for five regional Unified Program Integrity Contractors (UPIC) with the purpose of coordinating provider investigations across Medicare and Medicaid; improving collaboration with states; and increasing contractor accountability through coordinated oversight. CMS is also meeting with groups of states to clarify roles and responsibilities and discuss topics for new collaborative audits with the UPICs.

CMS also held sessions at the Medicaid Integrity Institute in 2017 to work with states on potential topics for new collaborative audits, including personal care services and managed care delivery systems. We will continue to monitor CMS's progress as it initiates and implements UPIC audits nationwide.

Medicaid: CMS Needs Better Data to Monitor the Provision of and Spending on Personal Care Services, GA0-17-169 (Washington, D.C.: Jan. 12, 2017).

Recommendation: To improve the collection of complete and consistent personal care services data and better ensure CMS can effectively monitor the states' provision of and spending on Medicaid personal care services, CMS should better ensure that personal care services data collected from states through T-MSIS and Medicaid Budget and Expenditure System (MBES) comply with CMS reporting requirements.

Action Needed: HHS concurred with this recommendation. In December 2017, CMS cited efforts related to claims data submitted by states through T-MSIS. Efforts included validation checks of person care service claims to ensure that key data are not missing or incorrect. In addition, CMS stated it was working with the states to address concerns that are identified with the quality of claims data submitted. However, as of August 2018, CMS had not addressed inaccurate state reporting through MBES; the agency stated that it is a priority for 2018. Complete implementation of our recommendation will better ensure state reporting of claims and expenditures is accurate and will allow CMS to effectively perform key management functions.

Recommendation: To improve the collection of complete and consistent personal care services data and better ensure CMS can effectively monitor the states' provision of and spending on Medicaid personal care services, CMS should develop plans for analyzing and using personal care services data for program management and oversight.

Action Needed: HHS concurred with this recommendation. As of August 2018, CMS stated that it is working with states to implement Electronic Visit Verification (EW) that will ensure the core elements of personal care service delivery in the home are being tracked. CMS has developed a process for states to submit data on their EW compliance by the January 1, 2020 deadline or to request a good faith exemption from the requirement until January 1, 2021. We will continue to monitor the implementation of this recommendation.

Medicaid: Program Oversight Hampered by Data Challenges, Underscoring Need for Continued Improvements, GA0-17-173 (Washington, D.C.: January 6, 2017).

Recommendation: The Administrator of CMS should take immedi'ate steps to assess and improve the data available for Medicaid program oversight, including, but not limited to, T-MSIS. Such steps could include (1) refining the overall data priority areas in T-MSIS to better identify those variables that are most critical for reducing improper payments, and (2) expediting efforts to assess and ensure the quality of these T-MSIS data.

Action Needed: HHS concurred with the recommendation. In July 2018, CMS noted that it had shifted its T-MSIS efforts to assessing and improving the quality of T-MSIS data, and expressed its commitment to working with states on improving their data submissions. As part of this effort, CMS identified 12 Top Priority Items for post-production data quality that all states should address. CMS told GAO that it reviews a state's data quality issues in these 12 areas and then works with the state on addressing them. The agency plans to expand its data quality monitoring review to be more comprehensive following discussions with a Technical Evaluation Panel to be held this summer. We will continue to monitor CMS's progress as it initiates these new data quality improvement activities.

Medicaid Program Integrity: Improved Guidance Needed to Better Support Efforts to Screen Managed Care Providers, GA0-16-402 (Washington, D.C.: Apri122, 2016).

Recommendation: The Acting Administrator of CMS should coordinate with other federal agencies, as necessary, to explore the use of an identifier that is relevant for the screening of MMC plan providers and common across databases used to screen MMC plan providers.

Action Needed: HHS concurred with the recommendation. In the final Medicaid Managed Care Rule 2390-F, CMS added a requirement that states and managed care plans add the National Plan and Provider Enumeration System (NPPES) to the list of databases required to be checked when enrolling providers. Individuals or organizations are identified in NPPES through the use of a National Provider Identifier (NPI). However, this NPI applies only to NPPES and is not used in other databases that states and managed care plans check when enrolling providers. To fully implement the recommendation, CMS should continue to explore the use of an identifier common across all relevant databases.

Medicaid: Federal Guidance Needed to Address Concerns About Distribution of Supplemental Payments, GA0-16-108 (Washington, D.C.: February 5, 2016).

Recommendation: To promote consistency in the distribution of supplemental payments among states and with CMS policy, the Administrator of CMS should issue written guidance clarifying its policy that requires a link between the distribution of supplemental payments and the provision of Medicaid-covered services.

Action Needed: HHS concurred with this recommendation. CMS has issued clarifying letters to some states, but has not issued written clarification to all states explaining that the distribution of supplemental payments be linked to the provision of Medicaid-covered services. CMS indicated that it anticipates issuing a proposed rule in October 2018 that would establish new reporting requirements for supplemental payments that may address this recommendation.

Recommendation: To promote consistency in the distribution of supplemental payments among states and with CMS policy, the Administrator of CMS should issue written guidance clarifying its policy that payments should not be made contingent on the availability of local funding.

Action Needed: HHS did not concur with this recommendation, although it did agree that the issue is a concern and stated it was considering additional options to address the issue. As of April2018, CMS has not taken action. In light of our finding that, among selected states reviewed, supplemental payments were often contingent on availability of local funding; we maintain that HHS should issue written guidance to all states communicating its policy prohibiting Medicaid payments contingent on the availability of local funding. To implement this recommendation, CMS should issue written guidance clarifying its policy.

Medicaid: Additional Efforts Needed to Ensure that State Spending is Appropriately Matched with Federal Funds, GA0-16-53 (Washington, D.C.: October 16, 2015).

Recommendation: To improve the effectiveness of its oversight of eligibility determinations, the Administrator of CMS should conduct reviews of federal Medicaid eligibility determinations to ascertain the accuracy of these determinations and institute corrective action plans where necessary.

Action Needed: HHS concurred with this recommendation. In July 2017, HHS issued its final rule on the Payment Error Rate Measurement (PERM) program, and stated that it would include reviews of federal eligibility determinations in states that have delegated that authority. In December 2017, HHS provided information noting that the first cycle of the revised PERM includes two states where there were federal eligibility determinations. The results will be reported in 2019. We will continue to monitor HHS's implementation of the revised PERM to determine if HHS is ascertaining the accuracy of federal eligibility determinations and taking corrective action where necessary.

Recommendation: To increase assurances that states receive an appropriate amount of federal matching funds, the Administrator of CMS should use the information obtained from state and federal eligibility reviews to inform the agency's review of expenditures for different eligibility groups in order to ensure that expenditures are reported correctly and matched appropriately.

Action Needed: HHS did not concur with this recommendation. As of August 2018, CMS indicated that it is establishing a process for sharing information between the eligibility and expenditure reviews. Once this process is established, we will determine whether these actions address the recommendation.

Medicaid: CMS Oversight of Provider Payments Is Hampered by Limited Data and Unclear Policy, GA0-15-322 (Washington, D.C.: April10, 2015).

Recommendation: To improve CMS's oversight of Medicaid payments, the Administrator of CMS should develop a policy establishing criteria for when such payments at the provider level are economical and efficient.

Recommendation: To improve CMS's oversight of Medicaid payments, the Administrator of CMS should, once criteria are developed, develop a process for identifying and reviewing payments to individual providers in order to determine whether they are economical and efficient.

Action Needed: HHS concurred with these recommendations. To fully address these recommendations, CMS would need to develop a policy establishing criteria for when Medicaid payments at the provider level are economical and efficient, and once criteria are developed, develop a process for identifying and reviewing payments to individual providers in order to determine whether they are economical and efficient CMS indicated that it anticipates issuing a proposed rule in October 2018 that would establish new reporting requirements for supplemental payments that may address these recommendations.

Medicaid Information Technology: CMS Supports Use of Program Integrity Systems but Should Require States to Determine Effectiveness, GA0-15-207 (Washington, D.C.: January 30, 2015).

Recommendation: To ensure that the federal government's and states' investments in information systems result in outcomes that are effective in supporting efforts to save funds through the prevention and detection of improper payments in the Medicaid program, the Secretary of Health and Human Services should direct the Administrator of CMS to require states to measure quantifiable benefits, such as cost reductions or avoidance, achieved as a result of operating information systems to help prevent and detect improper payments. Such measurement of benefits should reflect a consistent and repeatable approach and should be reported when requesting approval for matching federal funds to support ongoing operation and maintenance of systems that were implemented to support Medicaid program integrity purposes.

Action Needed: HHS initially concurred with this recommendation. However, in December 2017, CMS officials stated that they no longer concur with this recommendation. CMS noted that the agency is taking steps to reduce the regulatory and reporting burden for states and that requiring states to measure benefits achieved as a result of implementing systems for program integrity and other purposes is not feasible.

Unless CMS requires states to measure such benefits, it cannot determine whether the billions of dollars of federal funds spent to support the maintenance of the systems used by the states for program integrity purposes result in savings for the Medicaid program. As such, we continue to believe that steps should be taken by CMS to ensure financial benefits are achieved as a result of federal IT investment in states' continuing operation and maintenance of systems to support Medicaid program integrity efforts. In order to fully address this recommendation, HHS should direct the Administrator of CMS to require states to measure quantifiable benefits achieved as a result of operating information systems to help prevent and detect improper payments.

Medicaid Financing: States' *Increased Reliance on Funds from Health Care Providers and Local Governments Warrants Improved* CMS *Data Collection [Reissued on March 13, 2015],* GA0-14-627 (Washington, D.C.: July 29, 2014).

Recommendation: The Administrator of CMS should develop a data collection strategy that ensures that states report accurate and complete data on all sources of funds used to finance the nonfederal share of Medicaid payments. There are short- and long-term possibilities for pursuing the data collection strategy, including (1) in the short-term, as part of its ongoing initiative to annually collect data on Medicaid payments made to hospitals, nursing facilities, and other institutional providers, CMS could collect accurate and complete facility-specific data on the sources of funds used to finance the nonfederal share of the Medicaid payments, and (2) in the long-term, as part of its ongoing initiative to develop an enhanced Medicaid claims data system (T-MSIS), CMS could ensure that T-MSIS will be capable of capturing information on all sources of funds used to finance the nonfederal share of Medicaid payments, and, once the system becomes operational, ensure that states report this information for supplemental Medicaid payments and other high-risk Medicaid payments.

Action Needed: CMS did not initially concur with this recommendation. In April 2018, CMS officials told us that the agency has started to collect information about the source of funds used to finance the nonfederal share of Medicaid payments through T-MSIS. However, the agency has not yet planned how it will use the data it is collecting and T-MSIS limits states to reporting one source of the nonfederal share per payment. CMS also indicated that as part of its program integrity strategy released in June 2018, it will begin to conduct program audits focused on states' improper claiming of the federal match. Once CMS develops a plan for using the T-MSIS data it collects, begins conducting its planned audits, and prepares and releases a final rule on supplemental payment and financing oversight, GAO will be in a position to consider closing this recommendation.

Medicaid Demonstration Waivers: Approval Process Raises Cost Concerns and Lacks Transparency, GA0-13-384 (Washington, D.C.: June 25, 2013).

Recommendation: To improve the transparency of the process for reviewing and approving spending limits for comprehensive section 1115 demonstrations, the Secretary of Health and Human Services should update the agency's written budget neutrality policy to reflect actual criteria and processes used to develop and approve demonstration spending limits, and ensure the policy is readily available to state Medicaid directors and others.

Action Needed: HHS did not agree with this recommendation; however, the agency has recently taken some steps to establish spending limits and clarify approval criteria. For example, in 2017, GAO described how states have been allowed to accrue, in the context of inflated spending limits, unused spending authority and use it to finance expansions of demonstrations. One state that GAO reviewed was allowed to convert $8 billion in unspent federal spending authority into an incentive payment poolwithin its demonstration.[257] Under a policy implemented in 2016, HHS restricted the amount of unspent funds states can accrue for each year of a demonstration, and has also reduced the amount of unspent funds that states can carry forward to new demonstrations. For 10 demonstrations it has recently approved, HHS estimated that the new policy has reduced total demonstration spending limits by $109 billion for 2016 through 2018, the federal share of which is $62.9 billion. These limits reduce the effect, but do not specifically address all, of the questionable methods and assumptions that we have identified regarding how HHS sets demonstration spending limits.

Additionally, in a November 2017 informational bulletin released on CMS's website, CMS indicated that the agency will clarify expectations regarding its budget neutrality

---

[257] See GAO, *Medicaid Demonstrations: Federal Action Needed to Improve Oversight of Spending,* GA0-17-312 (Washington, D.C.: Apr. 3, 2017).

policy and may provide additional written guidance to states on both policy and methodology for demonstrating budget neutrality. In April 2018, CMS told us that it estimates that additional guidance will be issued by the end of calendar year 2018 that may address this recommendation.

Medicaid and SCHIP: Recent HHS Approvals of Demonstration Waiver Projects Raise Concerns, GA0-02-817 (Washington, D.C.: July 12, 2002).

Recommendation: To meet its fiduciary responsibility of ensuring that section 1115 waivers are budget neutral, we recommended that the Secretary of HHS better ensure that valid methods are used to demonstrate budget neutrality, by developing and implementing consistent criteria for consideration of section 1115 demonstration waiver proposals.

Action Needed: HHS disagreed with this recommendation. However, we have reiterated the need for increased attention to fiscal responsibility in the approval of the section 1115 Medicaid demonstrations in subsequent 2008 and 2013 reports (GA0-08-87 and GA0-13-384).[258] HHS has taken steps to change some aspects of methods used to determine budget neutrality and demonstration spending limits. In May 2016, HHS communicated four key changes to its budget neutrality policy. These changes addressed some, but not all of the questionable methods GAO identified in its reports.

In addition, in a November 20171nformational Bulletin, CMS communicated plans to clarify expectations regarding budget neutrality and to provide additional guidance on methodologies for demonstrating budget neutrality. In April 2018, CMS told us that it estimates that additional guidance will be issued by the end of calendar year 2018 that may address this recommendation.

We agreed to provide Senator McCaskill details about the data we used in a 2011 report on application coverage denials (on page 68 (lines 16-23) of transcript).

In our 2011 report, data from six select states, the American Medical Association, and the National Association of Insurance Commissioners were our primary sources to describe the data available on coverage denials-that is, denial of coverage for a medical service before it is provided or denial of payment for a service after it is provided.[259] We also reviewed information on the outcomes of complaints and appeals submitted by 35 states and the District of Columbia to HHS in their applications for Consumer Assistance Program grants, as well as data from the Department of Labor on complaints related to coverage denials for those with employer- sponsored coverage.

To describe the data available on denials of enrollment applications for individuals seeking to purchase insurance coverage, we reviewed data that HHS collected from 459 state-licensed insurers that offered coverage in the individual market on the number of

---

[258] See GAO, *Me.dicaid Demonstration Waivem: Recent HHS Approvals Continue to Raise Cost and Ovemight Concerns.* GA0-08-87 (Washington, D.C.: Jan. 31, 2008) and *Medicaid Demonstration Waivers: Approval Process Raises Cost Concerns and Lacks Transparency,* GA0-13-384 (Washington, D.C.: June 25. 2013).

[259] See GAO, *Private Health Insurance: Data on Application and Coverage Denials,* GA0-11-268 (Washington, D.C.: Mar. 16, 2011).

applications received and denied. The data included application denial rates by insurer for a 3-month period-January through March-in 2010, which was the only quarter of data that HHS had collected as of December 2010. To supplement the single calendar quarter of HHS data, we also collected data from insurance department officials in the six selected states. Additionally, we reviewed data from America's Health Insurance Plans on application denial rates.

We agreed to provide Senator McCaskill coverage denial detail from 2011 report (on page 71 (lines 4-5) of transcript).

In our 2011 report, coverage denial rates varied significantly across states, with aggregate rates of claim denials ranging from 11 percent to 24 percent across the three states that collected such data.[260] In addition, rates varied significantly across insurers, with data from one state indicating a range in claim denial rates from 6 percent to 40 percent across six large insurers operating in the state. There are several factors that may have contributed to the variation in rates across states and insurers, such as states varying in the types of denials they require insurers to report. Data also indicated that

- Coverage denials occurred for a variety of reasons, frequently for billing errors, such as duplicate claims or missing information on the claim, and eligibility issues, such as services being provided before coverage was initiated, and less often for judgments about the appropriateness of a service.
- Coverage denials, if appealed, were frequently reversed in the consumer's favor. For example, data from four of the six states on the outcomes of appeals filed with insurers indicated that 39 percent to 59 percent of appeals resulted in the insurer reversing its original coverage denial.

GAO U.S. Government Accountability Office
Comptroller General of the United States

August 17, 2018

The Honorable Ron Johnson
Chairman
Committee on Homeland Security and Governmental Affairs
U.S. Senate

Dear Chairman Johnson:

[260] See GAO, *Private Health Insurance: Data on Application and Coverage Denials,* GA0-11-268 (Washington, D.C.: Mar. 16, 2011).

This letter is in reference to the hearing of the U.S. Senate Committee on Homeland Security and Governmental Affairs entitled "Medicaid Fraud and Overpayments: Problems and Solutions" at which I testified on June 27, 2018.

Sincerely yours,

Gene L. Dodaro
Comptroller General of the United States

cc: The Honorable Claire McCaskill, Ranking Minority Member

GAO Response to Hearing Questions, Chairman Johnson and Ranking Member McCaskill, Committee on Homeland Security and Governmental Affairs, United States Senate, June 27, 2018, Hearing Entitled "Medicaid Fraud and Overpayments: Problems and Solutions"

1. The threat regarding rollback of protections on preexisting conditions is real. Has the Government Accountability Office begun any analysis of the impact of eliminating these protections?

In March 2011, GAO reported on health insurance application denial rates prior to the Patient Protection and Affordable Care Act (ACA) prohibition on denying coverage on the basis of preexisting conditions. GAO has not conducted any work relating to preexisting conditions, including reviewing any policy changes relating to preexisting conditions, since this time.

2. If the challenges against the ACA are successful, is it likely that we would return to a time when 25 percent of the health insurance companies in this country had denial rates of 40 percent or higher?

GAO issued a report in March 2011, which looked at health insurance application denial rates prior to the ACA prohibition on denying coverage on the basis of a preexisting condition.[261] GAO reported that the aggregate rate of application denials nationally was 19 percent, with 25 percent of insurance companies denying 40 percent or more of applications for individual coverage. Given those rates, if such a prohibition were eliminated, insurers could return to using application denials as a strategy to manage risk. It is important to note that the denial rates cited in GAO's report were for one

---

[261] See GAO, *Private Health Insurance: Data on Application and Coverage Denials,* GA0-11-268 (Washington, D.C.: Mar. 16, 2011).

calendar quarter and may have limited utility in providing a sufficiently complete benchmark for projecting any changes to denial rates.

It is also important to note that other aspects of ACA-as well as state laws and regulations-could affect application denial rates. For example, ACA included other provisions that reformed the individual market by introducing premium tax credits for those with low-incomes and providing federal risk adjustment payments. These policies change the financial incentives for health insurance companies and for individuals applying for coverage, and could affect the extent to which companies deny applications. State laws and regulations could also affect denial rates. For example, GAO's report noted that prior to the enactment of ACA six states prohibited insurers from denying applications on the basis of health status as of January 2010.

3. It has been over seven years since the provider screening and enrollment requirements took effect in March 2011. Why are states still failing to properly screen and enroll Medicaid providers?

States need to make significant changes to their provider enrollment and screening systems in order to come into compliance with the March 2011 requirements. The Centers for Medicare & Medicaid Services (CMS) has taken a variety of actions-such as issuing guidance and regulations, and offering assistance in screening providers using federal databases-to support states' efforts to improve provider screening and enrollment processes. However, GAO's work has identified various factors, such as fragmented information, lack of data sharing across states, and inconsistent practices that have affected CMS's and states' oversight of providers. For example, in April2016, GAO found that two selected states and 16 selected Medicaid managed care plans used information that was fragmented across 22 databases by 15 different federal agencies to screen providers, including databases that CMS did not identify for use for screening providers. To improve the effectiveness of states' and plans' Medicaid managed care plan provider screening efforts, GAO recommended that CMS consider additional databases used to screen providers and assess whether any of these databases should be added to the list of databases identified by CMS for screening purposes, in order to ensure that they are not paying providers determined to be ineligible to do business with the federal government.[262] HHS agreed with this recommendation, and in August 2018, implemented this recommendation. CMS provided GAO with its analysis of 22 databases that were reported to GAO as being used by Medicaid managed care plans to screen providers. It determined that several of the 22 databases were already in use by states and managed care plans and mentioned in CMS guidance. In its analysis, CMS concluded that

- 6 of the databases should be used for provider screening and 3 more contained information that was available from other databases.

---

[262] See GAO, *Medicaid Program Integrity: Improved Guidance Needed to Better Support Efforts to Screen Managed Care Providers,* GA0-16-402 (Washington, D.C.: April22, 2016).

- 12 of the databases should not be implemented into the screening process and is still considering one of the databases for inclusion in the screening process.

GAO is beginning work examining CMS's oversight of state efforts to implement and comply with Medicaid provider screening and enrollment requirements in ACA and the 21st Century Cures Act (Cures Act). GAO anticipates this work will be completed in 2019.

4. Would proper screening and enrollment of Medicaid Providers prevent improper payments and reduce the incidence of fraud in the Medicaid program?

Yes. Providers who are not appropriately enrolled in Medicaid are one of the largest causes of improper payments in the Medicaid program. Because provider actions can be a major factor behind improper payments, the integrity of the Medicaid program depends, in large part, on ensuring that only eligible providers participate in the program. Consequently, screening providers is important in preventing improper payments, including potential fraud and abuse.

In its fiscal year 2017 Agency Financial Report, the Department of Health and Human Services (HHS) stated that errors due to state non-compliance with provider screening, enrollment, and National Provider Identifier requirements, have been the main cause of improper payments in Medicaid fee-for-service since fiscal year 2014. Further, CMS does not assess provider eligibility as a part of estimating the improper payment rate in managed care; so the impact of ineligible providers in managed care on improper payments is unknown.

GAO's work in Medicaid has also identified potential program risks-including fraud-associated with how CMS and states have enrolled providers in Medicaid. In May 2015, GAO reported that hundreds of the approximately 881,000 Medicaid providers in four states were ineligible or potentially ineligible. These providers had suspended or revoked medical licenses, had invalid addresses, were identified as deceased in federal death files, or had been excluded from federal health care programs, including Medicaid.[263]

Comprehensive state screening and enrollment processes that prevent fraudulent providers from billing Medicaid are more efficient at protecting Medicaid funds than attempting to recover these funds once payments have been made.

5. Is CMS implementing methods to conduct proper screening and enrollment of Medicaid providers?

CMS has taken steps to enhance Medicaid provider screening and enrollment, in some cases addressing GAO's recommendations, including

[263] See GAO, *Medicaid: Additional Actions Needed to Help Improve Provider and Beneficiary Fraud Controls,* GA0-15-313 (Washington, D.C.: May 14, 2015).

- *Issuing regulations.* For example, in May 2016, CMS issued regulations that required states to screen and enroll providers under contract to managed care organizations (MCO), and terminate network providers upon notification.[264]
- *Issuing guidance.* Consistent with GAO's recommendations, CMS updated and issued its Medicare Provider Enrollment Compendium-eMS's manual on how state Medicaid agencies are expected to comply with federal regulations for screening providers.[265] Also, CMS issued a toolkit for sharing provider data, which includes information on how to access systems and retrieve CMS data from multiple sources.[266]
- *Providing access to federal databases.* CMS has taken steps to increase state access to federal databases to implement GAO's recommendations. For example, CMS provides full access to all pertinent information needed for screening Medicaid providers in Medicare's provider enrollment database-the Provider Enrollment, Chain and Ownership System (PECOS)-and, according to CMS officials, offers trainings on using this information.[267] Also, CMS signed an interagency agreement that provides states with access to the Social Security Administration's (SSA) Death Master File, made this file available to state officials, and provided assistance to states in accessing this file.[268]
- *Offering states an optional data compare service.* States may submit their Medicaid provider enrollment information to CMS and receive results about how that information compares to related data sources, such as Medicare enrollment records and HHS's Office of Inspector General (HHS-OIG) information on excluded providers.
- *Conducting site visits, outreach, and education.* According to CMS, the agency has conducted site visits to assist states with implementing Medicaid provider screening and enrollment requirements. Also, CMS reported providing education, outreach, and assistance to support and oversee state efforts.

In June 2018, CMS provided information on a new Medicaid program integrity strategy. This planned strategy includes many of the aforementioned steps, such as providing states with access to federal databases, and other steps, such as monitoring states' implementation of and compliance with Medicaid managed care final rules,

---

[264] These screening and enrollment requirements were later codified by the Cures Act and took effect January 1, 2018.

[265] See GA0-16-402.

[266] See GA0-15-313.

[267] PECOS is CMS's centralized database for Medicare enrollment information. PECOS maintains data from Medicare provider and supplier applications, including name, address, specialty area, licensure, and accreditations. PECOS also maintains information on the number of approved, denied, and rejected new enrollment applications, the number of deactivated or revoked existing enrollment records, and the number of enrollment records associated with providers and suppliers eligible to bill Medicare. See GA0-15-313.

[268] See GA0-16-402. CMS issued regulations designating four federal databases that states must use to screen providers, including SSA's Master Death File.

including program integrity safeguards such as screening and enrolling Medicaid managed care providers. Additionally, as part of this new strategy, CMS plans to pilot a process to screen Medicaid providers on behalf of states beginning in summer 2018. CMS officials told us that part of this pilot process will involve leveraging the existing data and process CMS uses to screen Medicare providers. According to agency officials, CMS plans to begin implementing this pilot process in a few states and then expand it to additional states. GAO plans to monitor the implementation of the strategy.

Finally, GAO is beginning work examining CMS's oversight of state efforts to implement and comply with Medicaid provider screening and enrollment requirements in ACA and the Cures Act. GAO anticipates this work will be completed in 2019.

6. What steps should CMS take to ensure that states comply with federal regulations requiring screening and enrollment of Medicaid providers?

CMS could improve its oversight of state compliance with federal regulations requiring screening and enrollment of Medicaid providers, and aid state program integrity generally by implementing a number of GAO recommendations, such as the following:

- To ensure that only eligible providers are enrolled in Medicaid, GAO made four recommendations in its April2016 report on provider screening in managed care.[269] One recommendation remains open, which HHS concurred with. To address this recommendation, CMS will need to explore the use of a common identifier for screening providers across databases.
- To ensure appropriate program integrity oversight in the territories including protecting territories' Medicaid programs from fraud, waste, and abuse, CMS should examine and select from a broad array of activities-such as establishing program oversight mechanisms, assisting in improving program information, and conducting program assessments-and develop cost-effective approaches.[270] HHS concurred with GAO's recommendation. In 2016, CMS communicated plans to review program integrity activities in the territories, and as of July 2018, the agency had conducted and issued a report for Puerto Rico. It has not released reports for other territories, nor has it implemented new program integrity activities and approaches for the territories, as GAO recommended.
- To better support states' efforts to reduce improper payments and communicate effective program integrity practices across the states, CMS should collaborate with states and take additional steps to collect and share promising state program integrity practices, among other actions.[271] Although HHS agreed with these

---

[269] See GA0-16-402.

[270] See GAO, *Medicaid and CHIP: Increased Funding in U.S. Tenitories Merits Improved Progrem Integrity Efforts,* GA0-16-324 (Washington, D.C.: AprilS, 2016).

[271] See GAO, *Medicaid Program Integrity: CMS Should Build on Current Oversight Efforts by Further Enhancing Collaboration with States.* GA0-17-277 (Washington, D.C.: March 15, 2017).

recommendations, as of July 2018, CMS had not fully addressed these recommendations.

- To fully align its fraud risk management efforts with the four components of the Fraud Risk Framework, CMS should (1) require and provide fraud-awareness training to its employees, (2) conduct fraud risk assessments, and (3) create an antifraud strategy for Medicaid, including an approach for evaluation.[272] HHS agreed with these recommendations. As of August 2018, CMS is developing annual fraud, waste, abuse training for all CMS employees. Additionally, CMS is working to apply the fraud risk framework to the Medicaid program more broadly.

7. What steps should CMS take to ensure that states are using Medicaid funds efficiently?

GAO's work on supplemental payments and Medicaid demonstrations offers insights on actions CMS-and in some cases, the Congress-could take to ensure more efficient use of Medicaid funds.

Supplemental Payments

Since 2004, GAO has made recommendations to CMS to improve the transparency and accountability of supplemental payments. For example, GAO has recommended that

- CMS develop a policy establishing criteria for determining whether Medicaid payments are economical and efficient, as required by law, as well as require provider-specific payment data needed to assess total Medicaid payments, including supplemental payments. GAO has reported on cases in which states made total Medicaid payments to individual providers-after accounting for supplemental payments-that were greatly in excess of Medicaid costs and raise questions about whether federal Medicaid funds were used for non-Medicaid purposes.[273] HHS agreed with this recommendation. In August 2018, CMS indicated that it anticipates issuing a proposed rule in early 2019 that would establish new reporting requirements for supplemental payments that may address GAO's concerns.[274]
- CMS take steps to ensure states report accurate and complete information on all sources of funds they use to finance the nonfederal share. GAO has reported on problematic financing and distribution methods that allow states to shift

---

[272] See GAO, *Medicare and Medicaid: CMS Needs to Fully Align* Its *Antifraud Efforts with the Fraud Risk Framework.* GA0-18-88 (Washington, D.C.: Dec. 5, 2017).

[273] See GAO, *Medicaid: CMS Oversight of Provider Payments Is Hampered by Limited Data and Unclear Policy,* GA0-15-322 (Washington, *D.C.:* Apr. 10, 2015).

[274] See HHS, Medicaid Supplemental Payment and Accountability, *Spring 2018 Unified Agenda of Federal Regulatory and Deregulatory Actions,* (CMS-2392-P), RIN 0938-AT50, accessed on July 27, 2018.

Medicaid program costs to the federal government and distort the distribution of supplemental payments.[275] HHS disagreed with and has not addressed GAO's recommendation, although the agency stated that it will examine efforts to improve data collection for oversight. Moreover, as part of its planned program integrity strategy released in June 2018, CMS indicated that it will begin to conduct program audits focused on states' improper claiming of the federal match. GAO will monitor CMS's audits to determine if they address the recommendation.

- CMS develop written guidance clarifying CMS's policies that non-disproportionate share hospital (OSH) supplemental payments should be linked to the provision of Medicaid services and not be contingent on the availability of local financing.[276] GAO has reported that distributing payments based on the ability of hospitals or their local governments to finance the nonfederal share may result in some hospitals with relatively low uncompensated care costs receiving large payments while other hospitals with larger uncompensated care costs, but less access to local funds, receiving smaller payments.[277] HHS agreed with this recommendation. In August 2018, CMS indicated that it anticipates issuing a proposed rule in early 2019 that would establish new reporting requirements for supplemental payments that may address GAO's concerns.

Congressional action may also be needed to implement GAO's recommendations. For example, in 2012, CMS officials said legislation was needed to implement reporting and auditing requirements for non-DHS supplemental payments. According to officials, legislation would allow the agency to institute requirements similar to those for DSH payments, such as requiring annual facility-specific reporting of non-OSH payment information, clarifying permissible methods for calculating non-DSH payment amounts, and requiring annual independent audits of state non-OSH payment calculations. GAO suggested that Congress consider requiring CMS to improve state reporting of non-OSH payments, including those made to individual facilities; provide guidance on permissible methods for calculating non-OSH payments; and require state reports and audits.[278]

---

[275] See GAO, *Medicaid Financing: States' Increased Reliance on Funds from Health Care Providers and Local Governments Warrants Improved CMS Data Collection (Reissued on March 13, 2015],* GA0-14-627 (Washington, D.C.: July 29, 2014).

[276] Two types of supplemental payments exist in Medicaid: (1) disproportionate share hospital (DSH) payments, which states are required to make to hospitals serving low-income and Medicaid patients to offset those providers' uncompensated care costs; and (2) non-DSH supplemental payments that states may, but are not required, to make to hospitals and other providers that, for example, serve high-cost Medicaid beneficiaries.

[277] See GAO, *Medicaid: Federal Guidance Needed to Address Concerns About Distribution of Supplemental Payments,* GA0-16-108 (Washington, D.C.: Feb. 5, 2016).

[278] See GAO, *Medicaid: More Transparency of and Accountability for Supplemental Payments Are Needed,* GA0-13-4e (Washington. D.C.: Nov. 26, 2012).

Medicaid Demonstrations

Since 2002, GAO has also made recommendations to improve the transparency and accountability of states' demonstration spending. For example, GAO has recommended that the Secretary of HHS

- ensure that valid methods are used to establish demonstration spending limits,[279] and
- update written policy to reflect the approval criteria and processes used to develop and approve demonstration spending limits, so that states' use of this flexibility does not inappropriately increase federal costs.[280]

HHS did not agree with these recommendations; however, the agency has recently taken some steps to establish spending limits and clarify approval criteria. For example, under a policy implemented in 2016, HHS restricted the amount of unspent funds states can accrue for each year of a demonstration, and has also reduced the amount of unspent funds that states can carry forward to new demonstrations. For 10 demonstrations it has recently approved, HHS estimated that the new policy has reduced total demonstration spending limits by $109 billion for 2016 through 2018, the federal share of which is $62.9 billion. These limits reduce the effect, but do not specifically address all, of the questionable methods and assumptions that GAO has identified regarding how HHS sets demonstration spending limits. To fully address the recommendations, HHS must update its written policy to reflect the criteria and processes used for determining spending limits. HHS expects to release additional guidance later in 2018 that may address GAO's concerns.

8. What obligations do states have to collect and report data from managed care organizations (MCO)?

Federal law requires states to collect and report to CMS managed care enrollee encounter data as specified by the Secretary of HHS.[281] In 2010, Congress added to this provision a requirement for states to report additional data elements that the Secretary deems necessary for program integrity oversight and administration, which states may report through CMS's new repository of national Medicaid data-the Transformed Medicaid Statistical Information System (T-MSIS).[282]

---

[279] See GAO, *Medicaid and SCHIP: Recent HHS Approvals* of *Demonstration Waiver Projects Raise Concerns,* GA0-02-817 (Washington, D.C.: July 12, 2002).

[280] See GAO, *Medicaid Demonstration Waivers: Approval Process Raises Cost Concerns and Lacks Transparency,* GA0-13-384 (Washington, D.C.: June 25, 2013).

[281] See 42 U.S.C. §§ 1396b(r)(1)(F) and 1396b(i)(25).

[282] See Patient Protection and Affordable Care Act, Pub. L. No. 111-148, § 6504, 124 Stat. 119, 776 (2010). To enforce these requirements, CMS may wrthhold federal matching payments for the use, maintenance or modification of automated data systems from states that fail to report required data. See 42 C.F.R. § 433.120 (2017). Additionally, CMS may withhold federal matching payments for medical assistance to managed care enrollees for whom states fail to report required encounter data. See 42 U.S.C. § 1396b(i)(25) and 42 C.F.R. § 438.818 (2017).

T-MSIS is designed to capture significantly more data from states and MCOs than previously collected, which should provide CMS and states with information to enhance their oversight efforts. Specifically, among other new information, T-MSIS requires states to report a new data file on managed care. The managed care file includes more detailed information on MCOs, such as type and name of managed care plans, covered eligibility groups, service areas, and reimbursement arrangements. In addition to identifying which MCOs are reporting encounter data as required, this file could help CMS's oversight by allowing the agency to identify excess plan profits and volatility of expenditures for some beneficiary groups across states.

CMS has issued guidance and other information to states on their data collection, validation, and reporting responsibilities. For example, CMS defines and periodically updates the required T-MSIS data elements and reporting formats through the T-MSIS data dictionary and provides supplementary guidance and best practices for states' encounter data activities on a website, the T-MSIS Coding Blog. Additionally, CMS announced specifications for reporting the expanded set of data through T-MSIS in a 2013 state Medicaid Director letter. However, as of December 2017, GAO has reported that the data collected by states GAO reviewed was not complete or comparable across states.[283]

In May 2016, CMS issued a managed care rule that included new reporting requirements, among other things. For example, states must validate that encounter data submitted by an MCO to the state are a complete and accurate representation of services provided to beneficiaries, and states must report to CMS after each MCO contract year an assessment of encounter data reporting by each MCO, among other topics. The rule also implements requirements that should improve the integrity of managed care data, such as independent audits of the encounter and financial data submitted by MCOs at least once every 3 years. However, the audits and annual assessments have not yet begun, and the validation requirement only became applicable recently-for contracts that began on or after July 1, 2017-so it is too early to know their actual impact on oversight.

9. Are the current reporting requirements sufficient, or are further steps necessary to compel compliance with current reporting regulations?

GAO has not conducted a systematic assessment of Medicaid program reporting requirements. However, GAO's work does show examples of areas where additional reporting would be beneficial to improving oversight. Some examples include the following:

- GAO has reported on the need for CMS to take steps to ensure that states report accurate and complete information on all sources of funds they use to finance the

[283] See GAO, *Medicaid: Further Action Needed to Expedite Use of National Data for Program Oversight,* GA0-18-70 (Washington, D.C.: Dec. 8, 2017).

nonfederal share.[284] HHS disagreed with and has not addressed GAO's recommendation. However, taking action is especially important because GAO's work has identified increased use of provider taxes and transfers from local government to finance the states' share of supplemental payments, which, although allowed under federal law, effectively shift Medicaid costs from the states to the federal government.

- GAO has made four recommendations to improve the reporting and use of data on the provision of personal care services-which are at a high risk for improper payments, including fraud.[285] CMS agreed with these recommendations and has implemented two. GAO maintains that taking action on the remaining two recommendations-ensuring state compliance with reporting requirements, and developing plans to use data for oversight-is important given that GAO's work has found that the data CMS collects to monitor the provision of these services were often not timely, complete, or consistent.
- GAO has begun work on a request that, in part, asks GAO to consider how program reporting requirements might be duplicative or outdated, and whether there are ways to streamline state reporting. GAO anticipates issuing the results of this work in 2019.

10. Has CMS ever withheld any federal funding from states that failed to comply with their obligation to collect and report MCO data to CMS?

GAO is not aware of any cases where CMS has withheld federal funds for these reasons; however, it has not been a focus of GAO's audit work.

11. What efforts, if any, is CMS undertaking to increase transparency and ensure that MCOs are spending taxpayer dollars properly and efficiently?

In July 2018, GAO reported that while CMS has initiated efforts to assist states with program integrity oversight for managed care, some efforts have been delayed and GAO identified gaps in oversight.[286] In that report, GAO reported the following:

- CMS established a new approach for conducting managed care audits; however, only a few audits have been conducted, with none initiated in the past 2 years. In part, this was due to impediments identified by states such as the lack of needed provisions in MCO contracts.

---

[284] See GAO, *Medicaid Financing: States' Increased Reliance on Funds from Health Care Providers and Local Governments Warrants Improved CMS Data Collection [Reissued on March 13, 2015],* GA0-14-627 (Washington, D.C.: July 29, 2014).

[285] See GAO, *Medicaid: CMS Needs Better Data to Monitor the Provision of and Spending on Personal Care Services,* GA0-17-169 (Washington, D.C.: Jan. 12, 2017).

[286] See GAO, *Medicaid Managed Care: Improvements Needed to Better Oversee Payment Risks,* GA0-18-528 (Washington, D.C.: July 26, 2018).

- CMS has updated standards for its periodic review of state capitation rates set for MCOs; however, overpayments to providers by MCOs were not consistently accounted for when determining future state payments to MCOs, which can result in states' payments to MCO's being too high.

GAO also has recommended actions CMS could take to ensure transparency and oversight of MCOs. GAO recommended that CMS (1) expedite issuing planned guidance on Medicaid managed care program integrity, (2) address impediments to managed care audits, and (3) ensure states account for overpayments in setting future MCO payment rates.[287] HHS agreed with GAO's recommendations; GAO will monitor the department's efforts to address them.

In June 2018, CMS announced its new planned Medicaid program integrity strategy. The information about this new strategy briefly describes several new and enhanced initiatives intended to create greater transparency in and accountability for Medicaid program integrity and reduce improper payments. Some of the new initiatives CMS plans to undertake include

- implementing targeted audits of some states' MCO financial reporting to include a review of high-risk vulnerabilities;
- optimizing T-MSIS data to allow it to be used for advanced analytics; and
- centralizing provider screening on a voluntary basis.

GAO will continue to monitor the agency's current, ongoing, and future efforts to oversee MCOs.

12. Administrator Verma has expressed an interest in rolling back the managed care rule announced in May 2016. What impact would this roll back have on CMS's ability to collect data from managed care organizations?

The Managed Care Rule, issued in May 2016, updated existing provisions and added new requirements that could strengthen the integrity of managed care payments. The following are examples of the updated provisions and new requirements under the rule:

- States must arrange for an independent audit of the accuracy, truthfulness, and completeness of the encounter and financial data submitted by MCOs, at least once every 3 years.
- Through contracts with MCOs, states must require MCOs to have a mechanism through which providers report and return overpayments to the MCOs. States must also require MCOs to promptly report any identified or recovered overpayments- specifying those that are potentially fraudulent-and submit an

[287] See GA0-18-528.

annual report on recovered overpayments to their state. States must use this information when setting actuarially sound capitation rates.

- Through contracts with MCOs, states must also require MCOs to report specific data, information, and documentation. In addition, the MCO's chief executive officer or authorized representative must certify the accuracy and completeness of the reported data, information, and documentation.
- State agencies must have monitoring systems that address all aspects of the managed care program, including information systems for encounter data reporting and program integrity, among other things. States must submit to CMS no later than 180 days after each contract year a report assessing a range of areas including encounter data reporting by each MCO, financial performance, and availability of services.

It is too early to know whether the rule will assure better oversight of MCO payments to providers and the data used to set future capitation rates, as the above requirements only recently became applicable-for contracts starting on or after July 1, 2017. That said, GAO's work has shown that oversight of managed care is currently lacking, which is concerning given the growth in managed care spending. The data collection and verification requirements in the rule are a promising step, especially since GAO and others have found that the data states are required to submit to CMS have, at times, been incomplete or have not been reported at all, particularly managed care encounter data.[288] If fully implemented, the rule may help with the identification and removal of overpayments and unallowable costs from the data used to set future capitation rates.

13. In the event that the managed care rule is rolled back, how might CMS move forward with ensuring the integrity of Medicaid?

CMS needs to take fundamental actions in three key areas to strengthen Medicaid oversight and better manage program risks:

1) Improve data. CMS needs to make sustained efforts to ensure that the data collected through T-MSIS are timely, complete, and comparable from all states, and useful for program oversight. This is particularly relevant to managed care as the managed care file in T-MSIS includes detailed information on MCOs, such as type and name of managed care plans, covered eligibility groups, service areas, and reimbursement arrangements. In addition to identifying which MCOs are reporting encounter data as required, this file could help CMS's oversight by allowing the agency to identify excess plan profits and volatility of expenditures for some beneficiary groups across states. Data are also needed for oversight of

---

[288] See GAO, *Medicaid: Program Oversight Hampered by Data Challenges, Underscoring Need for Continued Improvements,* GA0-17-173 (Washington D.C.: Jan. 6, 2017); and HHS-OIG, *NotAl/ States Reported Medicaid Managed* Care *Encounter Data as Required,* OEI-07-13-00120 (Washington, D.C.: July 2015).

supplemental payments and ensuring that demonstrations are meeting their stated goals.

2) Target fraud. CMS needs to conduct a fraud risk assessment for Medicaid, and design and implement a risk-based antifraud strategy for the program. A fraud risk assessment allows managers to fully consider fraud risks to their programs, analyze their likelihood and impact, and prioritize risks. Managers can then design and implement a strategy with specific control activities to mitigate these fraud risks, as well as design and implement an appropriate evaluation. Through these actions, CMS could better ensure that it is addressing the full portfolio of risks and strategically targeting the most-significant fraud risks facing Medicaid.
3) Collaborate. Oversight of the Medicaid program could be further improved through leveraging and coordinating program integrity efforts with state agencies, state auditors, and the HHS Inspector General. Collaborative audits-in which CMS's contractors and states work in partnership to audit Medicaid providers-are one beneficial collaborative approach. CMS has expanded the federal-state collaborative audits beyond fee-for-service, and has begun to engage states to participate in collaborative audits of MCOs and providers under contract to MCOs. In May 2018, GAO reported that collaborative audits of providers under contract to MCOs in three states identified substantial potential overpayments. Expanding collaborative audits in managed care will require commitment from and coordination with states. GAO has also found that state auditors and the HHS Inspector General offer additional oversight and information that can help identify program risks. For example, state auditors have conducted program integrity reviews to identify improper payments and deficiencies in the states' processes used to identify them. GAO believes that these reviews could provide insights into program weaknesses that CMS could learn from and potentially address nationally.

14. What is the current state of the T-MSIS database? When will CMS be prepared to launch the database and grant access to states?

As of June 2018, CMS reported that all states, the District of Columbia, and Puerto Rico were submitting T-MSIS data; however, the agency's efforts to ensure T-MSIS data comparability and quality are still evolving. Further, the agency has yet to articulate a specific plan and specific timeframes for using these data for program oversight. In a January 2017 report, GAO noted that without an improved focus on ensuring the accuracy of data-and setting priorities for the data that are most likely to improve program oversight-the effectiveness of T-MSIS could not be assured. GAO recommended that CMS take immediate steps to assess and improve the data available for Medicaid program oversight, including, but not limited to, T-MSIS data.[289] HHS agreed with this recommendation and noted in July 2018 that CMS has shifted its T-MSIS efforts to assessing and improving the quality of T-MSIS data, and expressed its commitment to working with states on improving their data submissions. These efforts are ongoing, and this recommendation remains open.

In a subsequent December 2017 report, while acknowledging the progress made in states' reporting of T-MSIS data, GAO identified concerns regarding the completeness of T-MSIS data across states, as well as the absence of an agency plan and related timeframes for using these data for program oversight.[290] GAO recommended that CMS, in partnership with the states, take additional steps to expedite the use of T-MSIS data for program oversight. Such steps should include, but are not limited to

- obtaining complete information from all states on unreported T-MSIS data elements and their plans to report applicable data elements;
- identifying and sharing information across states on known T-MSIS data limitations to improve data comparability; and
- implementing mechanisms, such as the Learning Collaborative, by which states can collaborate on an ongoing basis to improve the completeness, comparability, and utility of T-MSIS data.

GAO also recommended that CMS establish specific plans and associated time frames for using T-MSIS data for oversight. While HHS agreed with GAO's recommendations in these areas, and reported plans to outline a timeline for sharing T-MSIS data, CMS has not implemented the recommendations. GAO will continue to monitor CMS's progress and actions the agency takes to address them.

15. How many states are reporting the required T-MSIS data?

CMS noted that as of June 2018, all states, the District of Columbia, and Puerto Rico were submitting T-MSIS data. CMS added that it monitors ongoing monthly T-MSIS data submissions and works with the remaining U.S. territories not yet submitting data. However, as GAO reported in December 2017, concerns regarding the completeness and comparability of data across states remain.[291] In the 2017 report, GAO made several recommendations to CMS to improve the completeness and comparability of T-MSIS data; these recommendations remain open. Implementing the recommendations would help address the completeness and comparability concerns that GAO identified, which include the following.

---

[289] See GAO, *Medicaid: Program Oversight Hampered by Data Challenges, Underscoring Need for Continued Improvements,* GA0-17-173 (Washington, D.C.: Jan. 6, 2017).

[290] See GA0-18-70.

[291] See GA0-18-70.

- Completeness. GAO reported that six selected states in its review did not report 80 to 260 of the nearly 1,400 T-MSIS elements. The selected states provided a range of reasons for not reporting T-MSIS data elements, including that certain elements were contingent on federal or state actions; were too costly to report; or in some cases, were not applicable to their Medicaid programs and therefore were not required. Although CMS requires states to report all T-MSIS data elements applicable to their program, CMS officials said they did not specify a reporting deadline for states, and selected states' documentation to CMS did not always include the reasons they did not report certain elements, or whether or when they planned to report them.
- Comparability. GAO also reported concerns about the comparability of T-MSIS data across states that may limit the data's usefulness for oversight. Officials from most selected states cited the benefit of a national repository of T-MSIS data. Such a repository would allow them to compare their Medicaid program data-such as spending or utilization rates-to other states and potentially improve their oversight. However, concerns about comparability of the data make some states hesitant to use the data in this manner.

16. What is being done with that data now? Is it being used, or able to be used by CMS in its current form?

In July 2018, CMS noted that it had shifted its T-MSIS efforts to assessing and improving the quality of T-MSIS data, and expressed its commitment to working with states on improving their data submissions. As part of this effort, CMS identified 12 Top Priority Items (TPI) for post-production data quality that all states should address.[292] CMS told GAO that it reviews a state's data quality issues in these 12 areas and then works with the state on addressing them. The agency plans to expand its data quality monitoring review to be more comprehensive following discussions with a Technical Evaluation Panel to be held this summer.

CMS also noted in July 2018 that it reviews T-MSIS data using two data quality methods. The first is the T-MSIS system business rules review, which displays the results of the basic edits and identifies the obvious errors as the data are processed on the T-MSIS operational dashboard.[293] States are expected to address errors identified by the system business rules review. The second method reviews each state's data through inferential validation, which looks at patterns in the state's data and identifies "warnings" where data elements fall outside of a normal range. CMS told us that it is sharing these

---

[292] Examples of the 12 TPI include "Reasonableness of Eligible Counts," under which CMS compares the number of beneficiaries reported in T-MSIS to other Medicaid enrollment data; and "Linking Providers from Claims to Provider Files," under which CMS identifies providers included on T-MSIS claims files (Inpatient, Long-Term Care, Pharmacy and Other) that are not found in the T-MSIS Provider file.

[293] According to CMS, basic edits may include checking for valid data types (character, numeric, etc.) and valid data values.

data quality results with states during meetings as part of its ongoing data quality monitoring efforts and expects states to make corrections to address identified issues.

CMS continues to focus on efforts to improve the quality of T-MSIS data. In August 2018, CMS released a State Health Official letter noting that it expects states to resolve identified data quality issues related to the 12 TPI no later than 6 months of the letter's release. Further, CMS reported that it will request a corrective action plan from states that are unable to resolve issues identified with respect to the 12 TPis within the 6 month timeframe. According to the letter, CMS will expand the data quality review from the 12 TPis to a more comprehensive data quality approach later during 2018 and has set a timeframe of calendar year 2019 to have T-MSIS research-ready files available. Until these efforts are further along, the usefulness of T-MSIS data for CMS and state oversight efforts are limited. Further, as we reported in December 2017, CMS has yet to fully articulate specific plans for how it will use these data for oversight purposes. This remains the case today.

Office of Inspector General
Aug 10 2018

The Honorable Ron Johnson
Chairman
Committee on Homeland Security and Governmental Affairs
United States Senate
Washington, DC 20510

Dear Chairman Johnson:

I am writing in response to questions for the record from Ranking Member McCaskill following my testimony before the Committee on Homeland Security and Governmental Affairs on June 27, 2018, at the hearing entitled “Medicaid Fraud and Overpayments: Problems and Solutions.”

Sincerely,

Brian P. Ritchie
Assistant Inspector General

Enclosure:
Responses to Questions for the Record

HHS OIG Response to Post-Hearing Questions for the Record from Senator McCaskill, Submitted to Brian P. Ritchie, "Medicaid Fraud and Overpayments: Problems and Solutions"

Pre-Existing Conditions-Overall Impact

When enacted in 2010, the Affordable Care Act (ACA) reformed the health insurance market. These reforms eliminated annual and lifetime caps, required free preventive services, guaranteed coverage of maternity care, and allowed children to stay on their parents' insurance until age 26. Most importantly, for the first time, the ACA required insurance companies to provide health insurance to everyone, regardless of their medical conditions. UndeFthe ACA, insurance companies were prohibited from charging individuals more based on their health status.

Unfortunately, Republicans want to return to a health care system where insurers are free to deny people coverage for medical care when they need it most. A group of Republican Attorneys General have challenged the constitutionality of the ACA and the Department of Justice has said that they would no longer defend key provisions of the law.

1. If the Republicans are successful in challenging the constitutionality of the ACA, and the protections for individuals with pre-existing conditions are eliminated as a result, what impact will this have on as many as 130 million adults living with pre-existing conditions?

Our marketplace work, https://oig.hhs.gov/reports-and-publications/aca/, focused on topics related to HHS dollars and operations (for example, establishment grants, advance premium tax credits, and eligibility). We have not conducted work related to the Affordable Care Act (ACA) provision regarding coverage for individuals with pre-existing conditions. We therefore do not have any findings or recommendations relevant to the pre-existing condition requirements.

2. Allowing insurance companies to again discriminate on the basis of pre-existing conditions would create havoc on the health sector. Has the Department of Health and Human Services (HHS) Office of Inspector General (OIG) initiated any investigative work to examine the effects of removing pre-existing condition protections? Does HHS OIG intend to investigate this matter?

Our marketplace work, https://oig.hhs.gov/reports-and-publications/aca/. focused on topics related to HHS dollars and operations (for example, establishment grants, advance premium tax credits, and eligibility). We have not initiated work related to pre- existing condition protections. We have no plans to investigate this matter. We typically do not conduct reviews of the potential impact of pending changes but rather review programs as currently operating to ensure that they are meeting intended objectives. All new work is evaluated as part of our normal work planning process and undergoes a risk assessment and legal analysis to ensure we have jurisdiction.

Pre-Existing Conditions - Energy and Commerce Report

Republicans want to return to a time when insurance companies could discriminate against people based on their past medical conditions. Prior to the passage of the ACA, insurance companies could refuse to provide health insurance to any one- even children- because of their past medical history. Alternatively, insurers could offer individuals a skimpy policy and refuse to cover any medical treatment for a disclosed pre-existing condition. Finally, if an individual made one mistake on their forms- even a clerical mistake- insurers could rescind an individual's health insurance coverage when a person needed it the most.

In 2010, the House Energy and Commerce Committee investigated the extent of coverage denials and exclusions for pre-existing conditions in the individual health insurance market. The report analyzes data from the four largest for-profit health insurance companies, Aetna, Humana, UnitedHealth Group, and Well Point. In the three years prior to the passage of health reform, these four insurance companies denied over 600,000 individuals coverage because of pre-existing conditions.

3. If companies are allowed to deny health insurance coverage to individuals based on pre-existing conditions, is it likely that the four largest health insurers and others will deny coverage to more than half a million people based solely on pre-existing conditions?

Please see our response to question 1.

4. On average, the four companies denied coverage to one out of every seven applicants based on a pre-existing condition. If we removed the protections of the ACA, what would happen to those people with pre-existing conditions?

Please see our response to question 1.

5. The committee obtained a list of over 400 medical diagnoses that triggered a permanent denial of health insurance coverage to applicants. Can you explain your understanding of the types of medical conditions that used to trigger permanent denials of insurance?

Please see our response to question 1.

Pre-existing conditions that health insurers routinely declined to cover included, "[a]ny applicant who is a surgical candidate," "[a]ny female applicant currently pregnant," and "[a]ny applicant with a BMI [body mass index] of 39.0 or greater."

6. If companies are allowed to decline coverage for pre-existing conditions once again, is it likely that individuals with the conditions listed above will be denied coverage?

Please see our response to question 1.

T-MSIS

HHS OIG previously testified that "a quality national Medicaid dataset is essential to states' and the Federal Government's ability to effectively and collaboratively administer and ensure the integrity of Medicaid." To accomplish this, HHS OIG recommended that CMS set a deadline for when national T-MSIS data will be available for multi-state program integrity efforts.

7. As of August 2017, CMS had yet to outline how best to use T-MSIS data for program monitoring, oversight, and management. Has CMS articulated a specific plan and associated time frame for using T-MSIS data for oversight as GAO recommended?

To DIG's knowledge, CMS has not publicly articulated a specific time frame. The 2013 DIG recommendation that CMS establish a deadline for when T-MSIS data will be available for program analysis and other management functions remains open. We continue to follow up with CMS to monitor the status of this recommendation and promote its implementation. DIG notes that in June 2018, CMS announced efforts it is taking to improve program integrity in the Medicaid program. CMS's strategy is outlined here: https://www.medicaid.gov/state-resource-center/downloads/program-integrity-strategy-factsheet. pdf.

8. With the full implementation of T-MSIS as recommended, how much of a reduction in improper payments and fraud can we expect to see?

Having quality, useable national T-MSIS data is essential for program integrity and for CMS's, States', DIG's, and others' efforts to prevent, detect, and respond to fraud, waste, and abuse. While we cannot project exactly how many dollars may be saved through prevention of improper payments and fraud and through audit and investigative recoveries, we expect the positive return on investment to be substantial.

PRIVATE HEALTH INSURANCE: DATA ON APPLICATION AND COVERAGE DENIALS*

Why GAO Did This Study

The large percentage of Americans that rely on private health insurance for health care coverage could expand with enactment of the Patient Protection and Affordable Care Act (PPACA) of 2010. Until PPACA is fully implemented, some consumers seeking coverage can have their applications for enrollment denied, and those enrolled may face denials of coverage for specific medical services. PPACA required GAO to study the rates of such application and coverage denials. GAO reviewed the data available on denials of

1) applications for enrollment and
2) coverage for medical services.

GAO reviewed newly available nationwide data collected by the Department of Health and Human Services (HHS) from 459 insurers operating in the individual market on application denials from January through March 2010. GAO also reviewed a year or more of the available data from six states on the rates of application and coverage denials and the rates and outcomes of appeals related to coverage denials. The six states included all states identified by experts and in the literature as collecting data on the rates of application or coverage denials and together represented over 20 percent of private health insurance enrollment nationally. GAO conducted a literature review to identify studies related to application and coverage denials and reviewed data from selected studies. GAO interviewed HHS and state officials and researchers about factors to consider when interpreting the data.

What GAO Found

The available data indicated variation in application denial rates, and there are several issues to consider in interpreting those rates. Nationwide data collected by HHS from insurers showed that the aggregate application denial rate for the first quarter of 2010 was 19 percent, but that denial rates varied significantly across insurers. For example, just over a quarter of insurers had application denial rates from 0 percent to 15 percent while

* This is an edited, reformatted and augmented version of United States Government Accountability Office; Report to the Secretary of Health and Human Services and the Secretary of Labor, Publication No. GAO-11-268, dated March 2011.

another quarter of insurers had rates of 40 percent or higher. Data reported by Maryland—the only of the six states in GAO's review identified as collecting data on the incidence of application denials—indicated that variation in application denial rates across insurers has occurred for several years, with rates ranging from about 6 percent to over 30 percent in each of 3 years. The available data provided little information on the reasons that applications were denied. There are also several issues to consider when interpreting application denial rates. For example, the rates may not provide a clear estimate of the number of individuals that were ultimately able to secure coverage, as individuals can apply to multiple insurers, and the rates do not reflect applicants that have been offered coverage with a premium that is higher than the standard rate.

The available data from the six states in GAO's review and others indicated that the rates of coverage denials, including rates of denials of preauthorizations and claims, also varied significantly. The state data indicated that coverage denial rates varied significantly across states, with aggregate rates of claim denials ranging from 11 percent to 24 percent across the three states that collected such data. In addition, rates varied significantly across insurers, with data from one state indicating a range in claim denial rates from 6 percent to 40 percent across six large insurers operating in the state. There are several factors that may have contributed to the variation in rates across states and insurers, such as states varying in the types of denials they require insurers to report. The data also indicated that coverage denials occurred for a variety of reasons, frequently for billing errors, such as duplicate claims or missing information on the claim, and eligibility issues, such as services being provided before coverage was initiated, and less often for judgments about the appropriateness of a service. Further, the data GAO reviewed indicated that coverage denials, if appealed, were frequently reversed in the consumer's favor. For example, data from four of the six states on the outcomes of appeals filed with insurers indicated that 39 percent to 59 percent of appeals resulted in the insurer reversing its original coverage denial. Data from a national study conducted by a trade association for insurance companies on the outcomes of appeals filed with states for an independent, external review indicated that coverage denials were reversed about 40 percent of the time.

GAO provided a draft of the report to HHS and the Department of Labor (DOL). HHS agreed with GAO's findings, noting the need to improve the quality and scope of existing data, and suggested clarifications, which were incorporated. HHS and DOL also provided technical comments, which were incorporated as appropriate.

Abbreviations

AHIP	America's Health Insurance Plans
AMA	American Medical Association

DOL	Department of Labor
ERISA	Employee Retirement Income Security Act of 1974
HHS	Department of Health and Human Services
HIPAA	Health Insurance Portability and Accountability Act of 1996
HMO	health maintenance organization
HRP	high-risk health insurance pool
NAIC	National Association of Insurance Commissioners
PPACA	Patient Protection and Affordable Care Act
PPO	preferred provider organization

United States Government Accountability Office
Washington, DC 20548

March 16, 2011

The Honorable Kathleen Sebelius
Secretary of Health and Human Services

The Honorable Hilda L. Solis
Secretary of Labor

A large majority of Americans—nearly 64 percent as of 2009—rely on private insurance for health care coverage, most through employer- sponsored group health coverage.[294] With the enactment of the Patient Protection and Affordable Care Act (PPACA) in March 2010,[295] enrollment in private health insurance could expand significantly, particularly for individuals and families that do not have access to group coverage through their employer. While there are certain federal requirements protecting against the denial of applications for enrollment for individuals eligible for group coverage, until PPACA is fully implemented, these protections do not apply to some consumers seeking individual coverage from private health insurers.[296] In addition, once consumers are enrolled in either group or individual coverage, coverage can be denied for specific medical services, either through a denial of authorization of a service before it

[294] Private health insurance includes all forms of health insurance that are not funded by the government and may be purchased on an individual or group basis.

[295] Pub. L. No. 111-148, 124 Stat. 119 (Mar. 23, 2010), as amended by the Health Care and Education Reconciliation Act of 2010, Pub. L. No. 111-152, 124 Stat.1029 (Mar. 30, 2010).

[296] Throughout this chapter, the term "insurer" refers to commercial, state-licensed issuers of health insurance coverage and entities such as health maintenance organizations (HMO). Insurers can offer coverage in the group market, individual market, or both. In this chapter, the term "insurer" does not include self-funded group health plans where instead of purchasing health insurance from an insurance company an employer sets aside its own funds to pay for at least some of its employees' health care.

has been provided or payment for a service that has been delivered.[297] There are some national data on the extent to which applications for enrollment are being denied; however, there is not yet any comprehensive, national information on the extent to which coverage for medical services is being denied when consumers seek health care. The federal government plans to collect additional information on the extent of denials of applications for enrollment and coverage for medical services and the reasons for those denials, with the intent to make it easier for consumers to shop for coverage. According to experts, those data may also help with government oversight of private health insurance.

Oversight of private health insurance has been a responsibility of state departments of insurance, and states vary in what they require of insurers and the degree to which they track insurers' activities, including the extent to which insurers are denying applications and coverage. The federal government's role in the oversight of private health insurance has included, for example, the establishment of certain consumer protections for states to enforce. It also includes oversight of employer-based coverage performed by the Department of Labor (DOL). However, the federal government's role has expanded with the enactment of PPACA. PPACA required the Department of Health and Human Services (HHS) to begin collecting, monitoring, and publishing information on health insurance products. HHS began publishing data from insurers on denials of applications for enrollment in October 2010 and intends to collect data in the future on denials of coverage for medical services.

PPACA directed us to study denials of applications for enrollment and coverage for medical services by considering samples of data related to such denials, including the reasons for the denials and favorably resolved disputes resulting from the denials.[298] Specifically, we reviewed (1) the data available on denials of applications for enrollment and (2) the data available on denials of coverage for medical services.

To describe the data available on denials of applications for enrollment— referred to as application denials in this chapter—we reviewed federal, state, and other data including data on the rates of and reasons for such denials. First, we reviewed data recently collected by HHS from 459 insurers operating in the individual market in all 50 states and the District of Columbia.[299] The data included application denial rates by insurer for a 3-month period—January through March—in 2010.[300] To supplement the single calendar quarter of HHS data, we contacted insurance department officials in six states regarding data on application and coverage denials.[301] The six states include all the states identified by experts and in the literature as states that collect data from insurers on

[297] Throughout this chapter, we refer to denials of authorization for services not yet provided as "preauthorization denials" and denials of payment for services rendered as "claim denials."

[298] PPACA also directed that we submit our report to the Secretaries of HHS and DOL. Pub. L. No. 111-148, § 10107, 124 Stat. 911-2.

[299] The data were reported by state-licensed health insurers offering coverage in the individual market.

[300] This is the only quarter of data that HHS had collected as of December 2010.

[301] The six states we selected to contact were California, Connecticut, Florida, Maryland, New York, and Ohio.

the incidence of application denials, coverage denials, or both. Because we did not survey all states to determine whether they collect data on the incidence of application or coverage denials, or both, there may be other states that collect such data that were not known to experts or discussed in the literature.[302] Of the six states, we identified one, Maryland, that collected data on application denials. We reviewed data from Maryland for 2008, 2009, and the first half of 2010 on the rate of application denials by insurers operating in the individual market in that state. (See app. I for more information about our methodology for selecting states and the state data we reviewed.) We also conducted a structured literature review to identify studies related to application and coverage denials.[303] We determined that a study was directly relevant to our objective on application denial data if it included empirical analyses of the frequency of application denials. Through our review, we identified four studies that met our criteria. Two of these four studies, produced by America's Health Insurance Plans (AHIP), included data on application denial rates in 2006 and 2008, and we reviewed those data. (See app. II for a description of the literature review methodology and the list of studies identified through the review.) Finally, we interviewed officials from HHS, Maryland, and AHIP about factors to consider when interpreting the data. We also interviewed officials from three large insurance companies about the data they collect on application denials.[304]

To describe the data available on denials of coverage for medical services—referred to as coverage denials in this chapter—we reviewed state and other data, including data on the rates of and reasons for denials and the outcomes of appeals related to denials, such as disputes resolved in favor of consumers. First, of the same six states we contacted regarding application denial data, we reviewed the most recent year of data available on the rate of coverage denials from the four that reported collecting such data.[305] Second, we reviewed data on the outcomes of appeals related to coverage denials from all of the six states for the most recent year available. We also interviewed officials from departments of insurance and other departments involved in overseeing insurance or responding to appeals in the six states about considerations for interpreting the data. To supplement the information from selected states, we reviewed data reported by 49 states and the District of Columbia to the National Association of Insurance Commissioners (NAIC) on the number of complaints related to coverage denials resolved in 2009 and the

[302] For example, through the course of our work, we found that Texas requires certain insurers to report on the number of requests for preauthorization of coverage for proposed services that insurers declined.

[303] To conduct this review, we searched a number of reference databases, such as EconLit and Social SciSearch, for peer-reviewed, industry, or government studies published from January 2000 through July 2010. In addition, we checked the bibliographies of the studies and interviewed a number of experts regarding the research done on private health insurance denials to identify other relevant studies.

[304] The insurance companies we contacted offered coverage in both the individual and group markets and, according to AHIP, were among the 10 largest by enrollment, together accounting for nearly 26 million enrollees.

[305] The data obtained from states on the incidence of coverage denials were not broken out by the types of medical services being denied.

reasons for and outcomes of those complaints.[306] We also reviewed information on the outcomes of complaints and appeals submitted by 35 states and the District of Columbia to HHS in applications for Consumer Assistance Program grants.[307] As part of our literature review, we identified studies that included empirical analyses of the frequency of coverage denials, the reasons for such denials, the frequency of appeals of coverage denials, or the outcomes of such appeals. Through the review, we identified annual studies produced by the American Medical Association (AMA) in 2008, 2009, and 2010 that included data on the incidence and reasons for claim denials. We reviewed data from the 2010 study and interviewed AMA officials about factors to consider when interpreting the data. Finally, we reviewed data from DOL on complaints related to coverage denials for those with employer-sponsored coverage from fiscal year 2010, including the number and value of financial recoveries made by the department on behalf of consumers as a result of complaints.

To assess the reliability of the data we reviewed on the incidence of application and coverage denials, the reasons for such denials, and the outcomes of appeals and complaints related to those denials, we interviewed federal, state, and other officials about their efforts to ensure the quality of the data. This included discussing whether they required insurers to certify the accuracy of data reported on the incidence of application or coverage denials and what steps were taken to ensure the quality of data tracked by states and DOL on the outcomes of appeals and complaints related to denials. We also asked officials about the limitations of the data and reviewed any statements about data limitations in published reports of the data. We determined the data to be sufficiently reliable for the purposes of describing the (1) denial rates, (2) reasons for denials, and (3) outcomes of appeals related to denials indicated by the data; where relevant we stated the limitations of the data in the findings.

We conducted our performance audit from September 2010 through January 2011 in accordance with generally accepted government auditing standards. Those standards require that we plan and perform the audit to obtain sufficient, appropriate evidence to provide a reasonable basis for our findings and conclusions based on our audit objectives. We believe that the evidence obtained provides a reasonable basis for our findings and conclusions based on our audit objectives.

---

306 State regulators established NAIC to help promote effective insurance regulation, to encourage uniformity in approaches to regulation, and to help coordinate states' activities. Among other activities, NAIC collects data from state regulators on insurers, including complaints about insurer practices filed by consumers with states. We requested NAIC to provide us with data on the number of complaints reported by states that were related to coverage denials. The complaint data did not include information on the type of service for which coverage was denied.

307 Under PPACA, $30 million was appropriated to the Secretary of HHS for the award of federal grants to states to establish, expand, or provide support for offices of health insurance consumer assistance or health insurance ombudsmen programs. Pub. L. No. 111- 148, § 1002, 124 Stat. 138. To receive these grants, called Consumer Assistance Program grants, states must ensure that their programs assist consumers with such tasks as enrolling in health coverage and filing complaints and appeals. In the applications for the grants, HHS directed states to report on complaints and appeals. States varied in the data they included in their application and the time frames for those data.

Background

In 2009, approximately 156 million nonelderly individuals obtained health insurance through their employer and another 16.7 million purchased health insurance in the individual market. Of those with employer-sponsored group health plans, in 2009, 43 percent were covered under a fully insured plan where the employer pays a per-employee premium to an insurance company.[308] The remaining 57 percent were covered under self-funded plans where instead of purchasing health insurance from an insurance company the employer sets aside its own funds to pay for at least some of its employees' health care.[309]

Application Denials

Application denials result when an insurer determines that it will not offer coverage to an applicant either because the applicant does not meet eligibility requirements or because the insurer determines that the applicant is too high of a risk to insure. Underwriting is a process conducted by insurers to assess an applicant's health status and other risk factors to determine whether and on what terms to offer coverage to an applicant.

Many consumers are protected from having their application for enrollment denied. Consumers who obtain health coverage through their employment by enrolling in a group health plan sponsored by their employer have certain protections against application denials. For example, under federal law, individuals enrolling in group health plan coverage are protected from being denied enrollment because of their health status.[310] Under federal law, insurers also generally are prohibited from denying applications for

---

[308] Throughout this chapter, the term "group health plan" refers to employer-sponsored health plans, including both fully insured and self-funded plans.

[309] As of 2009, 85 percent of small employers, those with 3 to 199 employees, that offered health benefits were fully insured while 88 percent of large employers, those with 5,000 or more employees, offered self-funded plans. See The Kaiser Family Foundation and Health Research & Educational Trust, *Employer Health Benefits: 2009 Annual Survey* (2009).

[310] Group health plans and health insurance issuers offering group coverage are prohibited from implementing eligibility rules based on health-status-related factors defined as health status, medical condition, claims experience, receipt of health care, medical history, genetic information, evidence of insurability, or disability. See, for example, 42 U.S.C. § 300gg-1 (2006). PPACA extends this prohibition to health insurance issuers offering coverage in the individual market for plan years beginning on or after January 1, 2014. Pub. L. No. 111-148, § 1201(4), 124 Stat. 156.

Health insurance issuers that offer coverage in the small group market in a state generally are required to accept every small employer that applies for health coverage in that state. In addition, issuers cannot deny an application for enrollment by individuals employed by such employers due to health-status-related factors if the individuals apply when they are first eligible. See 42 U.S.C. § 300gg-11 (2006). For plan years beginning on or after January 1, 2014, PPACA requires health insurance issuers offering group or individual coverage in a state to accept every employer and individual that applies for coverage in that state, subject to certain requirements. Pub. L. No. 111-148, § 1201(4), 124 Stat. 156.

individual health coverage for certain individuals leaving group health plan coverage and applying for coverage in the individual market.[311]

Currently, some consumers who apply for private health insurance through the individual market can have their applications denied for eligibility reasons or as a result of underwriting. For example, applications filed by some consumers with preexisting health conditions can be denied, unless prohibited by state or federal law.[312] Additionally, insurers may accept the application but offer coverage at a premium level that is higher than the standard rate or that excludes coverage for certain benefits. The options for appealing application denials in the individual market can be limited to filing a complaint with the state department of insurance.

However, in 35 states, individuals who—due to a preexisting health condition—have been denied enrollment or charged higher premiums in the individual market are typically eligible for coverage through high-risk health insurance pools (HRP).[313] Additionally, as required under PPACA, individuals who have preexisting health conditions and have been uninsured for 6 months are eligible for enrollment in a temporary national HRP program.[314]

Coverage Denials

Coverage for medical services can be denied before or after the service has been provided, either through denial of preauthorization requests or denial of claims for payment. As a condition for coverage of some services, providers or consumers are required to request authorization prior to providing or receiving the service. Preauthorization denials occur when a determination is made that (1) the consumer is not

---

[311] Health insurance issuers offering individual coverage are prohibited from denying coverage for individuals who (1) have had at least 18 months of prior creditable coverage with no break of more than 63 days; (2) have exhausted any available continuation of coverage; (3) are uninsured and are not eligible for other group coverage, Medicare, or Medicaid; and (4) did not lose group coverage because of the nonpayment of premiums or fraud. See 42 U.S.C. § 300gg-41 (2006). As referenced above, PPACA requires health insurance issuers to guarantee coverage to all individuals seeking coverage in that state for plan years beginning on or after January 1, 2014, subject to certain requirements.

[312] According to data from the Kaiser Family Foundation, as of January 2010, six states have guaranteed issue requirements that prohibit any insurer from denying coverage to an individual based on their current medical conditions or risk of poor health. Another seven states have guaranteed issue requirements that only apply to certain insurance plans or during limited times during the year.
As referenced above, in certain circumstances, federal law also protects consumers seeking individual coverage from application denials. For example, health insurance issuers cannot deny applications for eligible consumers who had prior group or other coverage.

[313] See GAO, *Health Insurance: Enrollment, Benefits, Funding, and Other Characteristics of State High-Risk Health Insurance Pools*, GAO-09-730R (Washington, D.C.: July 22, 2009).

[314] The temporary national HRP program will terminate in 2014. Pub. L. No. 111-148, § 1101, 124 Stat. 141. As referenced above, for plan years beginning on or after January 1, 2014, PPACA prohibits health insurance issuers offering individual coverage from implementing eligibility rules based on health status-related factors and requires health insurance issuers offering individual coverage to accept every individual in the state who applies for coverage, subject to certain requirements. In addition, PPACA prohibits group health plans and insurers offering group and individual coverage from excluding coverage for pre- existing health conditions. This prohibition is generally effective for plan years beginning on or after January 1, 2014 for adults and plan years beginning on or after September 23, 2010 for individuals under age 19. Pub. L. No. 111-148, § 1201(2), 10103(e), (f), 124 Stat. 154, 895.

eligible to receive the requested service, for example, because the service is not covered under the individual's policy, or (2) the service is not appropriate, meaning that it is not medically necessary or is experimental or investigational. Denials of claims occur for various reasons. Claims may be denied for billing reasons, such as the provider failing to include a piece of required information on the claim, such as documentation that the provider received preauthorization for a service, or submitting a duplicate claim. Claims may also be denied because of eligibility issues. For example, a claim may be submitted for a service provided before an individual's coverage began or after it was terminated, or a claim may be submitted for a service that has been excluded from coverage under an individual's policy. Another reason for denials reported by some insurers is that the individual has not met the cost-sharing requirements of his or her policy, such as the required deductible. Finally, claim denials can occur when a determination is made that the service provided was not appropriate, specifically that the service was not medically necessary or was experimental or investigational. Depending on the reason for a claim denial, either the provider or the consumer may bear the financial responsibility for the denied coverage amount. Claims that are denied because of such billing errors as the provider not providing a required piece of information can be resubmitted and ultimately paid.

For claim denials, the full claim may be denied or, if the claim contained multiple lines, such as a surgery with charges for multiple procedures and supplies, only certain lines of the claim may be denied. How insurers and self-funded group health plans track claim denials and the reasons for denials may vary. For example, AMA officials noted that there is no guidebook for how reason codes should be assigned to claim denials. Officials noted that denials are often assigned the code for the most general reason even though the denial may be for a more specific reason.

Consumers have several avenues available to dispute coverage denials. First, consumers can file an appeal of a denial with the insurer or self-funded group health plan for review, referred to as an internal appeal. Internal appeals can result in the denial being upheld or reversed. In addition, consumers in most states can have their appeal reviewed by an external party, such as an independent medical review panel established by the state.[315] These appeals, referred to as external appeals, can also result in denials being reversed and in states recovering funds for consumers for the cost of the denied service. State external appeal options may only be available once the consumer has exhausted the internal appeal process or for consumers with certain types of coverage.

Historically, those with self-funded group health plans generally did not have access to an external appeal process, but consumers could file suit against a health plan in court to challenge a denial. PPACA, however, required that group health plans, including self-

[315] According to research completed by AHIP, as of January 2006, 44 states and the District of Columbia operated external review programs. Such programs are generally available to consumers purchasing coverage from insurers regulated by states.

funded plans, provide access to an external appeal process that meets federal standards for plan years beginning on or after September 2010.[316] Finally, consumers may file complaints regarding coverage denials with the state, generally the department of insurance, or, for those with group health plans, with DOL.

Filing a complaint can be a less formal mechanism for disputing a coverage denial than filing an appeal; however, complaints can result in reversals of denials and in financial recoveries for consumers.

State and Federal Oversight of Private Health Insurance

States have responsibility for regulating private health insurance, including insurers operating in the individual market and the fully insured group market. In overseeing insurer activity, states vary in the data they require insurers to submit on denials and internal appeals of denials. According to NAIC officials, few states require insurers to report data regularly on the frequency of denials and internal appeals, and NAIC has not issued any model laws or regulations that include requirements for insurers to report such data. States also may use data on complaints and external appeals to identify trends in the practices of insurers and target examinations of specific insurers' practices. Nearly all states and the District of Columbia regularly report complaint data, which includes information on the numbers of, reasons for, and outcomes of complaints, to NAIC.

Historically, the federal government's role in oversight of private health insurance has included establishing requirements for states to enforce. For example, the Health Insurance Portability and Accountability Act of 1996 (HIPAA) established consumer protections on access, portability, and renewability of coverage.[317] In addition, with respect to group health plans, the federal government enforces disclosure, reporting, fiduciary, and claims-filing requirements under the Employee Retirement Income Security Act of 1974 (ERISA).[318] DOL conducts a number of efforts to enforce the

---

[316] Under PPACA and implementing regulations, group health plans and health insurance issuers offering group or individual coverage, subject to certain exceptions, must comply with a state external review process that, at a minimum, includes consumer protections identified in the NAIC Uniform External Review Model Act. If a state external review process does not incorporate these consumer protections or a self-insured group health plan is not required to comply with the state external review process, then the health plan must follow a federal external review process. Pub. L. No. 111-148, §§ 1001(5), 10101(g), 124 Stat. 137, 887; *Interim Final Rules for Group Health Plans and Health Insurance Issuers Relating to Internal Claims and Appeals and External Review Processes under PPACA*, 75 Fed. Reg. 43,330 (July 23, 2010).

[317] For example, with respect to those leaving group coverage and applying for coverage in the individual market, HIPAA prohibited health insurance issuers from denying coverage for individuals who (1) have had at least 18 months of prior creditable coverage with no break of more than 63 days; (2) have exhausted any available continuation of coverage; (3) are uninsured and are not eligible for other group coverage, Medicare, or Medicaid; and (4) did not lose group coverage because of the nonpayment of premiums or fraud. See 42 U.S.C. § 300gg-41 (2006).

[318] ERISA established certain federal requirements that apply when employers offer their employees, retirees, and dependents employee benefit plans that include health coverage, retirement plans such as pensions, and other benefits such as life insurance. See Pub. L. No. 93-406, 88 Stat. 829 (1974). ERISA requirements generally apply regardless of the size of the business, although some requirements are streamlined for smaller employers. ERISA imposes certain reporting and disclosure requirements, fiduciary obligations, and requirements for claims-filing procedures. ERISA is enforced through DOL's Employee Benefits Security

ERISA requirements. For example, the department conducts civil investigations that can result in corrective actions, such as monetary recoveries for consumers who are enrolled in employment-based plans. In addition to these formal methods, DOL also works to resolve complaints filed with the department. These efforts are considered informal resolutions, although complaints can also serve as a trigger for formal enforcement actions.

PPACA expanded the federal oversight role by requiring HHS to begin collecting, monitoring, and publishing data from certain insurers. Specifically, PPACA required the establishment of an internet Web site through which individuals can identify affordable health insurance coverage options in their state.[319] To implement this requirement, in May 2010, HHS issued an interim final rule requiring insurers in the individual and small group markets to submit data to HHS on their products, including data on the number of enrollees, geographic availability of the products, and customer service contact information, by May 21, 2010, and annually after that.[320] In July 2010, HHS began publishing these data on the new Web site, which is designed for individuals and small businesses to obtain information on coverage options available in their state. In October 2010, HHS began posting additional data collected from insurers, including data on the percentage of applications denied for each product offered in the individual market. The interim final rule also required insurers to submit other data, such as data on the percentage of claims denied in the individual and small group markets, and the number and outcomes of appeals of denials to insure, pay claims, and provide preauthorization, in accordance with guidance to be issued by HHS. As of December 2010, HHS had not issued any guidance on reporting these additional data.

Federal, State, and Other Data Indicated Variation in Application Denial Rates and Provided Little Information on the Reasons for Denials

Nationwide data from HHS showed variation in application denial rates across insurers operating in the individual market. Specifically, data collected by HHS from 459 state-licensed insurers on the number of applications received and denied from January through March 2010 indicated that, while the aggregate rate of application denials was 19 percent nationally, the rate varied significantly across insurers. For example, just over a quarter of insurers had application denial rates from 0 percent to 15 percent while another

---

Administration. PPACA expands upon ERISA's requirements for claims- filing procedures by applying new standards for internal claims appeals and for external claims review processes, as referenced above. Pub. L. No. 111-148, §§ 1001(5), 10101(g), 137, 887.

[319] Pub. L. No. 111-148, §§ 1103, 10102(b), 124 Stat. 146, 892. The Web site is www.healthcare.gov.

[320] Health Care Reform Insurance Web Portal Requirements, 75 Fed. Reg. 24,470 (May, 5, 2010).

quarter of insurers had rates of 40 percent or higher.[321] However, the insurers with rates of 40 percent or higher reported fewer applications. See Table 5 for additional information on the range in application denial rates across insurers.

Table 5. Range of application denial rates among state-licensed insurers, based on HHS data, January-March 2010

Application denial rates (percentage of applications denied)	Number of insurers reporting rates in range[a]	Number of applications received[b]
0 to 15	132	499,239
16 to 23	102	471,878
24 to 39	113	230,846
40 or higher	112[c]	57,923

Source: GAO analysis of HHS data.

[a]Data were reported to HHS by 459 state-licensed insurers operating in 50 states and the District of Columbia. Data on insurers operating in states with guaranteed issue requirements that prohibit any insurer from denying coverage to an individual based on his or her current medical conditions or risk of poor health were included in the analysis.

[b]Insurers were instructed to report the number of applications received for products offering comprehensive medical coverage. HHS officials told us that they identified instances where insurers included data on applications for more limited products, such as one that covers only hospital services. The application data may also include applications for products being sold for only a portion of the 3-month period.

[c]The data indicated that two insurers had denial rates of 100 percent and each of these insurers reported receiving one application in the 3-month reporting period.

HHS officials noted that the data the department collected on application denials, which represent a single calendar quarter of applications, are only a starting point. They told us that as insurers report additional quarters of data, the value and usefulness of the data will increase. In addition, officials said that they have taken steps to ensure the accuracy of the data and noted that the accuracy of these data is critical to HHS, because no other source of information on private health insurance has a complete catalog of insurers operating in the individual market and what products those insurers are selling.

Data reported by Maryland—the only state we identified as collecting data on the incidence of application denials—indicated that variation in application denial rates across insurers operating in the state's individual market has occurred in that state for several years. Maryland data showed that the range of application denial rates across insurers was 26 percentage points or more in each of three reporting periods, 2008, 2009, and the first half of 2010. (See Table 6 for the range in denial rates in the data reported by Maryland.)

[321] The data indicated that two insurers had denial rates of 100 percent and each of these insurers reported receiving one application in the 3-month reporting period.

Table 6. Range in application denial rates across insurers licensed in Maryland, 2008-2010

Data year	Range in application denial rates (percentage of applications denied)	Number of insurers represented in the data	Number of applications received	Aggregate application denial rate (percentage)
2008	6 to 34	11	98,612	14
2009	7 to 33	11	107,617	14
2010 (first half)	6 to 45	11	47,791	16

Source: GAO analysis of data from Maryland.

Note: Data are from 2008, 2009, and the first two quarters of calendar year 2010 and reported by insurers to Maryland.

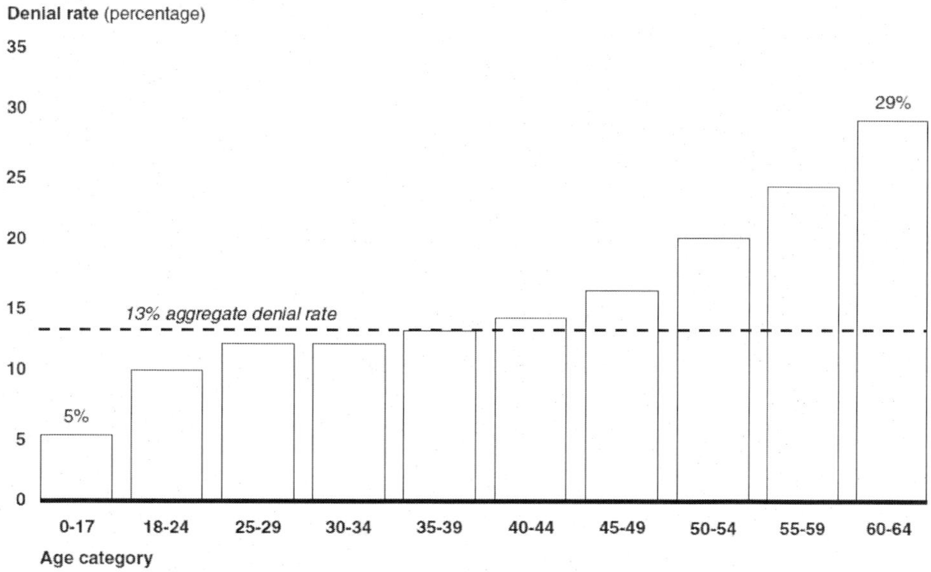

Source: GAO analysis of data reported by AHIP.

Note: Data are from AHIP, Individual Health Insurance 2009: A Comprehensive Survey of Premiums, Availability, and Benefits (Washington, D.C.: 2009).

Figure 3. Application Denial Rates by Age Group for 2008, as Reported by AHIP.

Data reported in studies by AHIP also showed variation in application denial rates. The AHIP data illustrated that application denial rates varied across age groups, with denial rates increasing as the age of the primary applicant increased. In 2008, when AHIP data showed that 13 percent of all medically underwritten applications were denied,[322] in general the denial rate progressively increased as the applicant's age increased, from a low of 5 percent for applicants under 18 years of age to a high of 29 percent for

[322] In 2008, according to AHIP data, 84 percent of applications were medically underwritten and 16 percent were not medically underwritten. Just over 1 percent of applications were denied before going through medical underwriting, and those denials were unrelated to the applicant's health status.

applicants from 60 to 64 years of age.[323] Similar variation in AHIP application denial rates was seen in data from 2006.[324] (See Figure 3.)

The available data on application denial rates provided little information on the reasons that applications were denied. For instance, the HHS and Maryland data did not include any information on the reasons for application denials. The AHIP data, however, provided limited information. Specifically, AHIP's data showed that a higher percentage of applications were denied because of the applicant's health status than for nonmedical reasons, such as the plan not being offered in the applicant's geographic area. AHIP data showed that in 2008, of the 1.8 million applications for enrollment that insurers either denied or made offers of coverage, 1 percent were denied for nonmedical reasons and 12 percent were denied after underwriting when the applicant's health status and other risk factors were assessed. According to an AHIP official, applications that were denied after underwriting were presumably denied because the applicant's medical questionnaire responses were beyond the insurer's threshold for issuing a policy.

There are several issues to consider when interpreting application denial rates. First, application denial rates may not provide a clear estimate of the number of individuals that were ultimately able to secure health coverage, because individuals may submit applications with more than one insurer and be denied by one insurer but offered enrollment by another. Second, denial rates also do not reflect applications that have been withdrawn. For example, AHIP data for 2008 indicated that 8 percent of applicants withdrew their applications before underwriting occurred. Experts also noted that some individuals may not submit applications for health coverage because they believe or have been advised, for example by an insurance agent, that their application would likely be denied. Third, an insurer's denial rates may be affected by requirements of the states in which the insurer operates. For example, officials from one insurance company explained that for applicants in the state for which they are the insurer of last resort, state law prohibits them from denying applications for enrollment based on the health status of the applicant.[325] Officials told us that a denial can occur only for nonmedical eligibility reasons, which the AHIP data indicate are far less frequent.

Another consideration when interpreting application denial rates is that the rates do not reflect applications that have been accepted by an insurer but for coverage with a premium that is higher than the standard rate or with exclusions for coverage of specified services. Data from HHS, Maryland, and AHIP all indicated that some portion of

---

[323] America's Health Insurance Plans, *Individual Health Insurance 2009: A Comprehensive Survey of Premiums, Availability, and Benefits* (Washington, D.C.: 2009). (See app. II for references to the AHIP study and other studies with information on application denial rates identified through our literature review.)

[324] America's Health Insurance Plans, *Individual Health Insurance 2006–2007: A Comprehensive Survey of Premiums, Availability, and Benefits* (Washington, D.C.: 2007).

[325] According to data from the Kaiser Family Foundation, as of January 2010, four states— Michigan, Pennsylvania, Rhode Island, and Virginia—and the District of Columbia have insurers of last resort, which are insurers that typically accept consumers with health conditions that prevent those consumers from obtaining coverage in the individual market.

applicants received offers at a premium that was higher than the standard rate. For example, the HHS data demonstrated that from January through March of 2010, about 20 percent of individual market applicants were offered coverage with premiums higher than the standard rate. Maryland data also indicated that for the first half of 2010, 8 percent of applicants were offered either coverage with premiums higher than the standard rate or coverage that excluded specified health conditions. Finally, AHIP data from 2008 showed that 34 percent of offers for coverage were for coverage at a higher premium rate. The AHIP data also showed that 6 percent of offers for coverage were for coverage that excluded specified health conditions.

State and Other Data Indicated That Coverage Denial Rates and the Reasons for Denials Vary and That Denials, If Appealed, Are Often Reversed

Data from selected states and others indicated that the rates of coverage denials, including denials for preauthorizations and claims, varied significantly, and a number of factors may have contributed to that variation. The data also indicated that coverage denials occurred for a variety of reasons, frequently for billing errors and eligibility issues and less often for judgments about the appropriateness of a service. Further, the data we reviewed indicated that coverage denials, if appealed, were frequently reversed in the consumer's favor and that appeals and complaints related to coverage denials sometimes resulted in financial recoveries for consumers.

State and Other Data Indicated Wide-Ranging Coverage Denial Rates, and a Number of Factors May Have Contributed to This Variation

State data that we reviewed showed that rates of coverage denials by insurers operating in the group and individual markets varied significantly across states. Specifically, aggregate claim denial rates for the three states that we identified as collecting such data ranged from 11 percent in Ohio in 2009 to 24 percent in California in the same year.[326] Data reported by the remaining state, Maryland, indicated a claim denial rate of 16 percent in 2007.[327] A fourth state, Connecticut, collected data on a different measure, preauthorization denials, and these data indicated a denial rate of 14 percent in

[326] The Ohio data included the number of electronically submitted claims paid and denied in the first and third quarters of calendar year 2009 and represented all insurers licensed in Ohio. The California data included the number of claims received and denied by six of the largest managed care insurers licensed in the state, each with enrollment in 2009 of over 400,000. We obtained these data from the Department of Managed Health Care's Web site from June through September 2010 (www.wpso.dmhc.ca.gov/fe/search).

[327] The Maryland data were obtained from the Maryland Insurance Administration's *Report on Semi-Annual Claims Data Filing for Calendar Years 2005-2007* and represented data for calendar year 2007 from 41 insurers licensed in the state.

2009.[328] In addition, claim denial rates indicated by AMA data—3 percent during 2 months of 2010—varied from coverage denial rates in the four states.[329]

Several factors may have contributed to the variation in rates across the four states and the AMA data. For example, Ohio and AMA data were based on denials of electronic claims.[330] AMA officials told us that providers with electronic billing systems and insurers that accept electronic claims are more sophisticated in terms of billing management, and therefore the denial rates calculated by AMA may be lower than rates of denials for all claims, including both electronic and paper-based. In another example, Maryland's rate was calculated using data for categories of denials that accounted for about 90 percent of all claims denied. In contrast, according to California officials, California's data represented all claim denials.[331] Differences in the time frames for the data may have also contributed to the variation. AMA officials noted that their data were from a 2-month period of the year (February through March) when there was less contractual activity, such as open enrollment periods, and when denials related to meeting deductible requirements—which according to officials from one insurance company can be significant—have already been resolved. In contrast, data from the four states, except Ohio, covered a full year and therefore reflect all denials for the year, including those related to enrollment and deductible issues. See Table 7 for the rates of coverage denials indicated by state data and a description of the characteristics of the data, some of which may have contributed to the variation in rates.

In addition to variation across states in aggregated rates, state and other data also indicated that coverage denial rates varied significantly across insurers. For example, the California data indicated that in 2009 claim denial rates ranged from 6 percent to 40 percent across six of the largest managed care organizations operating in the state. Similarly, preauthorization denial rates in Connecticut varied across 21 insurers, with rates among the seven largest insurers ranging from 4 percent to 29 percent in 2009. Somewhat narrower variation across insurers was also evident in the AMA data, with

---

[328] The Connecticut data were obtained from the Connecticut Insurance Department's *Consumer Report Card on Health Insurance Carriers in Connecticut* and represented data for calendar year 2009 from 21 managed care insurers licensed in the state.

[329] The data were reported to GAO by AMA and represented claims from February 1, 2010, through March 31, 2010. The data indicated the total number of claim lines—charges for specific services included in the claim—that were denied. AMA defines a denial as a claim line where the amount allowed and the amount billed were equal, but the amount paid was $0. Though not included in the claim denial rate, AMA also reported data indicating that 5 percent of claim lines were edited, that is, the claim lines were automatically reduced to a payment of $0 by the insurer's payment system. According to AMA officials, both claim-line denials and claim-line edits result in no payment for the service, and therefore are denials from the perspective of the provider. The data on claim lines denied and edited were used as the basis for rates reported in AMA's *2010 National Health Insurer Report Card.* See citations to the 2010 report card and previous AMA report cards as well as other studies related to coverage denials in app. II.

[330] Providers can submit paper or electronic claims. According to Ohio and AMA officials, electronic claims represented roughly 70 to 80 percent of their total claims activity.

[331] California officials told us they currently require plans to report on their full "inventory" of denials but the state is revising its claim denial reporting instructions to clarify the denials that should be included and excluded from the numbers reported.

claim denial rates in 2010 that ranged from less than 1 percent to over 4 percent across the seven insurers represented in those data.[332]

Table 7. Rates of claim or preauthorization denials across states in GAO's review and characteristics of the state data

State	Rate of claim or preauthorization denials	Data year[a]	Characteristics of the data
Ohio	11 percent across all insurers licensed in the state	2009	Data limited to denials of electronic claims in the first and third quarters of the fiscal year[b]
Connecticut	14 percent across 21 managed care organizations licensed in the state	2009	Data were limited to denials of preauthorization for services and did not include data on denials of claims[c]
Maryland	16 percent across 41 insurers licensed in the state	2007	Data were limited to 16 categories of denials of claims, representing 90 percent of total claim denials[d]
California	24 percent across six of the largest managed care organizations licensed in the state	2009	Data were limited to denials of claims and reflected each insurer's inventory of denials, which means that some insurers may have reported denials for government- sponsored health coverage, such as Medicaid[e]

Source: GAO analysis of data reported by insurers to states.

[a]The data years cited represent calendar years and the data reflect the most recent complete year of data available.

[b]Data were reported to GAO by the Ohio Department of Insurance.

[c]Data were obtained from Connecticut's *Consumer Report Card on Health Insurance Carriers in Connecticut* (Hartford, Conn.: 2010).

[d]Data were obtained from the Maryland Insurance Administration's *Report on Semi-Annual Claims Data Filing for Calendar Years 2005-2007* (Baltimore, Md.: 2009).

[e]Data were obtained from the Department of Managed Health Care's Web site from June through September 2010 (www.wpso.dmhc.ca.gov/fe/search).

State and other officials told us about several factors that may have contributed to the variation across insurers and make it difficult to compare data across insurers. First, California officials told us that insurers may interpret a state's reporting requirements differently and noted that some insurers may count certain claims transactions as denials that the state would not consider a denial. This was evidenced by discussions with one insurer who told us that if asked to report the number of claims denied, some insurers might include claims where the service was approved but the insurer paid nothing because the member was liable for the charge, which California officials would not characterize as a denial. Officials from the insurer said that their current overall denial rate is 27 percent, but it would be 18 percent if member liability denials were excluded. Officials from California and AMA also indicated that circumstances unique to an insurer may affect their denial rate. For example, California officials told us one insurer's denials rose sharply in a month because providers were submitting claims to the insurer's HMO

[332] According to officials, the AMA claim data included data for insured products offered by the companies represented and self-insured products administered by the companies.

when they should have gone to the preferred provider organization (PPO). Rather than transferring the claims, the HMO denied all of them, and then the PPO paid the claims shortly after that.

State and Other Data Indicated That Coverage Denials Occurred for Various Reasons and That Denials, if Appealed, Were Frequently Reversed

According to state and other data, coverage denials occurred for various reasons. For example:

- Claim denials were often made for billing errors such as duplicate claims and missing information on the claim. For example, data from Maryland showed that the most prevalent reason for claim denials in 2007 was duplicate claim submissions, accounting for 32 percent of all denials.[333] Among six of the largest managed care organizations in California, the four that reported on the most prevalent reasons for claim denials in 2009 all reported duplicate claims as one of those reasons. With regard to claims missing required information, the 2010 AMA data indicated that five of the seven insurers represented in the data made 15 percent or more of denials on the basis that the claim was missing information, such as documentation of preauthorization. Data from Maryland showed that 74 percent of denied claims did not meet the state's criteria for "clean" claims, those claims that include all of the required information needed for processing.[334]
- Denials of claims also frequently resulted from eligibility issues. For example, for six of the seven insurers in the 2010 AMA data, over 20 percent of claim denials occurred as a result of eligibility issues such as services being provided before coverage was initiated or after coverage was terminated.
- Insurers also denied preauthorizations and claims as a result of judgments about the appropriateness of the service, such as that the service was not medically necessary or was experimental or investigational, although less frequently than for billing errors and eligibility issues. Data from Maryland showed that in 2007 insurers denied nearly 40,000 preauthorizations or claims because they

---

[333] The calendar year 2007 data were obtained from the Maryland Insurance Administration's *Report on Semi-Annual Claims Data Filing for Calendar Years 2005-2007*.

[334] Maryland reports the total claim denial rate, as well as a denial rate for "clean claims"— those health care claims submitted by a health care provider on one of two widely used industry standard billing forms and that also include all of the essential information needed by a plan for processing—in their Semi-Annual Claims Data Filing Reports.

determined the services were not medically necessary.[335] This was a relatively small number compared to the 6.3 million claim denials reported in the same year.[336] The 2010 AMA data showed that only one of the seven insurers denied claims on the basis that services were not appropriate, specifically that the service was experimental or investigational, with about 9 percent of denials made for that reason.[337] NAIC data on complaints filed with states in 2009 also provided some information on coverage denials related to the appropriateness of services. Specifically, the data showed that of the approximately 14,000 complaints related to coverage denials, at least 8 percent were related to the insurer's determination that the service was not medically necessary and 2 percent were related to the determination that the service was experimental.

State and other data indicated that coverage denials, if appealed, were frequently reversed in the consumer's favor.[338] The data from the four states that we identified as collecting data on the outcomes of internal appeals filed with insurers indicated that at least 39 percent of internal appeals resulted in the insurer reversing its original coverage denial.

Officials from two insurance companies explained that denials are frequently reversed because the consumer or provider submits additional information, such as the consumer's medical records. Officials from one of these insurance companies also explained that because insurers receive additional information through the appeals process, reversals of denials are expected even when the company is using accepted medical criteria to make the initial assessment of the appropriateness of the service; and regulators are sometimes concerned when few appeals result in reversals of denials. See Table 8 for a summary of the outcomes of internal appeals reported by insurers to Connecticut, Maryland, New York, and Ohio.

---

[335] The data were obtained from The Maryland Insurance Administration's *2007 Report on the Health Care Appeals & Grievances Law.*

[336] The data were obtained from the Maryland Insurance Administration's *Report on Semi- Annual Claims Data Filing for Calendar Years 2005-2007.*

[337] The data on the reasons for claim denials reflect the reasons assigned by the insurer that denied the claim. According to AMA officials, there is no requirement that insurers assign the most specific reason for the claim denial, and they sometimes assign more general reasons. For example, although a denial may have occurred because the insurer determined a service was not medically necessary, the insurer may document that the claim was denied because the service was not covered, which could be for reasons other than that the service was not medically necessary.

[338] Reversals of coverage denials were limited to denials for which an appeal was initiated. The data we reviewed did not allow for a systematic calculation of an "appeal rate"—the number of coverage denials for which an appeal was initiated—for several reasons, including different data sources or data years for denials and appeals data. Data from Ohio did provide limited information; specifically, for the first quarter of calendar year 2010, Ohio data indicated that 0.5 percent of claim denials were internally appealed.

Table 8. Number and outcomes of internal appeals filed with insurers across states in GAO's review

State	Type of insurer reporting[a]	Data year[b]	Number of internal appeals	Percentage of internal appeals where initial determination was reversed
Connecticut[c]	HMOs	2009	1,932	53
	Indemnity managed care organizations	2009	1,797	59
Maryland[d]	HMOs, nonprofit health service plans, and commercial insurers	2009	4,844	50
New York[e]	HMOs	2009	5,968	39
	Commercial insurers	2009	71,787	47
	Nonprofit indemnity insurers	2009	8,946	48
Ohio[f]	All insurers	2010 (1st quarter)	6,434	48

Source: GAO analysis of data reported by insurers to states.

[a]The types of insurers reported in this column are the categories used by each state and may not be comparable across states.

[b]The data years cited represent calendar years and reflect the most recent complete year of data available, unless indicated otherwise.

[c]Data were obtained from Connecticut's *Consumer Report Card on Health Insurance Carriers in Connecticut* (Hartford, Conn.: 2010). The reversal rates represent the aggregate reversal rates for 6 HMOs and 15 indemnity managed care organizations.

[d]Data were obtained from the Maryland Insurance Administration's *2009 Report on the Health Care Appeals & Grievances Law* (Baltimore, Md.: 2010).

[e]Data were obtained from the *2010 New York Consumer Guide to Health Insurers* (Albany, N.Y.: 2010). The reversal rates represent the aggregate reversal rates for 12 HMOs, 28 commercial insurers, and 5 nonprofit indemnity insurers.

[f]Data were reported to GAO by Ohio and represent internal appeals filed by all insurers licensed in Ohio.

Data on the results of appeals filed with states for external review also indicated that denials were frequently reversed. A study conducted by AHIP on 37 states' external appeal programs showed that for 2003 and 2004, about 40 percent of external appeals resulted in denials being reversed.[339] More recent data from the six states we contacted indicated similar rates of denials being reversed upon external appeal. See Table 9 for a summary of the outcomes of external appeals indicated by state data.

The data on the outcomes of external appeals also indicated that the rate at which denials are reversed, if appealed, may vary depending on the reason for the denial and the type of service denied. For example, one study identified through our literature review looked at 740 external appeal decisions in California in 2001 and 2002. The study showed that appeals resulted in denials being reversed in 42 percent of cases where the denial resulted from the determination that services were not medically necessary and 20 percent of cases where services were determined to be experimental and investigational.[340]

---

[339] America's Health Insurance Plans, Update on State External Review (Washington, D.C.: 2006).

[340] C. R. Gresenz and D. M. Studdert, "External Review of Coverage Denials by Managed Care Organizations in California" (RAND Institute for Civil Justice, Santa Monica, Calif.: 2005). See app. II for the list of studies

Table 9. Number and outcomes of appeals submitted for external review across states in GAO's review

State	Types of insurers for which denials were appealed[a]	Data year[b]	Number of external appeals resolved	Percentage of appeals where insurer determination was reversed or revised
California[c]	Managed care organizations with enrollment over 400,000	2009	1,606	54
Connecticut[d]	Managed care organizations	2009	184	40
Florida[e]	Managed care organizations	State fiscal year 2010	186	49
Maryland[f]	HMOs, nonprofit health service plans, and commercial insurers	2009	915	54
New York[g]	HMOs	2009	570	38
	Commercial insurers	2009	812	42
	Nonprofit indemnity insurers	2009	395	41
Ohio[h]	Traditional health insurers, PPOs, HMOs, and Public Employee Health Benefit Plans	2008	311	23

Source: GAO analysis of data reported by states.

[a]The types of insurers reported in this column are the categories used by each state and may not be comparable across states.

[b]The data years cited represent calendar years unless indicated otherwise, and the data reflect the most recent complete year of data available.

[c]Data were obtained from the California Department of Managed Health Care's *2009 Independent Medical Review and Complaint Results* report.

[d]Data were reported to GAO by the Connecticut Insurance Department.

[e]Data were reported to GAO by the Florida Agency for Health Care Administration.

[f]Data were obtained from the Maryland Insurance Administration's *2009 Report on the Health Care Appeals & Grievances Law* (Baltimore, Md: 2010).

[g]Data were obtained from the *2010 New York Consumer Guide to Health Insurers* (Albany, N.Y.: 2010). The reversal rates represent the aggregate reversal rates across 12 HMOs, 28 commercial insurers, and 5 nonprofit indemnity insurers.

[h]Data were obtained from the Ohio Department of Insurance's *Patient Protection Act Report for the Year 2008* (Columbus, Ohio: 2009). The data represent external reviews for denials because the service was not appropriate and denials for contractual reasons, which were less frequently reversed than denials because the service was not appropriate.

Further, the study showed that reversals of denials were more likely for certain services, such as gastric bypass surgery, stem cell transplants, and breast reduction surgery, than for other services, such as residential behavioral health care. Data from Florida also indicated variation in outcomes of external appeals based on the reason for the denial and the type of service denied. For example, for state fiscal year 2010, denials were reversed in 49 percent of cases where the denial resulted from the determination that services were not medically necessary and in 60 percent of cases where the service was deemed experimental or investigational, although there were fewer appeals of coverage

---

that included external appeal data by the reason for the denial being appealed and the type of service being denied.

denials for this reason.[341] Further, the data showed that appeals were more likely to result in a denial being reversed when the denial was for diagnostic testing and pharmaceuticals than for other services, such as cosmetic surgery and durable medical equipment.

Finally, federal and state data indicated that appeals and complaints related to coverage denials sometimes resulted in financial recoveries for consumers. According to data from DOL, more than 9,600 complaints related to coverage denials by group health plans resulted in about 500 recoveries of payments totaling nearly $7 million in fiscal year 2010. Data reported by states to HHS in applications for the Consumer Assistance Program grants also documented that complaints and appeals resulted in recoveries.[342] Specifically, 21 of the 35 states submitting applications reported financial recoveries. For example, Maryland reported recovering more than $1.4 million for consumers in fiscal year 2009 as a result of internal appeals. NAIC data on complaints filed with states also gave some indication of recoveries. For example, NAIC's 2009 data indicated that of the approximately 14,000 complaints related to coverage denials, over 4 percent resulted in an outcome where money or benefits were returned to the consumer and about 7 percent resulted in the insurer paying more of a claim than was initially paid.

AGENCY COMMENTS AND OUR EVALUATION

HHS provided us with written comments on a draft version of this chapter. These comments are reprinted in appendix III. HHS agreed with our findings, noting in particular the need to improve the quality and scope of existing data, and suggested clarifications, which we incorporated. HHS and DOL also provided technical comments to the draft report, which we incorporated as appropriate.

In its written comments, HHS emphasized the importance—for policymakers, regulators, and consumers—of data on health insurance application and coverage denials. HHS noted that data on application and coverage denials can help increase transparency in the private health insurance market and that these data can also provide an important baseline measure for evaluating the impact of changes resulting from PPACA. In its comments, HHS also noted that data collection on application and coverage denials has been uneven across insurers, plans, and states and that very little information is available to help analysts understand the causes or sources of variation in the data that are available. According to HHS, more effort is needed to improve the quality and scope of

---

[341] Data were reported to GAO by the Florida Agency for Health Care Administration. Maryland's data, obtained from the Maryland Insurance Administration's *2009 Report on the Health Care Appeals & Grievances Law,* also included some information on external appeals by the type of service being denied.

[342] In October 2010, HHS awarded nearly $30 million in Consumer Assistance Program grants to 35 states and the District of Columbia. States receiving the grants are required to begin reporting data 6 months after the award notice on the number of inquiries filed with the state about health coverage, the reasons for the inquiries, and the outcomes of the inquiries.

existing data collection to give policymakers and regulators better and richer data to evaluate health insurance plan practices and market changes and to produce measures that may be useful to consumers when they are shopping for insurance.

In its written comments, HHS also identified a limitation to our data that needed some clarification. Specifically, HHS pointed out—correctly—that while our draft report provided information on the percentage of claims that were denied, as well as data on the outcomes of internal appeals and external reviews of denied claims, our draft report did not provide data on the frequency with which claim denials are appealed by consumers. These data were not included in the report because the data we reviewed did not allow for a systematic calculation of an "appeal rate"—the number of coverage denials for which an appeal was initiated—for several reasons, including different sources or years of denials and appeals data we reviewed. In response to HHS' comments, we added language to the report clarifying this limitation. For context, we also added information on the appeal rate from one quarter for one state—the only information we identified on internal claims appeal rates. HHS also noted that the statement in our draft report that "denials are frequently reversed" upon appeal may be confusing, because readers may assume a large number of claim denials are ultimately overturned. We revised the language in our draft report to prevent this misinterpretation of our data, by stating that coverage denials, if appealed, were frequently reversed in the consumer's favor.

We are sending copies of this chapter to the Secretaries of HHS and DOL, the congressional committees of jurisdiction, and other interested parties.

John E. Dicken
Director, Health Care

Appendix I: Methodology for Selecting States and State Data Reviewed by GAO

In order to describe the data on denials of applications for enrollment and coverage of medical services, we contacted six states to interview officials and to obtain data the states collect and track on denials and appeals related to denials. The six states we selected included states identified in the literature, through searches of state insurance department Web sites, or in interviews with experts as a state collecting data on the incidence of application or coverage denials.[343] These also included states that collect or track data on appeals related to coverage denials reviewed by insurers (internal appeals)

[343] Because we did not survey all states to determine whether they collect data on the incidence of application or coverage denials, there may be other states that collect such data that were not known to experts or discussed in the literature. For example, through the course of our work, we found that Texas requires certain insurers to report on the number of requests for verification of coverage for proposed services that insurers declined.

or reviewed by external parties (external appeals). The six states accounted for at least 20 percent of national enrollment in private health insurance.

Table 9. Information on denial data collected by and private health insurance enrollment for states in GAO's review

State	Reported collecting data on the incidence of application denials	Reported collecting data on the incidence of coverage denials	Reported collecting data on internal appeals, including outcomes	Reported collecting data on external appeals, including outcomes	Total number of people enrolled in private health insurance in 2008 (in thousands)	Percentage of national enrollment
California		√		√	22,848	11.4
Connecticut		√	√	√	2,575	1.3
Florida				√	11,129	5.5
Maryland	√	√	√	√	4,171	2.1
New York			√	√	12,567	6.3
Ohio		√	√	√	8,109	4.0

Source: GAO summary of state and U.S. Census Bureau data.

Note: Table includes data that officials from selected states reported collecting. U.S. Census Bureau data are from the bureau's Current Population Survey, 2009 Annual Social and Economic Supplement.

Once we selected the states, we asked officials from each state whether they collected the following types of data: (1) incidence of application denials; (2) incidence of coverage denials, including incidence of denials of preauthorizations and claims; (3) incidence and outcomes of appeals reviewed by insurers (that is, internal appeals); and (4) incidence and outcomes of appeals reviewed by external parties (that is, external appeals). If state officials reported collecting the data, we reviewed at least the most recent year of data available. We reviewed data from one state on the incidence of application denials, from four states on the incidence of coverage denials, from four states on the number and outcomes of internal appeals, and from all six states on the number and outcomes of external appeals. (See Table 9.)

APPENDIX II: METHODOLOGY FOR AND STUDIES IDENTIFIED BY STRUCTURED LITERATURE REVIEW

To identify research that examined private health insurance denials, including the incidence of denials of applications for enrollment and of coverage for medical services (i.e., "coverage denials") and the incidence and outcomes of appeal related to coverage denials, we conducted a structured literature review. This review resulted in 24 studies that we determined to be relevant to our objectives. To conduct this review, we searched

23 reference databases for articles or studies published from January 2000 through July 2010,[344] using a combination of search terms, such as “denial” and “insurer.”[345] We determined that a study was directly relevant to our objectives if it: (1) included empirical analysis related to the incidence of application denials, the incidence of coverage denials, or the incidence and outcomes of appeals related to such denials; and (2) analyzed, at minimum, denial or appeal data from an entire state or two or more insurers. In addition to searching the reference databases, we checked the bibliographies of the relevant studies to identify other potentially relevant research and interviewed several private health insurance experts about research done on denials.

Table 10. Index of studies examining private health insurance denials, by topic

Topic	Study numbers	Total number of studies
Frequency of denials of applications for enrollment	2, 3, 11, 20	4
Frequency of denials of coverage for medical services	5, 6, 7, 10, 16, 17, 19, 22, 24	9
Reasons for denials of coverage	5, 6, 7, 17, 19	5
Outcomes of appeals related to denials of coverage	1, 4, 8, 9, 12, 13, 14, 15, 18, 21, 23, 24	12
By reason for denial being appealed	9, 12, 13, 23	4
By type of service being denied	9, 13, 23	3

Source: GAO.

We identified 24 studies in the literature that included empirical analyses examining (1) the frequency of denials of applications for enrollment or (2) the frequency of or reasons for denials of coverage for medical services and outcomes of appeals related to such denials. Table 10 identifies the number of studies that address these topics, with some studies addressing more than one topic.

The 24 studies that GAO identified in the literature are as follows:

1) American Association of Health Plans. *Independent Medical Review of Health Plan Coverage Decisions: Empowering Consumers with Solutions*. Washington, D.C., 2001.

---

[344] The 23 databases were BIOSIS Previews, NTIS: National Technical Information Service, Social SciSearch, ABI/INFORM, Gale Group PROMT, SciSearch: a Cited Reference Science Database, Pharmaceutical News Index, EMCare, Elsevier BIOBASE, EMBASE, Gale Group Business A.R.T.S., General Science Abstracts, Wilson Applied Science & Technology Abstracts, EconLit, Readers’ Guide Abstracts, Wilson Social Sciences Abstracts, Gale Group Trade & Industry Database, Gale Group Legal Resource Index , MEDLINE, CANCERLIT, EMBASE Alert, Periodical Abstracts PlusText, and Wilson Business Abstracts.

[345] We searched the reference databases for the terms “denial” or “refusal” and “health plan,” “insurer,” “carrier,” or “issuer” with all of the following combinations of terms: (1) “application” or “enrollment;” (2) “coverage,” “claim,” or “preauthorization;” and (3) “complaint,” “appeal,” or “dispute” and “coverage,” “claim,” “service,” or “preauthorization.”

2) America's Health Insurance Plans. *Individual Health Insurance 2009: A Comprehensive Survey of Premiums, Availability, and Benefits.* Washington, D.C., 2009.
3) ——. *Individual Health Insurance 2006–2007: A Comprehensive Survey of Premiums, Availability, and Benefits*. Washington, D.C., 2007.
4) ——. *Update on State External Review Programs*. Washington, D.C., 2006.
5) American Medical Association. *2010 National Health Insurer Report Card.* Chicago, Ill., 2010.
6) ——. *2009 National Health Insurer Report Card.* Chicago, Ill., 2009.
7) ——. *2008 National Health Insurer Report Card.* Chicago, Ill., 2008.
8) California Healthcare Foundation. *Independent Medical Review Experiences in California, Phase I: Cases of Investigational/Experimental Treatments*. Prepared by the Institute for Medical Quality for the California Healthcare Foundation, Oakland, Calif., 2002.
9) Chuang, K. H., W. M. Aubry, and R. A. Dudley. "Independent Medical Review of Health Plan Coverage Denials: Early Trends." *Health Affairs*, vol. 23, no. 6 (November/December 2004), 163-169.
10) Collins, S. R., J. L. Kriss, M. M. Doty, and S. D. Rustgi. *Losing Ground: How the Loss of Adequate Health Insurance is Burdening Working Families: Findings from the Commonwealth Fund Biennial Health Insurance Surveys*, 2001–2007. New York, N.Y., 2008.
11) Doty, M. M., S. R. Collins, J. L. Nicholson, and S. D. Rustgi. *Failure to Protect: Why the Individual Insurance Market is not a Viable Option for Most U.S. Families. Findings from the Commonwealth Fund Biennial Health Insurance Survey*, 2007. New York, N.Y., 2009.
12) Foote, S. B., B. A. Virnig, L. Bockstedt, and Z. Lomax. "External Review of Health Plan Denials of Mental Health Services: Lessons from Minnesota." *Administration and Policy in Mental Health and Mental Health Services Research*, vol. 34 (2007), 38-44.
13) Gresenz, C. R., and D. M. Studdert. *External Review of Coverage Denials by Managed Care Organizations in California.* Working Paper No. WR-264-ICJ, RAND Institute for Civil Justice, Santa Monica, Calif., 2005.
14) Gresenz, C. R., D. M. Studdert, N. Campbell, and D. R. Hensler. "Patients In Conflict With Managed Care: A Profile of Appeals in Two HMOs." *Health Affairs*, vol. 21, no. 4 (July/August 2002), 189-196.

15) Gresenz, C. R., and D. M. Studdert. "Disputes over Coverage of Emergency Department Services: A Study of Two Health Maintenance Organizations." *Annals of Emergency Medicine*, vol. 43, no. 2 (February 2004), 155-162.
16) Kaiser Family Foundation / Harvard School of Public Health. *National Survey on Consumer Experiences With and Attitudes Toward Health Plans: Key Findings.* Washington, D.C., 2001.
17) Kapur, K., C. R. Gresenz, and D. M. Studdert. "Managed Care: Utilization Review in Action at Two Capitated Medical Groups." *Health Affairs*, Web exclusive (2003), W3-275-282.
18) Karp, N., and E. Wood. *Understanding Health Plan Dispute Resolution Practices*, Washington. D.C., 2000.
19) Pearson, S. D. "Patient Reports of Coverage Denial: Association with Ratings of Health Plan Quality and Trust in Physician." *The American Journal of Managed Care* (March 2003), 238-244.
20) Pollitz, K., R. Sorian, and K. Thomas. How Accessible is Individual Health Insurance for consumers in less-than-perfect health? *Prepared for the Henry J. Kaiser Family Foundation,* Menlo Park, Calif., 2001.
21) Pollitz, K., J. Crowley, K. Lucia, and E. Bangit. Assessing State External Review Programs and the Effects of Pending Federal Patients' Rights Legislation. *Prepared for the Henry J. Kaiser Family Foundation*, Menlo Park, Calif., 2002.
22) Schauffler, H. H., S. McMenamin, J. Cubanski, and H. S. Hanley. "Differences in the Kinds of Problems Consumers Report in Staff/Group Health Maintenance Organizations, Independent Practice Association/Network Health Maintenance Organizations, and Preferred Provider Organizations in California." *Medical Care*, vol. 39, no. 1 (2001), 15-25.
23) Studdert, D. M., and C. R. Gresenz. "Enrollee Appeals of Preservice Coverage Denials at 2 Health Maintenance Organizations." *The Journal of the American Medical Association*, vol. 289, no. 7 (Feb. 19, 2003), 864-870.
24) Young, G. P., J. Ellis, J. Becher, C. Yeh, J. Kovar, and M. A. Levitt. "Managed Care Gatekeeping, Emergency Medicine Coding, and Insurance Reimbursement Outcomes for 980 Emergency Department Visits from Four States Nationwide." *Annals of Emergency Medicine*, vol. 39, no. 1 (January 2002), 24-30.

APPENDIX III: COMMENTS FROM THE DEPARTMENT OF HEALTH AND HUMAN SERVICES

DEPARTMENT OF HEALTH & HUMAN SERVICES

OFFICE OF THE SECRETARY

Assistant Secretary for Legislation
Washington, DC 20201

FEB 16 2011

John E. Dicken
Director, Health Care
U.S. Government Accountability Office
441 G Street N.W.
Washington, DC 20548

Dear Mr. Dicken:

Attached are comments on the U.S. Government Accountability Office's (GAO) draft report entitled, "PRIVATE HEALTH INSURANCE: Data on Application and Coverage Denials" (GAO 11-268).

The Department appreciates the opportunity to review this report prior to publication.

Sincerely,

Jim R. Esquea
Assistant Secretary for Legislation

GENERAL COMMENTS OF THE DEPARTMENT OF HEALTH AND HUMAN SERVICES (HHS) ON THE GOVERNMENT ACCOUNTABILITY OFFICE'S (GAO) DRAFT REPORT ENTITLED, "PRIVATE HEALTH INSURANCE: DATA ON APPLICATION AND COVERAGE DENIALS" (GAO-11-268)

The Department appreciates the opportunity to review and comment on this draft report.

The Affordable Care Act (ACA) of 2010 required GAO to study the rates of such application and coverage denials. GAO reviewed the data available on denials of the applications of enrollment and coverage for medical services.

We would like to emphasize the importance—for policy makers, regulators and consumers—of the data presented in your report, and make note of Center for Consumer Information and Insurance Oversight's (CCIIO) role in improving and expanding data collection on application and coverage denials to help bring about increased transparency in private health insurance.

We would like to also bring your attention to an important piece of data not included in your analysis. Although GAO's draft report provides information on the percentage of claims that are denied by private health insurance plans, as well as data on the outcomes of internal appeals and external review of denied claims, it does not provide data on the frequency with which claims denials are appealed by consumers. This letter offers views on why the gap matters and what might be done to close that data gap. It also highlights HHS' role, together with our Federal partners in the Departments of Labor (DoL) and Treasury, in crafting federal regulations to both create more uniform federal protections for internal appeals and external review and enforce notice requirements so that consumers are aware of their appeal rights, as required by the ACA.

Why the Data on Application and Coverage Denials Matter

Data on application and coverage denials help increase transparency in private health insurance. However, more effort is needed to improve the quality and scope of existing data collections to give policymakers and regulators better and richer data to evaluate health insurance plan practices and market changes, and to produce measures that may be useful to consumers when they are shopping for insurance.

The GAO's draft report makes it abundantly clear that data collection on application and coverage denials have been uneven across insurers and plans and across states. The report also reveals that very little information is available to help analysts understand the causes or sources of variation in the data that are available. For example, the GAO analyzed data—collected by CCIIO and displayed in the individual market plan finder on HealthCare.gov—on applications denials by plans in the individual health insurance market. The data perform an important function—alerting consumers to the uncertainty that goes along with applying for private coverage in the current market. The data also provide an important baseline measure for evaluating the impact of the ACA. We should, for example, expect to see a sharp reduction in these application denials over time, since denials for pre-existing conditions will be a thing of the past after 2014.

Similarly, the GAO's analysis of claims denials primarily serves to illustrate that there is variation across issuers. Unfortunately, not much more can be said about these data. Although the data illustrate wide variation in the reported rate of claims denial, the GAO was unable to describe the sources or significance of that variation. Further, it is possible that the states that do provide data are also the states with stronger appeals protections such that the reported rates are not representative of the national picture.

The GAO report also reveals that the scope of existing data collection needs to be expanded to assure transparency across the health insurance market.

How Often Do Consumers Appeal Claims Denials and What Obstacles Do They Face?

Together with our Federal partners in DOL and Treasury, HHS has crafted Federal regulations to create more uniform Federal protections for internal appeals and external review and to implement improved notice requirements for consumers. In order for the Departments to provide oversight for those new protections, data on the rate at which claims denials are appealed (and the outcomes of those internal appeals and external reviews) are needed.

ACA directed the GAO to study data on denials including denials where a "health plan later approves such coverage." Unfortunately, due to the limitations of existing data collections, the GAO, with one small exception, was not able to report data on the frequency with which claims denials are appealed in any segment of the market. Consequently, the GAO risks confusion when it states that "denials are frequently reversed." Readers may reasonably assume that a large percentage of claim denials are ultimately overturned (with a consumer receiving a previously denied benefit payment). It is unclear that this is the case, especially in the pre-ACA patchwork of appeals protections. For example, in its own discussion, the GAO seems to suggest that reversals and recoveries for consumers may be rare, citing a favorable outcome for a plan enrollee in 5.2 percent of reported cases (i.e., the GAO reports that recoveries were made in 500 cases out of 9,600 complaints about benefit denials received by the DOL from enrollees in self-funded plans).

Systematic, standardized and richer data collection on claims denials and appeals is needed across market segments –in both the commercially insured market and in self-funded group plans—to provide transparency for consumers and meaningful information for policymakers.

APPENDIX IV

One Hundred Eleventh Congress
Congress of the United States
House of Representatives
Committee on Energy and Commerce
Memorandum
October 12, 2010

To: Members of the Committee on Energy and Commerce
From: Chairmen Henry A. Waxman and Bart Stupak
Re: Coverage Denials for Pre-Existing Conditions in the Individual Health Insurance Market

Since March 2010, the Committee has been investigating the extent of coverage denials and exclusions for pre-existing conditions in the individual health insurance market. This memorandum summarizes what we have learned in the investigation. We have found (1) the four largest for-profit health insurance companies denied over 600,000 individuals coverage because of pre-existing conditions in the three years before passage of health reform and (2) the number of coverage denials increased significantly each year.

The insurance company practices described in this memorandum are those that exist in today's market. In all likelihood, they would continue unabated in the absence of federal health reform legislation. One of the major benefits of the Affordable Care Act, which was signed into law on March 23, 2010, is a ban on the practice of denying coverage based on pre-existing conditions.

Key findings in our investigation are:

- From 2007 through 2009, the four largest for-profit health insurance companies, Aetna, Humana, UnitedHealth Group, and WellPoint, refused to issue health insurance coverage to more than 651,000 people based on their prior medical history. On average, the four companies denied coverage to one out of every seven applicants based on a pre-existing condition. One of the four companies maintained a list of over 400 medical diagnoses that triggered a permanent denial of health insurance coverage to applicants.
- From 2007 through 2009, the number of people denied coverage for pre-existing conditions increased at a rapid rate. The number of individuals denied coverage by Aetna, Humana, UnitedHealth Group, and WellPoint increased from 172,400 in 2007 to 257,100 in 2009, an increase of 49%. During the same period, applications for enrollment increased by only 16%.
- From 2007 through 2009, Aetna, Humana, UnitedHealth Group, and WellPoint refused to pay 212,800 claims for medical treatment due to pre-existing conditions. In some cases, the companies offered health insurance to individuals with pre-existing conditions, but used medical riders to exclude coverage or increase deductibles for the pre-existing conditions. In the case of one of the companies, nearly 15% of the company's customers in the individual market in 2010 had policies with riders limiting coverage or increasing deductibles for certain medical conditions.
- Each company had business plans that relied on using pre-existing conditions to limit the amount of money paid for medical claims. In one document, executives devised a plan for "strategic growth" in the individual market that identified areas of opportunity to be "improved pre-existing exclusion processes, tighter condition and large claim review, [and] tighter underwriting guidelines." Other internal corporate documents show that insurance company executives were considering practices such as lengthening the look-back period, assessing separate deductibles specifically for identified pre-existing conditions, denying payments for prescription drugs related to pre-existing conditions, linking

additional claims to pre-existing conditions exclusions, and narrowing the definition of prior creditable insurance coverage.

The Affordable Care Act signed into law by President Obama prohibits the use of pre-existing conditions to deny coverage or claims. For children, this provision becomes effective for policies issued on or after September 23, 2010. For everyone else, the ban on the use of pre-existing conditions takes effect on January 1, 2014. As a result, health insurance companies will no longer be able to deny coverage to people due to their medical history. The companies also will not be permitted to exclude medical coverage for treatments related to pre-existing conditions, and they will not be allowed to charge higher premiums based on covering individuals with pre-existing conditions.

Purpose and Methodology of the Investigation

While most Americans receive health insurance coverage through group plans sponsored by their employers, millions of people who cannot obtain health insurance through their employers and do not qualify for government programs such as Medicare or Medicaid can obtain health insurance only through the individual market. In 2008, approximately 15.7 million adults under 65 received their health care coverage through individual health insurance policies.[346] In the individual health insurance market, companies screen applicants for pre-existing medical conditions prior to providing insurance coverage. Health insurance companies use information about pre-existing conditions to deny insurance coverage outright, charge higher premiums, or exclude coverage for medical claims related to the pre-existing conditions.

In early 2010, before passage of the Affordable Care Act, we initiated an investigation into insurance company practices relating to pre-existing conditions. On March 2, 2010, the Committee wrote the four largest for-profit health insurance companies – Aetna, Humana, UnitedHealth Group, and WellPoint – to request information about rejection of insurance coverage and denial of claims related to pre-existing conditions in the individual health insurance market.[347] Collectively, these four companies covered 2.8 million people in the individual health insurance market in 2009.[348]

---

[346] Kaiser Family Foundation, *Health Insurance Coverage in America, 2008* (Oct. 9, 2009).

[347] Letter from Henry A. Waxman, Chairman, Committee on Energy and Commerce, and Bart Stupak, Chairman, Subcommittee on Oversight and Investigations, Committee on Energy and Commerce, to Angela Braly, President and Chief Executive Officer, WellPoint, Inc., Stephen Hemsley, President and Chief Executive Officer, UnitedHealth Group, Michael McCallister, President and Chief Executive Officer, Humana, Inc., and Ronald Williams, Chairman and Chief Executive Officer, Aetna (Mar. 2, 2010).

[348] National Association of Insurance Commissioners, *Individual and Group Comprehensive Major Medical by Legal Entity* (Apr. 7, 2010).

The Committee sought documentation on the insurers' practices related to pre-existing conditions, including "internal communications, including e-mail, to or from senior corporate management" and "presentations to senior corporate management."[349] The Committee also requested information on the total number of denials of medical claims payments and the rejection of health insurance coverage due to pre-existing conditions over the last five years.[350] All companies voluntarily provided the information requested. In total, the Committee received over 68,000 pages of documents from the companies.

This memorandum is based on the information and documents provided to the Committee. It provides new insights into how the largest for-profit health insurance companies used pre-existing conditions to deny coverage and claims. Without passage of the Affordable Care Act, the practices described in the memorandum could have continued unchecked.

Findings

Coverage Denials

From 2007 to 2009, the four largest for-profit health insurance companies, Aetna, Humana, UnitedHealth Group, and WellPoint, refused to provide health insurance coverage to more than 651,000 people based on their prior medical history.[351]

A year-by-year analysis shows a significant increase in the number of coverage denials each year. The insurance companies denied coverage to 172,400 people in 2007 and 221,400 people in 2008. By 2009, the number of individuals denied coverage rose to 257,100.[352] Between 2007 and 2009, the number of people denied coverage for pre-existing conditions increased 49%.

During the same period, applications for insurance coverage at the four companies increased by only 16%. See Figure 1.

---

349 Letter from Henry A. Waxman, Chairman, Committee on Energy and Commerce, and Bart Stupak, Chairman, Subcommittee on Oversight and Investigations, Committee on Energy and Commerce, to Angela Braly, President and Chief Executive Officer, WellPoint, Inc., Stephen Hemsley, President and Chief Executive Officer, UnitedHealth Group, Michael McCallister, President and Chief Executive Officer, Humana, Inc., and Ronald Williams, Chairman and Chief Executive Officer, Aetna (Mar. 2, 2010).

350 *Id.*

351 Letter from Counsel, Aetna, to Henry A. Waxman, Chairman, Committee on Energy and Commerce, and Bart Stupak, Chairman, Subcommittee on Oversight and Investigations, Committee on Energy and Commerce (Mar. 26, 2010); Letter from Counsel, Humana, Inc., to Henry A. Waxman, Chairman, Committee on Energy and Commerce, and Bart Stupak, Chairman, Subcommittee on Oversight and Investigations, Committee on Energy and Commerce (Mar. 12, 2010); Letter from Counsel, UnitedHealth Group, to Henry A. Waxman, Chairman, Committee on Energy and Commerce, and Bart Stupak, Chairman, Subcommittee on Oversight and Investigations, Committee on Energy and Commerce (Mar. 19, 2010); and Letter from Counsel, WellPoint, Inc., to Henry A. Waxman, Chairman, Committee on Energy and Commerce, and Bart Stupak, Chairman, Subcommittee on Oversight and Investigations, Committee on Energy and Commerce (Mar. 12, 2010).

352 *Id.*

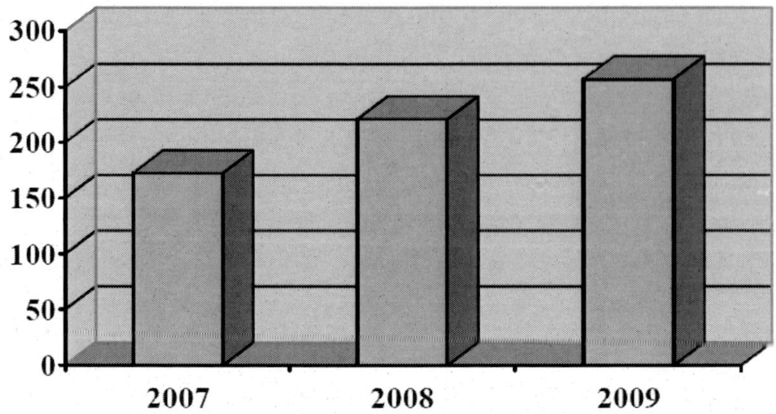

Figure 1. Coverage Denials in the Individual Health Insurance Market (in thousands).

A significant percentage of applicants for insurance were denied coverage for pre-existing conditions. In 2007, these four insurance companies denied coverage to 11.9% of applicants; and in 2008, they denied coverage to 13.8% of applicants. By 2009, Aetna, Humana, UnitedHealth Group, and WellPoint denied health insurance coverage to 15.3% of their applicants in the individual market due to pre-existing conditions. On average, the four companies denied coverage to one out of every seven applicants based on a pre-existing condition.

The actual number of coverage denials is likely to be significantly higher than reported by the companies. The companies do not report as denials individuals who are discouraged from applying for coverage by insurance agents because of their pre-existing conditions. A document from one company states that one-third of its applicants do not obtain coverage because of pre-existing conditions.[353] This estimate may reflect the actual denial rate when individuals who are discouraged from submitting formal applications are taken into account.

In addition, one of the four companies provided information to the Committee from only one of its subsidiaries, which represents only 32% of the company's individual health insurance business.[354]

The documents reveal that the health insurance companies denied individuals insurance coverage based on an extensive list of medical conditions. One of the companies maintains a list of 425 medical diagnoses that it used to decline health insurance coverage permanently to many applicants.[355] These diagnoses include common conditions, such as pregnancy, angina, diabetes, and heart disease.[356] A recent Families USA study found that 57.2 million people under the age of 65 suffer from at least one

---

[353] *Articulating Health Care Value Strategy for Individual Business* (Jan. 6, 2009).

[354] National Association of Insurance Commissioners, *Individual and Group Comprehensive Major Medical by Legal Entity* (Apr. 7, 2010).

[355] Underwriting Guide concerning health products (undated).

[356] *Id.*

diagnosed condition that could put them at risk for denial of coverage based on pre-existing conditions if they tried to purchase individual health insurance as a new subscriber.[357]

For certain medical conditions, companies routinely denied health insurance coverage without an internal review. In 2006, one of the companies distributed an inter-office memorandum that included a list of medical categories that "no longer require a review for declination."[358] A set of 14 categories followed, including:

- "Any applicant who is a surgical candidate."
- "Any female applicant currently pregnant."
- "Any female applicant who has been treated for infertility within 5 years."
- "Any applicant with a BMI [body mass index] of 39.0 or greater."[359]

The insurance companies declined coverage for applicants of all ages due to pre-existing conditions. Although young people generally enjoy better health, the companies routinely denied health insurance coverage for individuals under the age of 30. Internal correspondence shows that in some instances "[f]or . . . plans for individuals, between 9 and 10 percent of individuals between the ages of 18 and 30 are declined coverage during the application process."[360]

Claims Denials

In some instances, health insurance companies offer insurance to individuals with pre-existing conditions, but add riders to their policies denying payment for claims relating to those conditions or imposing additional deductibles. This was a practice commonly used by the four companies. From 2007 through 2009, Aetna, Humana, UnitedHealth Group, and WellPoint refused to pay 212,800 claims for medical treatment due to pre-existing conditions.[361]

The four companies denied 67,200 claims in 2007 and 74,650 in 2008. In 2009, the four health insurance companies refused to pay over 70,900 medical claims of individuals they insured due to pre-existing conditions.[362]

---

[357] Families USA, *Health Reform: Help for Americans with Pre-Existing Conditions* (May 2010).

[358] Inter-Office Memorandum from [redacted] to Distribution (Aug. 29, 2006).

[359] *Id.*

[360] E-mail from [redacted] to [redacted] (Aug. 28, 2007).

[361] Letter from Counsel, Aetna, to Henry A. Waxman, Chairman, Committee on Energy and Commerce, and Bart Stupak, Chairman, Subcommittee on Oversight and Investigations, Committee on Energy and Commerce (Mar. 26, 2010); Letter from Counsel, Humana, Inc., to Henry A. Waxman, Chairman, Committee on Energy and Commerce, and Bart Stupak, Chairman, Subcommittee on Oversight and Investigations, Committee on Energy and Commerce (Mar. 12, 2010); Letter from Counsel, UnitedHealth Group, to Henry A. Waxman, Chairman, Committee on Energy and Commerce, and Bart Stupak, Chairman, Subcommittee on Oversight and Investigations, Committee on Energy and Commerce (Mar. 19, 2010); and Letter from Counsel, WellPoint, Inc., to Henry A. Waxman, Chairman, Committee on Energy and Commerce, and Bart Stupak, Chairman, Subcommittee on Oversight and Investigations, Committee on Energy and Commerce (Aug. 31, 2010).

[362] *Id.*

One company excluded treatment or assessed additional deductible charges for 14.7% of its customers in the individual market.[363] The top four riders used by this company excluded coverage or increased deductibles for Caesarean deliveries, back disorders, psychiatric or psychological disorders, and outpatient treatment for cholesterol issues.[364]

Business Plans

Documents obtained by the Committee show that the companies' business plans included using pre-existing conditions to limit the amount of money paid for medical claims. Executives at one company, for example, devised a plan for "strategic growth" in the individual market that would "[r]e-position all new customer segment's pricing, products, and risk profile to gradually enhance profit profile of the book and . . . ultimately improve[e] price levels."[365] Areas of opportunity included: "improved pre-existing exclusion processes, tighter condition and large claim review, [and] tighter underwriting guidelines."[366]

At another company, executives identified key issues confronting the individual market. One document states: "Lack of attention to risk management, decreased ability to use pre-existing claim denials and rescind policies, and maternity policies have led to first year loss ratios climbing from less than 50% five years ago to over 65% today."[367] To lessen the company's financial losses, a senior executive recommended that the company should "[e]nsure Pre-existing condition[s] are administered effectively to the extent allowed by law."[368]

In one training presentation to insurance brokers, executives at a third company explained: "Insurance is a Gamble."[369] The training materials included the following statements about the company's approach to the health insurance business:

- "Because U.S. insurance has such high maximum limits, selling insurance is like gambling."
- "When we sell someone an insurance policy, we are betting that their total medical costs for the year will be less than they paid us in premiums."
- "We try to 'win' our bets by accurately assessing their medical risk and charging the right premiums."[370]

---

[363] E-mail from [redacted] to [redacted] (Feb. 8, 2010).
[364] *Id.*
[365] *Consumer Segment 2010 – 2012 Strategy Round 1* (Mar. 20, 2009).
[366] *Id.*
[367] *[State] 2010 Plan Information for Board Presentation* (Jan. 2010).
[368] *Id.*
[369] *The Importance of Insurance, and Your Role in Helping People Get It* (undated).
[370] *Id.*

The documents received by the Committee indicate that prior to passage of health reform, the insurance companies were considering ways to expand the use of pre-existing conditions to avoid paying for a broader class of medical claims. Internal corporate documents show that high-level executives considered practices such as:

- *Increasing the look-back period on pre-existing conditions*: When an individual applies for health insurance, the company will "look back" at the applicant's prior medical history for a certain period of time to identify pre-existing conditions that could provide a justification to deny coverage. State laws govern the length of the look-back period. According to documents obtained by the Committee, it appears that in July 2009, executives at one insurer held a meeting during which they discussed lengthening the look-back period for pre-existing conditions.[371] In a presentation circulated in advance of the meeting, the company's look-back guidelines were compared to the maximum legal limits in each state.[372]
- *Assessing separate deductibles specifically for identified pre-existing conditions*: In a presentation concerning risk assessments in the individual health insurance market, executives at another company were provided a "[p]re-ex opportunity overview."[373] Among a number of "additional potential opportunities [that] should be examined," the presenter highlighted "the introduction of condition specific deductibles" as a future improvement to be considered.[374]
- *Denying payments for prescription drugs related to pre-existing conditions*: Executives for a third company have recently introduced a project to withhold insurance reimbursement for prescription drugs if the medication is used to treat pre-existing conditions. A presentation in January 2010, explained: "We are proposing a pilot that enforces any medications used to treat pre-existing conditions be excluded for all members that do not have prior creditable coverage, as per Policy specifications."[375]
- *Linking additional claims to pre-existing conditions exclusions*: During an internal evaluation of the individual business, executives at the fourth company discussed "[c]ontrol[ling] cost by conducting Pre-Existing Condition Investigations."[376] As part of this dialogue, executives emphasized the importance to "[l]ink related claims to Pre-Existing Condition investigations"

[371] E-mail from [redacted] to [redacted] et al. (July 23, 2009).
[372] *Id.*
[373] *[Redacted] Claim Accuracy and Risk management assessment* (undated).
[374] *Id.*
[375] E-mail from [redacted] to [redacted] (Jan. 5, 2010).
[376] E-mail from [redacted] to [redacted] et al. (Nov. 10, 2005).

and "[i]dentify claims that should be linked to a Pre-Existing Condition investigation."[377]

- *Narrowing the definition of prior creditable coverage*: Prior creditable coverage is a period of past health insurance coverage that can shorten the length of time a new insurer can exclude insurance coverage of pre-existing conditions. Internal documents reveal that executives at one of the companies considered changing "the definition of prior creditable coverage to exclude prior individual coverage."[378]

Effect of Health Reform

The Affordable Care Act, which was enacted on March 23, 2010, will significantly reform insurance company practices relating to pre-existing conditions.

Effective January 1, 2014, insurance companies in the individual market will no longer be allowed to deny policy enrollment based on a person's health status, including pre-existing conditions.[379] Additionally, the Act will bar health insurers from charging higher premiums to people who have pre-existing conditions. By 2014, health insurance companies selling coverage in the individual market will be allowed to set their rates based only on geography, whether the plan covers an individual or family, age, and tobacco use. Insurance companies will no longer use medical histories to calculate premium rates.[380]

For children, these reforms are effective earlier. The law prohibits pre-existing condition claims exclusions for children under the age of 19 for new policies starting in September 2010.[381]

In addition, the Affordable Care Act established a new Pre-existing Condition Insurance Plan administered by the Department of Health and Human Services. This temporary program provides health insurance to individuals who currently are unable to obtain insurance due to their medical history. Enrollees must have been uninsured for at least six months due to a medical condition and be a United States citizen or reside legally in this country. This insurance plan will exist until the Act's comprehensive pre-existing condition reforms go into effect in 2014.[382]

[377] *Id.*
[378] E-mail from [redacted] to [redacted] (Apr. 27, 2009).
[379] The Patient Protection and Affordable Care Act, Pub. L. 111-148 § 1201 (2010).
[380] *Id.*
[381] *Id.* at § 1255.
[382] *Id.* at § 1101.

Conclusion

Our investigation examined practices concerning pre-existing conditions in the individual health insurance market. The investigation has revealed that from 2007 through 2009, the four largest for-profit health insurance companies, Aetna, Humana, UnitedHealth Group, and WellPoint, denied health insurance coverage to more than 651,000 people based on their prior medical history. During the same period, the four companies refused to pay 212,800 claims for medical treatment related to pre-existing conditions. Internal company documents show that this increasing use of pre-existing conditions to deny or limit coverage would have continued unabated if Congress had not passed health reform legislation.

In: Medicaid: Fraud, Payments and Beneficiaries
Editor: Nadia M. Hedegaard
ISBN: 978-1-53617-666-7

Chapter 2

MEDICAID: EFFORTS TO IDENTIFY, PREDICT, OR MANAGE HIGH-EXPENDITURE BENEFICIARIES*

United States Government Accountability Office

ABBREVIATIONS

ACO	accountable care organization
CMS	Centers for Medicare & Medicaid Services
MCO	managed care organization

WHY GAO DID THIS STUDY

Medicaid, a joint federal-state health care financing program, is one of the nation's largest sources of health care coverage for low-income and medically needy individuals. A 2016 report published by the National Governors Association noted that high-expenditure Medicaid beneficiaries typically have poorly managed chronic conditions and a host of unmet social needs that result in potentially preventable use of costly services, such as emergency department visits. The report also noted that identifying and better managing those beneficiaries are key to reducing costs and improving outcomes.

GAO was asked to examine state and federal efforts to manage costs and improve care coordination for high- expenditure Medicaid beneficiaries. This chapter describes (1) approaches selected states used to identify or predict high-expenditure Medicaid

* This is an edited, reformatted and augmented version of United States Government Accountability Office; Report to Congressional Committees, Accessible Version, Publication No. GAO-19-569, dated August 2019.

beneficiaries; (2) strategies selected states used to manage beneficiaries' health care costs while ensuring quality of care; and (3) resources CMS provided to states to help them identify, predict, or better manage high- expenditure beneficiaries.

GAO interviewed officials from CMS, as well as Medicaid officials from a nongeneralizable sample of seven states (Indiana, Nevada, Pennsylvania, South Carolina, South Dakota, Vermont, and Washington) and five MCOs. States were selected for variation in their total Medicaid enrollment, enrollment in Medicaid managed care, percentage of state population living in rural settings, and percentage of state population with disabilities. MCOs were selected based on state suggestions, and varied in terms of whether they operated nationally or on a state or regional basis.

What GAO Found

GAO previously reported that in fiscal years 2009 through 2011, the most expensive 5 percent of Medicaid beneficiaries accounted for nearly half of the expenditures for all beneficiaries; others have also found that a small percentage of beneficiaries account for a disproportionately large share of Medicaid program expenditures. These high-expenditure beneficiaries are an extremely diverse population with varying needs. GAO found that the seven selected states identified or predicted high-expenditure Medicaid beneficiaries using statistics and other approaches. For example, states used risk scores, which estimate an individual beneficiary's expected health care expenditures relative to the average expenditures for beneficiaries in the group. Other approaches included examining service utilization data to identify statistical outliers and using diagnoses, service utilization and claims expenditure thresholds, or clinical judgment to identify or predict high-expenditure beneficiaries.

To manage costs and ensure quality of care for high-expenditure beneficiaries, the seven selected states used care management and other strategies.

- Care management. All the selected states provided care management— providing various types of assistance such as coordinating care across different providers to manage physical and mental health conditions more effectively—for beneficiaries in their fee-for-service delivery systems. Five of the states also contracted with managed care organizations (MCO) to deliver services for a fixed payment and required the MCOs to ensure the provision of care management services to high-expenditure beneficiaries.
- Other strategies. Some of the seven selected states used additional strategies to manage care for high-expenditure beneficiaries. For example, Indiana officials described a program to restrict, or "lock in," a beneficiary who has demonstrated a pattern of high utilization to a single primary care provider, hospital, and

pharmacy, if other efforts to change the beneficiary's high utilization were unsuccessful.

The Centers for Medicare & Medicaid Services (CMS), which oversees the Medicaid program at the federal level, offered optional tools and other resources to support states' efforts to identify or better manage high-expenditure beneficiaries. For example, CMS officials said states received access to resources and technical assistance on establishing health home programs— which seek to better coordinate care for those with chronic conditions—including how to focus on high-expenditure beneficiaries. CMS officials noted that they supported 23 states' and the District of Columbia's health home programs. CMS also offered several resources that, while not designed specifically to target high- expenditure beneficiaries, have been used to support states in identifying or better managing their care. For example, CMS's Medicaid Innovation Accelerator Program offered targeted technical support to states' Medicaid agencies in building their data analytic capacity as they designed and implemented delivery system reforms, which could be used to identify high-expenditure beneficiaries. Officials in two selected states reported that these tools were beneficial for managing the health care costs associated with high-expenditure beneficiaries. HHS provided technical comments, which GAO incorporated as appropriate.

August 13, 2019

The Honorable Charles E. Grassley
Chairman
Committee on Finance
United States Senate

The Honorable Greg Walden
Republican Leader
Committee on Energy and Commerce
House of Representatives

The Honorable Michael C. Burgess
Republican Leader
Subcommittee on Health
Committee on Energy and Commerce
House of Representatives

Medicaid, a joint federal-state health care financing program, is one of the nation's largest sources of health care coverage for low-income and medically needy individuals.

In fiscal year 2018, Medicaid covered an estimated 75 million beneficiaries and expenditures totaling about $629 billion. Annual expenditures are projected to reach $1 trillion by 2026 and are placing a growing strain on federal and state budgets.[1]

We and others have found that a small percentage of beneficiaries account for a disproportionately large share of Medicaid program expenditures.[2] These high-expenditure Medicaid beneficiaries are an extremely diverse population with varying medical, behavioral, and psychosocial needs. For example, some high-expenditure Medicaid beneficiaries may have chronic conditions, such as diabetes or behavioral health issues; some may be children staying in a hospital or elderly receiving long term services and supports; some may need housing or food assistance. A 2016 report published by the National Governors Association noted that high-expenditure Medicaid beneficiaries typically have multiple poorly managed chronic conditions and a host of unmet social needs that result in potentially preventable use of costly services, such as emergency department visits.[3] That same report noted that key components of reducing costs and improving outcomes include identifying high-expenditure beneficiaries whose needs are best served through well- coordinated services and linking those beneficiaries to appropriate providers. Although federal Medicaid regulations do not require states to identify high-expenditure beneficiaries, some states have taken steps to do so.

In the context of these issues, you asked us to examine state and federal efforts to manage costs and improve care coordination for high- expenditure Medicaid beneficiaries. This chapter describes

1. approaches selected states used to identify or predict high- expenditure Medicaid beneficiaries;
2. strategies selected states used to manage the health care costs while ensuring quality of care for such beneficiaries; and
3. resources the Centers for Medicare & Medicaid Services (CMS) provided to states to help them identify, predict, or better manage high-expenditure Medicaid beneficiaries.

To answer all three questions, we interviewed officials from a nongeneralizable sample of seven state Medicaid agencies; specifically, Indiana, Nevada, Pennsylvania, South Carolina, South Dakota, Vermont, and Washington. We selected these states to

---

[1] See Department of Health and Human Services, Centers for Medicare & Medicaid Services, Office of the Actuary, *2017 Actuarial Report on the Financial Outlook for Medicaid* (Washington, D.C.: 2018).

[2] For example, see GAO, *Medicaid: Demographics and Service Usage of Certain High- Expenditure Beneficiaries*, GAO-14-176 (Washington, D.C.: Feb. 19, 2014); and *Medicaid: A Small Share of Enrollees Consistently Accounted for a Large Share of Expenditures*, GAO-15-460 (Washington, D.C.: May 8, 2018); as well as S. A. Pires, K. E. Grimes, K. D. Allen, T. Gilmer, and R. M. Mahadevan, *Examining Children's Behavioral Health Service Utilization and Expenditures* (Hamilton, N.J.: Center for Health Care Strategies, Inc., 2013).

[3] See S. Wilkniss and C. Kelleher, *Medicaid High-Need, High-Cost Programs: Promising Practices for Evaluation Metrics* (Washington, D.C.: National Governors Association Center for Best Practices, 2016).

obtain variation in (1) their total Medicaid enrollment as of July 2016; (2) the degree to which the state's Medicaid population was enrolled in managed care as of July 2016; (3) the percentage of the state's total population living in rural settings based on 2010 Census data; and (4) the percentage of the state population with disabilities based on the 2017-2018 Area Health Resource File.[4] We also interviewed officials from a nongeneralizable sample of five managed care organizations (MCO) in five of the selected states (Indiana, Nevada, Pennsylvania, South Carolina, and Washington); Vermont's all-payer accountable care organization (ACO); and officials from CMS and its contractors.[5] We selected these MCOs after asking the officials from each of the five state Medicaid agencies to identify which of their Medicaid MCOs might be able to provide good examples of practices related to our objectives. We then selected the organizations to provide us with variation in whether they operated nationally or on a state or regional basis. South Dakota does not use managed care, so we only spoke with state officials. In conducting this work, we relied on officials from states and organizations to explain how they identified, predicted, or managed beneficiaries they considered to be high-expenditure, and their definitions and responses varied widely. For the purpose of this chapter, we use the term "high-expenditure" to refer to beneficiaries who account for a disproportionately large share of Medicaid expenditures, or are at risk for doing so in the future.

We conducted this performance audit from August 2018 through September 2019 in accordance with generally accepted government auditing standards. Those standards require that we plan and perform the audit to obtain sufficient, appropriate evidence to provide a reasonable basis for our findings and conclusions based on our audit objectives. We believe that the evidence obtained provides a reasonable basis for our findings and conclusions based on our audit objectives.

BACKGROUND

At the federal level, CMS, within the Department of Health and Human Services, is responsible for overseeing the design and operation of states' Medicaid programs, and states administer their respective Medicaid programs' day-to-day operations. As a comprehensive health benefit program for vulnerable populations, each state Medicaid program, by law, must cover certain categories of individuals and provide a broad array of benefits. Within these requirements, however, states have significant flexibility to design and implement their programs, resulting in more than 50 distinct state-based

---

[4] The Area Health Resource File is a federal data set comprised of data collected from more than 50 sources and contains thousands of variables related to health care access at the county level.

[5] An MCO is an organization that contracts with the state to provide health care services to Medicaid beneficiaries. An ACO is a group of coordinated health care providers that are held responsible for the care of a group of patients.

programs. These variations in design have implications for program eligibility and services offered, as well as for how expenditures are reported and services delivered.

Medicaid Service Delivery

In administering their own programs, states may provide Medicaid services under a fee-for-service delivery model or a managed care service delivery model. Under a fee-for-service model, states make payments directly to providers for services provided, and the federal government generally matches state expenditures for such services on the basis of a statutory formula. Under a managed care model, states pay MCOs a capitation payment, which is a fixed periodic payment per beneficiary enrolled in an MCO—typically, per member per month. MCOs pay health care providers for the services delivered to enrollees.[6] In contrast, ACOs are organizations of health care providers and suppliers that come together voluntarily to provide coordinated care to patients with the goal of reducing spending while improving quality. States vary in terms of the types of managed care arrangements used, the populations enrolled, and the parts of the state covered by managed care.

Service Utilization and Expenditures

We previously reported that a small share of beneficiaries in each state collectively accounted for a disproportionately large share of total Medicaid expenditures.[7] We found that in fiscal years 2009 through 2011, the most expensive 5 percent of Medicaid beneficiaries consistently accounted for almost half of the expenditures for all Medicaid beneficiaries (See Figure 1).

---

[6] States may have different types of Medicaid managed care arrangements, some of which have a limited benefit package or do not assume financial risk for the services provided.

Except as otherwise noted, in this chapter, we are referring to comprehensive, risk-based managed care, which is the most common managed care arrangement. An MCO contracts with a state to provide comprehensive health care services through its network of providers, is responsible for ensuring access to Medicaid services, and is at financial risk for the cost of providing those services.

[7] See GAO, *Medicaid: Demographics and Service Usage of Certain High-Expenditure Beneficiaries*, GAO-14-176 (Washington, D.C.: Feb. 19, 2014), which reported findings based on 2009 data for dually eligible beneficiaries and for those who were only enrolled in Medicaid; and *Medicaid: A Small Share of Enrollees Consistently Accounted for a Large Share of Expenditures*, GAO-15-460 (Washington, D.C.: May 8, 2018), which reported findings based on data from 2009 through 2011 for those who were only enrolled in Medicaid.

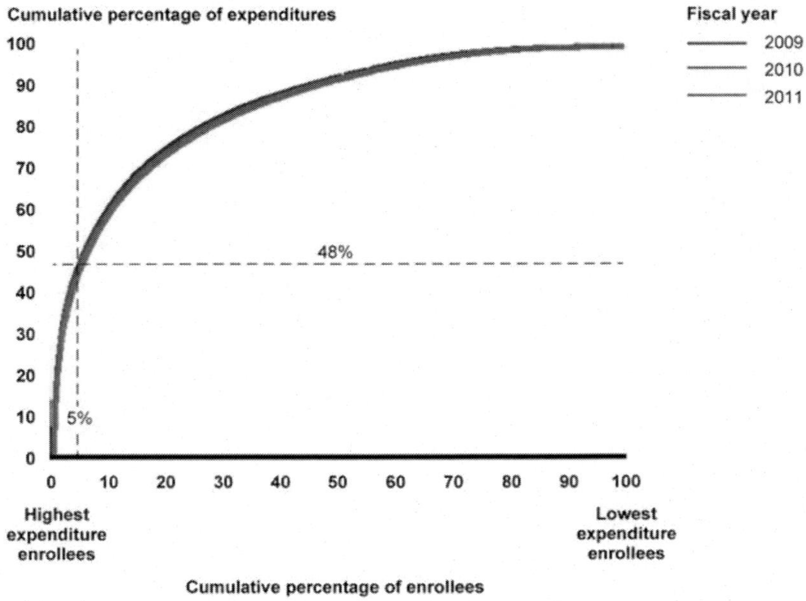

Source: GAO analysis of data from the Centers for Medicare & Medicaid Services. | GAO-19-569.

Figure 1. Distribution of Medicaid Expenditures Among Beneficiaries Only Enrolled in Medicaid, Fiscal Years 2009 through 2011.

Examining beneficiaries who were enrolled only in Medicaid, we also found that the most expensive 5 percent of beneficiaries were much more likely to have certain conditions—such as asthma, diabetes, and behavioral health conditions—than all other beneficiaries enrolled only in Medicaid. Examining 2009 data, we found that about 65 percent of the total expenditures for high-expenditure beneficiaries enrolled only in Medicaid were for hospital services and long-term services and supports, with the remaining 35 percent of expenditures for drugs, payments to managed care organizations and premium assistance, and non-hospital acute care.

Other studies have also found similar patterns of service utilization and expenditures within the Medicaid population. For example, a January 2018 report noted that while beneficiaries who are dually eligible for Medicare and Medicaid constituted about 15 percent of Medicaid beneficiaries in 2013, they accounted for nearly one-third of Medicaid spending.[8] A study examining data on children's use of behavioral health services in Medicaid found that in 2005, about 10 percent of children in Medicaid

[8] Some Medicaid beneficiaries are also eligible for Medicare—a federally financed health insurance program for persons 65 years of age or over, certain individuals with disabilities, and individuals with end-stage renal disease—and are characterized as "dually eligible." While dually eligible beneficiaries are diverse in terms of health care needs and service utilization, they include many with extensive health needs and high health care costs. See Medicare Payment Advisory Commission and Medicaid and Children's Health Insurance Program Payment and Access Commission, *Data Book: Beneficiaries Dually Eligible for Medicare and Medicaid* (Washington, D.C.: January 2018).

received behavioral health services, but those services accounted for about 38 percent of spending on the overall Medicaid child population.[9]

Care Management

Care management programs can be used as efforts to manage the cost and quality of health care services delivered to high-expenditure Medicaid populations, with the aim of improving outcomes and achieving cost savings. Generally, care management programs seek to assist consumers manage physical and mental health conditions more effectively, for example, by assessing patient needs and coordinating care across different providers. The general goal of care management is to achieve an optimal level of wellness and improve coordination of care while providing cost effective, non-duplicative services. Specific definitions for care management and other related terms such as care coordination, case management, and disease management vary. For the purpose of this chapter, we use care management to refer to these activities unless otherwise specified.

SELECTED STATES IDENTIFIED OR PREDICTED HIGH- EXPENDITURE MEDICAID BENEFICIARIES USING STATISTICS AND OTHER APPROACHES

Through interviews with officials, we found that all seven selected states, five MCOs, and the ACO took at least one approach to identify or predict high-expenditure beneficiaries, and some took more than one approach. State officials said they used these approaches to identify or predict high-expenditure beneficiaries among different segments of their Medicaid populations, such as beneficiaries in fee-for-service delivery systems or those with certain chronic conditions. The approaches were as follows:

Risk Scores

Officials from most state agencies, MCOs, and the ACO said they used risk scores to identify or predict high-expenditure beneficiaries.[10] Officials from four of the seven

---

[9] See S. A. Pires, *Examining Children's Behavioral Health Service Utilization and Expenditures*.

[10] A risk score is the ratio of expected—or predicted—health care expenditures for that beneficiary relative to the average health care expenditures for all beneficiaries in a reference population (e.g., adults in Medicaid who qualify for coverage based on a disability). For example, a beneficiary with a risk score of 1.05 would have expected expenditures that were 5 percent greater than the average beneficiary, who is assigned a risk score of 1.00.

selected states, four MCOs, and the ACO said they used software or hired vendors who computed beneficiaries' risk scores based on Medicaid service utilization data.[11] Washington state officials said that in addition to Medicaid service utilization data, they used utilization data from Medicare Parts A, B, and D to compute risk scores for their dual-eligible population.[12] Officials also discussed using the risk scores they computed in different ways. For example, Washington officials said they considered beneficiaries with a risk score of 1.5 or greater to be high expenditure, and they used that risk score as one of the eligibility criteria that must be met to receive certain care management services. In contrast, officials from an MCO in Nevada said they considered risk scores alongside other contextual information, such as the recent diagnosis of a chronic condition, to predict whether the beneficiary would likely generate high expenditures in the future and should be assigned care management services. Officials from three states, an MCO in South Carolina, and the ACO we interviewed said their software or vendors identified or predicted high-expenditure beneficiaries by using the risk scores they computed to stratify beneficiaries into risk tiers, such as low, medium, and high risk.[13]

Statistical Outliers

Officials from South Carolina's state Medicaid agency and two MCOs from Pennsylvania and Washington said they identified high-expenditure beneficiaries by examining service utilization data to identify statistical outliers or trends. Officials from the two MCOs said they looked for statistical outliers for various types of service utilization, such as emergency department visits, inpatient stays, and pharmacy use. Officials from South Carolina said they built internal software tools to help them easily examine service utilization for various subsets of beneficiaries and services. These officials said they looked for beneficiaries whose utilization appeared to be significantly higher or lower compared with other beneficiaries with similar characteristics, such as among children with Type 1 diabetes or among children in foster care. The officials also said that after they identified those outliers, they examined the reasons for those beneficiaries' utilization patterns to better understand why those beneficiaries were outliers and to take corrective action if appropriate.

The officials explained that they did not simply focus on a discrete list of beneficiaries with the highest overall expenditures, because many of those beneficiaries

[11] The four states were Nevada, South Dakota, Vermont, and Washington. The four MCOs were from Indiana, Nevada, Pennsylvania, and South Carolina.

[12] Medicare consists of Parts A, B, C, and the Part D prescription drug program. Parts A and B, which generally cover physician and hospital services, are known as traditional Medicare or Medicare fee-for-service. Medicare Part C, also known as Medicare Advantage, is a private plan alternative to traditional Medicare, and generally covers all traditional Medicare services.

[13] The three states were Nevada, South Dakota, and Vermont. Risk tiering assigns beneficiaries to distinct risk levels or categories based on multiple factors, including case complexity and cost.

have medical needs that are inherently expensive and cannot be meaningfully improved through intervention.

Diagnoses

Officials from three of the seven state Medicaid agencies and four MCOs said they identified high-expenditure beneficiaries based on diagnoses or other group categorization.[14] Officials commonly said they used chronic conditions, such as end-stage renal disease, the human immunodeficiency virus or acquired immune deficiency syndrome, chronic obstructive pulmonary disease, diabetes, or Hepatitis C. Pennsylvania officials said their list was developed based on clinical experience.

Officials from South Carolina said their list of diagnoses was based on a review of conditions associated with high expenditures.

Service Utilization and Claims Expenditure Thresholds

Officials from two state Medicaid agencies—Indiana and Nevada—and all five MCOs said they identified high-expenditure beneficiaries as beneficiaries who exceed certain service utilization or claims expenditure thresholds.[15] Indiana officials said they used service utilization thresholds, such as visiting the emergency room six or more times in the past 6 months. Nevada officials said one of their programs identified high-expenditure beneficiaries as those whose treatment costs exceeded $100,000 over a 12-month period. Officials from the five MCOs offered varying thresholds, such as claims exceeding $100,000 over a 6-month period; claims exceeding $40,000 during a state fiscal year; or stays in a neonatal intensive care unit exceeding 15 days.

Clinical Judgment

Officials from two state Medicaid agencies—Nevada and Pennsylvania— four MCOs, and the ACO said they relied on clinical judgment to decide whether a beneficiary was likely to be high expenditure.[16] Officials from one MCO in Washington said the MCO conducted health assessments of new members to obtain a baseline understanding of their clinical states, which were then used to stratify beneficiaries and

---

[14] The three states were Pennsylvania, South Carolina, and South Dakota. The four MCOs were from Indiana, Nevada, Pennsylvania, and Washington.

[15] The five MCOs were from Indiana, Nevada, Pennsylvania, South Carolina, and Washington.

[16] The four MCOs were from Indiana, Nevada, Pennsylvania, and Washington.

identify appropriate staff to address their needs. Similarly, officials from Pennsylvania and three MCOs said clinical reviews of beneficiaries' needs or histories were triggered by providers, caregivers, or self-referrals for care management or other services. Officials from the ACO said that while risk scores made initial predictions about beneficiaries' risk for generating high expenditures, those predictions could be overridden by clinical judgment.

SELECTED STATES USED CARE MANAGEMENT AND OTHER STRATEGIES TO MANAGE COSTS FOR HIGH- EXPENDITURE MEDICAID BENEFICIARIES

Officials from all seven selected states, all five MCOs, and the ACO we interviewed said they used care management to manage the costs and quality of care for high-expenditure Medicaid beneficiaries. In addition, some states used other strategies, such as strategies involving coverage policies, payment incentives, and restrictions on the number of providers certain beneficiaries could use. Across states that evaluated these efforts to manage costs and quality of care, results were mixed.

All Selected States Used Care Management to Manage Costs for High-Expenditure Medicaid Beneficiaries

Officials from all of the seven state Medicaid agencies we interviewed reported that they provided care management for high-expenditure beneficiaries in their fee-for-service delivery systems, for example, by assessing patient needs and coordinating care across providers, in an attempt to manage costs and ensure quality care. Further, the six selected states with MCOs or ACOs required these organizations to provide care management to high-expenditure beneficiaries enrolled in managed care. Officials also reported barriers to their efforts to provide care management.

Care Management in Fee-for-Service Medicaid

Officials from all of the seven state Medicaid agencies we interviewed reported that they provided care management for high-expenditure beneficiaries in their fee-for-service delivery system, to manage the cost and quality of their care. The organization and scope of the care management programs they described vary in some cases. For example:

- Pennsylvania provided care management for beneficiaries in fee-for- service through the state's "intensive case management" unit, a unit of providers that contact beneficiaries by phone to ensure that they get the care they need. Care management is provided to newly enrolled Medicaid beneficiaries who are identified as high-expenditure until the beneficiary selects a managed care plan, typically within 30 days, and to certain other beneficiaries.[17] State officials said that of the approximately 150,000 beneficiaries in fee-for-service, they provide care management to about 1,000 each month.
- Nevada implemented mandatory care management services for high- expenditure fee-for-service beneficiaries in rural areas of the state through a contract with a care management organization, which was paid to reach out to high-expenditure beneficiaries, assess their needs, and connect them with their medical providers.[18] The organization delivered care management through regional care teams geographically located in beneficiaries' communities, which coordinated with the beneficiaries' providers to implement personalized care plans and manage follow-up appointments and services. High-expenditure beneficiaries were assigned to one of eight care management programs based on the beneficiary's qualifying condition, such as whether they had cancer, chronic kidney disease, or a mental health diagnosis.
- South Dakota implemented a health home program in 2013, which paid local primary care clinics, community mental health centers, and Indian Health Service facilities to provide care management to high- expenditure Medicaid beneficiaries.[19] Each clinic or center had a care coordinator who reached out to high-expenditure beneficiaries to initiate care management and connect them with their primary care providers. These beneficiaries were placed in one of four categories indicating the level of care coordination they needed based on the severity of their illness and risk of future costs. The program helped beneficiaries create a care plan, set goals to address their particular care needs, and manage their conditions. In state fiscal year 2018, around 5,800 recipients received services through more than 100 health home clinics in South Dakota.[20]

---

[17] Care management was also provided to high-expenditure beneficiaries dually eligible for Medicaid and Medicare, a group that was not historically eligible for managed care in Pennsylvania, but is beginning to be enrolled in managed care, according to state officials.

[18] The Care Management Organization was not a risk-based managed care organization, in that it was not at risk for the cost of medical care provided to these beneficiaries. In Nevada, beneficiaries in the two most populous counties are generally enrolled in managed care, and those in other counties are in fee-for-service.

[19] In 2010, the Patient Protection and Affordable Care Act established a state option to provide health homes for Medicaid enrollees with chronic conditions, beginning January 1, 2011, which is called the Health Home State Plan Option. Health homes integrate physical and behavioral health (both mental health and substance abuse) and long-term services and supports for high-need, high-cost Medicaid populations. See Pub. L. No. 111-148, § 2703, 124 Stat. 119, 319 (codified as amended at 42 U.S.C. § 1396w-4).

[20] See South Dakota Department of Social Services, *South Dakota Medicaid Report, SFY18* (November, 2018).

- Washington State also implemented a health home program in 2013 in which care management activities were coordinated through "lead" entities, such as Area Agencies on Aging and other community-based organizations.[21] These entities established networks of care coordination organizations representing primary care, mental health, long term care, chemical dependency providers, and specialty providers. The lead entities conducted outreach to high-expenditure beneficiaries to connect them with a care manager, who might be a nurse, physician assistant, social worker, behavioral health professional, or chemical dependency professional.[22]

Care Management in Managed Care

State Medicaid officials who have MCOs and ACOs within their states said that they required these organizations to provide care management to high-expenditure beneficiaries to manage the cost and quality of their care.[23] Examples of states' care management requirements included steps such as beneficiary and provider outreach, conducting screenings or health assessments, and developing care plans (see sidebar). Some requirements specified the minimum frequency for conducting outreach and what information and data must be reported to the state regarding care management activities (see sidebar).

Indiana's Requirements for Care Management of High-Expenditure Beneficiaries in Managed Care Organizations (MCO)

- For specified diseases, the MCO must make a variety of disease management tools available, including care management.
- Beneficiaries with excessive utilization or under-utilization for conditions other than those specified diseases in the contract must also be eligible for disease management services.
- The MCO must contact beneficiaries via telephone and in person, as indicated by their need. Care managers must engage in care conferences with beneficiaries' health care providers, as necessary.
- Clinicians must develop the beneficiary's care plan, and care plans must be reviewed by the medical director.
- The MCO's care management services must involve the active management of the beneficiary and his or her group of health care providers, including physicians, medical equipment, transportation, and pharmacy.
- The MCO must submit quarterly reports providing data on care management.

Source: GAO analysis of state documentation Hoosier Healthwise and Healthy Indiana Plan MCE Policies and Procedures Manual, Published February 8, 2018.| GAO-19-569.

---

[21] Area Agencies on Aging are public or private nonprofit agencies designated by states to coordinate services at the regional and local level that help older adults, including social and nutrition services supported by federal funds authorized under the Older Americans Act of 1965, as amended. See 42 U.S.C. § 3001, et seq.

[22] Washington's Health Homes Program was incorporated into the state's Managed Fee- for-Service model demonstration under the Financial Alignment Initiative, a program created by CMS to test integrated care models for dually eligible beneficiaries.

[23] The states with MCOs were Indiana, Nevada, Pennsylvania, South Carolina, and Washington, and the state with an ACO was Vermont.

Examples of State Requirements for Managed Care Organizations (MCO) Related to Contacting High-Expenditure Beneficiaries and Reporting to the State

Contacting Beneficiaries:

- The accountable care organization must communicate with beneficiaries at least four times per year. (Vermont Medicaid)
- At least half of the encounters with beneficiaries must be face-to-face. (Pennsylvania Medicaid Community Based Care Management)
- The MCO shall document at least three attempts to conduct the initial health needs assessment screening. (Nevada Medicaid).

Reporting to the State:

- The MCOs must submit reports on how beneficiaries are categorized for different levels of care coordination. (Indiana Medicaid)
- MCOs must submit reports on beneficiaries with inpatient costs of over $50,000, on a quarterly basis. (Nevada Medicaid)

Source: GAO analysis of information from interviews of officials with selected state Medicaid agencies and MCOs. | GAO-19-569.

Officials from the MCOs and the ACO that we interviewed in these six states confirmed that they provided care management to high- expenditure beneficiaries. MCO and ACO officials described various aspects of their care management programs. For example:

- According to officials from an Indiana MCO, the MCO operated different care management programs for high-expenditure beneficiaries depending on their clinical condition or other characteristics. Examples include programs for beneficiaries with certain chronic conditions (such as diabetes, congestive heart failure, and asthma), programs for beneficiaries with complex medical conditions who are at high risk of not following their prescribed treatment, and programs for pregnant women with identified conditions that put them at high risk for poor outcomes.
- Officials from the South Carolina MCO told us that the MCO had a standard model of care management for high-risk beneficiaries, but each clinical department in the MCO—for example, Obstetrics or Cardiology—established specific plans for care management within their area of care. Care managers in these departments—nurses or social workers—were responsible for coordinating with a beneficiary's primary care provider to ensure that the beneficiary is appropriately referred to specialists. Care managers can contact beneficiaries by phone, but they are also based in the community, such as at hospitals and state mental health clinics.

- Officials from the ACO in Vermont said that the ACO paid providers that were part of their network—such as primary care offices, home health agencies, and mental health agencies—to serve as beneficiaries' care managers. Beneficiaries select one provider to be their "lead care coordinator" based on who they have the strongest relationship and trust with, and this provider receives enhanced payments from the ACO to support coordination with other providers in the beneficiary's care team. Care team members communicate with each other through a software tool provided by the ACO, which maintains updated information on beneficiaries' conditions and the care received.

Barriers to Care Management for High-Expenditure Beneficiaries

Officials we spoke to from the selected states, MCOs, and the ACO identified barriers to implementing care management for some high- expenditure Medicaid beneficiaries, including the inability to contact beneficiaries, the lack of social supports—that are part of what is referred to as "social determinants of health"—and shortages of providers or care management staff in rural areas.[24]

Addressing Social Determinants of Health

Officials at most of the selected states, managed care organizations (MCO), and the accountable care organization said they took steps to help beneficiaries address social determinants of health, for example, by gathering data to identify which beneficiaries needed help with social supports, helping beneficiaries obtain transportation to medical appointments, assisting beneficiaries in accessing social services, providing short-term housing, and meeting other needs.

For example, officials from one MCO described a beneficiary with diabetes, who, despite consistently filling his prescription and adhering to his care plan, regularly visited the emergency department in insulin shock. Through outreach they discovered that the beneficiary could not appropriately store his prescribed insulin, which needed to be refrigerated, because his home did not have running electricity or a refrigerator. The MCO identified resources in the community to provide a refrigerator and restore electricity.

Source: GAO analysis of information from interviews of officials with selected state Medicaid agencies and MCOs. | GAO-19-569.

- Difficulties contacting beneficiaries. The lack of valid contact information can result from missing or outdated information, transiency and homelessness, and beneficiary reliance on cell phones with limited minutes. Officials described efforts they had taken to address this barrier, including asking pharmacies to confirm and get updated information when beneficiaries pick up prescriptions;

[24] Social determinants of health include factors like socioeconomic status, education, neighborhood and physical environment, employment, and social support networks, as well as access to health care. Addressing these is important for improving health and reducing longstanding disparities in health and health care.

using e- mail, which officials stated is more consistent than physical addresses; and conducting direct outreach in emergency rooms.

- Social determinants of health. The effectiveness of care management in addressing the health needs of high-expenditure beneficiaries can be hindered by the lack of social supports. Officials said that in order to help beneficiaries manage their medical needs, care managers sometimes needed to address these social determinants of health, such as lack of transportation to medical appointments, lack of stable housing, and inconsistent access to food and other basic resources (see sidebar). At the same time, states and MCOs can face challenges to addressing social determinants of health, such as lack of data on social determinants of health and a lack of understanding about the effect of social determinants of health on health care utilization, which if available could help bolster program investments in those areas.[25]
- Staff shortages in rural areas. Efforts to provide care management and medical services can be hindered by staff shortages in rural areas. Officials with one state Medicaid agency's health home program said there was a shortage of individuals in rural areas willing to provide care management to high-expenditure beneficiaries. MCO officials in another state said their ability to care for beneficiaries in rural areas was also affected by a shortage of care managers.

In Addition to Care Management, Some Selected States Used Other Strategies to Manage High-Expenditure Beneficiaries

Other strategies, in addition to care management, reported by selected states—South Carolina, Nevada, Pennsylvania, and Indiana—to manage the cost and care for high-expenditure Medicaid beneficiaries included coverage policy changes, payment incentives, and restrictions on the use of providers.

Coverage Policy Changes

South Carolina Medicaid officials said that in certain cases they reviewed their coverage policy to see if changes could reduce costs and improve health outcomes for high-expenditure beneficiaries. For example, according to officials, the state had a small number of high-expenditure beneficiaries with Type 1 diabetes that officials thought could benefit from continuous glucose monitoring, which was not covered by their state Medicaid program. The officials said that they wrote a proposal into their state budget

[25] While there are certain Medicaid program options available to states that allow them to address some aspects of social determinants of health for beneficiaries, there are also restrictions on the use of Medicaid funds for certain purposes. For example, states generally cannot use Medicaid funds to pay for room and board, but they can provide referral to community and social support services.

and drafted state plan amendment language to address this, though they noted that the proposal had not been implemented as of January 2019.

Payment Incentives

Medicaid officials in Nevada and Pennsylvania described efforts to use payment incentives to manage costs for high- expenditure beneficiaries.

- Nevada officials told us that the state's arrangement with its care management organization for high-expenditure beneficiaries included payment incentives related to reductions in cost, as well as performance on certain quality measures, such as immunization rates and treatments for specific conditions such as asthma, coronary artery disease, and heart failure. However, state officials said that they faced difficulties measuring these outcomes. The care management organization did not receive incentive payments for the first year of operation of the program (2014-2015) and state officials said they did not have results on incentive payments for subsequent years.
- Pennsylvania officials told us that in response to the high cost of drugs to treat Hepatitis C, Pennsylvania's Medicaid agency created a risk-sharing arrangement with MCOs that had high-expenditure beneficiaries with Hepatitis C. According to state officials, the MCOs were required to submit their enrollees' Hepatitis C test scores to show whether beneficiaries were obtaining treatment and experiencing improvement. The state then allocated additional funds to MCOs that demonstrated positive quality outcomes, thus saving the cost of re-treating beneficiaries who failed to follow through on treatment.
- The Pennsylvania officials also told us that the state provided payment incentives to MCOs in its Integrated Care Plan Program, in which physical health and behavioral health MCOs coordinate with each other in the care of high-expenditure beneficiaries with persistent serious mental illness, such as schizophrenia, depression, or psychosis.[26] To quality for incentive payments, these MCOs had to create an integrated care plan for each beneficiary with a qualifying condition. The state's Medicaid agency identified outcome measures that MCOs were held accountable to in calendar year 2018 related to emergency department utilization, inpatient admissions, inpatient readmissions, prescription medication adherence, and engagement in treatment for substance use disorders. As metrics improved, MCOs become eligible for incentives. According to state officials, Pennsylvania allocated $10 million for Integrated Care Plan program incentive payments for calendar year 2018.

---

[26] Pennsylvania's state Medicaid agency contracts with limited benefit plans that provide a narrow set of benefits such as behavioral health services.

Restrictions on the Use of Providers

Indiana Medicaid officials described their program to address over-utilization of services by certain high-expenditure beneficiaries who may be engaged in doctor or pharmacy shopping—a strategy of using multiple providers that results in over-utilization or improper utilization of prescription drugs or other services. According to the officials, if other efforts to address a beneficiary's over-utilization fail over a 2- to 4-month period, the beneficiary may be enrolled in Indiana's Right Choices Program. This program restricts, or "locks in," the beneficiary to a single physician, pharmacy, and hospital. Officials said that this program has helped to ensure that the provider is aware of the beneficiary's history and has proven effective in getting beneficiaries to change their behavior. In addition to using the program for Medicaid beneficiaries enrolled in fee- for-service, MCOs are provided with a report of their beneficiaries who have high-utilization levels so that the MCO can determine if any of these beneficiaries should be enrolled in the program.

Across Selected States that Assessed the Effect of their Strategies on Medicaid Expenditures and Other Outcomes, Results Were Mixed

While some of the selected state Medicaid agencies reported that their efforts to manage costs and care for high-expenditure beneficiaries showed positive results, officials in other states reported mixed or inconclusive findings. Medicaid officials in four states—Pennsylvania, South Dakota, Vermont, and Washington—said their assessment of efforts to manage costs and care for high-expenditure beneficiaries showed positive results, such as cost savings or reductions in the use of expensive services.

- Pennsylvania Medicaid officials said that their Integrated Care Plan Program for high-expenditure beneficiaries with persistent serious mental illness resulted in improvements in utilization, including reductions in inpatient hospitalizations and readmissions.
- South Dakota Medicaid officials found that for 2017, health home participants cost $204 less per month than the comparison group, and experienced an 8 percent decline in emergency room visits from the prior year compared with a 10 percent increase in emergency room visits for the comparison group.[27] The state estimated $7.7 million in costs were avoided.
- Vermont Medicaid officials analyzed utilization of high-expenditure beneficiaries in care management before and after they enrolled. The state

[27] See Department of Social Services of South Dakota, *The State of the South Dakota Health Home Program CY 2017,* accessed April 30, 2019, https://dss.sd.gov/docs/healthhome/financial_analysis_word.pdf.

reported in 2018 that the rate of inpatient visits per thousand beneficiaries decreased from 600 to 393, and the annual rate of emergency visits per thousand beneficiaries decreased from 1,536 to 1,003.[28]

- An independent evaluation of a demonstration program for dually eligible beneficiaries in Washington that incorporated its Health Homes program found $107 million in Medicare cost savings over its first 42 months.[29] As part of the state's Financial Alignment Initiative, part of those savings went to the state Medicaid program.
- In contrast with the results reported by the four states, officials from Indiana and Nevada Medicaid agencies reported mixed or inconclusive findings related to the impact on cost or quality of their programs for high- expenditure Medicaid beneficiaries.
- Officials with Indiana's Medicaid agency told us that an assessment of the Right Choices Program found relatively low cost savings generally, with the exception of pharmacy costs, where the program curbed excessive drug use among beneficiaries with substance use disorders and led to cost savings.
- Nevada Medicaid officials said that their fee-for-service care management organization appeared to achieve some cost savings, but had little effect on quality of care after the program was implemented in 2013. They also said that it was difficult to determine the true effect of the program, because the state implemented several other cost savings policies at the same time as the care management organization. Nevada let the program expire in 2018 and is researching other potential ways to manage high-expenditure beneficiaries in the state's fee-for-service program.

CMS Offered Optional Tools and Technical Assistance That Could Be Used To Identify or Better Manage High-Expenditure Medicaid Beneficiaries

CMS offered optional tools, as well as technical assistance and other educational resources that state Medicaid agencies used to identify or better manage high-expenditure beneficiaries.

---

[28] See State of Vermont Agency of Human Services, *Global Commitment to Health 11-W- 00194/1, Annual Report for Demonstration Year 2017, January 1, 2017 to December 31, 2017* (March 29, 2018). The decline in utilization rates occurred between the 6-month period January to June 2016 and the 6-month period January to June 2017.

[29] See RTI International, Report for Washington Health Home Managed Fee-for-Service (MFFS) Final Demonstration Year 2 and Preliminary Demonstration Year 3 Medicare Savings Estimates: Medicare-Medicaid Financial Alignment Initiative, prepared for the Centers for Medicare & Medicaid Services (November 2018).

CMS Offered Tools That Could Help States Manage High- Expenditure Medicaid Beneficiaries

CMS's optional tools included the Health Home State Plan Option and the Financial Alignment Initiative, though these are not specifically designed for the purpose of identifying and managing high-expenditure beneficiaries. Medicaid officials in two selected states said that these programs improved their efforts to manage care for their high-expenditure beneficiaries.

Health Home State Plan Option

The Medicaid Health Home State Plan Option, authorized under the Patient Protection and Affordable Care Act, allowed states to design health home programs to provide comprehensive care coordination for Medicaid beneficiaries with chronic conditions.[30] CMS officials we spoke with said the states who chose the option received access to resources including planning funds and technical assistance from CMS. For example, CMS issued a brief illustrating how states could focus their health home programs on high-expenditure beneficiaries. CMS officials noted that they supported 23 states' and the District of Columbia's health home programs. Among the state officials we interviewed, South Dakota Medicaid officials said that when they were establishing their health home program, CMS was helpful in connecting them with other states that had created similar programs so that they could learn from other states' experiences. South Dakota Medicaid officials stated they would like CMS to continue to bring health home program managers from several states together to discuss their successes, challenges, and innovations. Nevada Medicaid officials stated they were considering establishing a health home program.

Financial Alignment Initiative

For the Financial Alignment Initiative, CMS oversaw efforts by states to implement improvements in Medicaid service delivery aimed at achieving savings for both Medicare and Medicaid, with one state we spoke with using the initiative to target high-expenditure beneficiaries. As noted earlier, Washington established its Health Homes demonstration program for dually eligible beneficiaries in association with the Financial Alignment Initiative. Washington targeted the demonstration to high-cost, high-risk Medicare-Medicaid beneficiaries based on the principle that focusing intensive care coordination on beneficiaries with the greatest need provided the greatest potential for improved health outcomes and cost savings. Washington's Financial Alignment Initiative

---

[30] States receive an enhanced Federal Medical Assistance Percentage for specific health home services defined in statute. The enhanced match does not apply to the underlying Medicaid services also provided to beneficiaries enrolled in a health home. The enhanced match is only available for the first eight quarters that the program is in effect. See 42 U.S.C. § 1396w-4(c)(1).

demonstration was approved through 2020, and Washington officials stated they are hoping to get an extension, because it has yielded cost savings for both Medicaid and Medicare.[31] A feature of the Financial Alignment Initiative is that any cost savings achieved by the program are split between the state Medicaid program and Medicare.

CMS Provided Technical Assistance and Educational Resources to Help States Identify and Manage Care for High-Expenditure Medicaid Beneficiaries

CMS also offered state Medicaid agencies access to several resources that, while not designed specifically to target high-expenditure beneficiaries, have been used to support states in identifying or better managing care for this population. These resources included the Medicaid Innovation Accelerator Program, the State Data Resource Center, and the Medicare-Medicaid Data Integration Initiative.

Medicaid Innovation Accelerator Program

The Medicaid Innovation Accelerator Program is funded by the Center for Medicare and Medicaid Innovation and run by the Center for Medicaid and CHIP Services, both within CMS. The goals of the program were to improve care for Medicaid beneficiaries and reduce costs by supporting states in their ongoing payment and delivery system reforms through targeted technical support. The program offered participating states targeted technical support to Medicaid agencies in building their data analytic capacity as they design and implement delivery system reforms for high-expenditure beneficiaries, one of the program's focus areas.[32] The program worked with five states on issues such as identifying and stratifying beneficiaries with complex care needs and high costs, designing effective care management strategies, and incorporating social determinants of health into program design activities.[33] In addition to working directly with five states, the program also offered a national webinar series under the broader topic of Medicaid Beneficiaries with Complex Care Needs and High Costs. The webinar series covered a variety of topics, including a webinar titled "Identification and Stratification of Medicaid Beneficiaries with Complex Care Needs and High Costs," which provided information about different approaches to targeting and assessing the needs of this population. Vermont Medicaid officials we spoke with said it would be helpful to have more

---

[31] As of April 24, 2019, CMS was accepting new applications for Financial Alignment Initiative demonstrations.

[32] The Medicaid Innovation Accelerator Program's other program focus areas include reducing substance use disorders, promoting community integration through long-term services and supports; and supporting physical and mental health integration.

[33] See CMS, Medicaid Innovation Accelerator Program, *Beneficiaries with Complex Care Needs and High Costs* (Baltimore, Md.: Oct. 31, 2016). The five states discussed were New Jersey, Oregon, Texas, Virginia, and the District of Columbia.

information about how social determinants of health impact beneficiaries' ability to manage their own care. CMS hosted other webinars on various technical support and data analytics topics for states. Among the state Medicaid officials we interviewed, Nevada officials mentioned participating in the Innovation Accelerator Program.

State Data Resource Center

State Medicaid agencies have traditionally been hampered in managing the Medicaid portion of care for dually eligible beneficiaries, because they lacked data on the Medicare services these beneficiaries receive, such as hospitalizations, physician visits, prescription drugs, and skilled nursing facility stays. To address this challenge, CMS established the State Data Resource Center to facilitate state access to and use of Medicare data on dually eligible beneficiaries. Through the program, states had access to technical advisors when working with CMS Medicare data, which have allowed states to better predict and identify high-expenditure dually eligible Medicaid beneficiaries, CMS officials told us. The officials said the State Data Resource Center provided states with learning opportunities through webinars and monthly "Medicare Data Workgroup" calls, during which states shared their data use experiences. CMS officials and CMS contractors we spoke with said 29 states have received Medicare data, including all 10 states that participated in the Financial Alignment Initiative, though not all had projects specifically linked to high- expenditure Medicaid beneficiaries. CMS officials said all states had some contact with the State Data Resource Center, whether through data inquiries or participation in webinars.

Medicare-Medicaid Data Integration Initiative

The Medicare-Medicaid Coordination Office and the Center for Medicaid and CHIP Services' Medicaid Innovation Accelerator Program, both within CMS, jointly sponsored the Medicare-Medicaid Data Integration Initiative. The initiative assisted states with integrating Medicare and Medicaid data in order to enhance care coordination and reduce costs for the dually eligible population, which may have included high-expenditure Medicaid beneficiaries. CMS officials we spoke with said the Medicare-Medicaid Data Integration Initiative had assisted 10 states—five participating in the Financial Alignment Initiative (Colorado, Minnesota, Ohio, Rhode Island, and Virginia) and five participating in the Medicaid Innovation Accelerator Program from October 2015 to March 2019 (Alabama, the District of Columbia, New Hampshire, New Jersey, and Pennsylvania).

AGENCY COMMENTS

We provided a draft of this product to the Department of Health and Human Services for review. The department provided technical comments, which we incorporated as appropriate.

As agreed with your office, unless you publicly announce the contents of this chapter earlier, we plan no further distribution until 30 days from the report date. At that time, we will send copies to the appropriate congressional committees, the Secretary of Health and Human Services, and other interested parties.

Carolyn L. Yocom
Director, Health Care

In: Medicaid: Fraud, Payments and Beneficiaries
Editor: Nadia M. Hedegaard
ISBN: 978-1-53617-666-7

Chapter 3

MEDICAID PAYMENT: CMS HAS NOT OVERSEEN STATES' IMPLEMENTATION OF CHANGES TO THIRD-PARTY LIABILITY*

United States Government Accountability Office

ABBREVIATIONS

CHIP	Children's Health Insurance Program
CMS	Centers for Medicare & Medicaid Services
CSE	child support enforcement
HHS	Department of Health and Human Services
MCO	managed care organization
MMIS	Medicaid Management Information System

WHY GAO DID THIS STUDY

The Medicaid program is typically the payer of last resort. The Bipartisan Budget Act of 2018 changed the Medicaid third-party liability payment requirements for prenatal care services, pediatric preventive services, and services provided to CSE beneficiaries. Before the act, in the case of these three services, states were generally required to pay

* This is an edited, reformatted and augmented version of United States Government Accountability Office; Report to Congressional Requesters, Publication No. GAO-19-601, dated August 2019.

providers for services delivered to Medicaid beneficiaries and then obtain any payments from liable third parties.

The Bipartisan Budget Act of 2018 also included a provision for GAO to study the potential effects of these changes. In this chapter, GAO (1) describes the status of selected states' implementation of Medicaid third-party liability changes; (2) evaluates CMS's implementation and oversight of the Medicaid third-party liability changes; and (3) describes stakeholders' views of the possible effects of these changes on providers and beneficiaries. GAO conducted interviews with state Medicaid agencies and provider associations in nine selected states, which were selected by taking into consideration Medicaid spending and stakeholder recommendations, among other factors. GAO also conducted interviews with national experts in Medicaid, national organizations representing beneficiaries and providers, and officials from CMS.

What GAO Recommends

GAO is recommending that CMS (1) ensure that its guidance to states on third-party liability requirements reflects current law, and (2) determine the extent to which state Medicaid programs are meeting federal third-party liability requirements. The Department of Health and Human Services concurred with these recommendations.

What GAO Found

Medicaid officials in the nine selected states GAO reviewed described being in various stages of implementing third-party liability changes as required by law. These changes affect whether health care providers must seek payment from a liable third party, such as private insurance, before the state Medicaid agency pays for services. The changes apply to prenatal care services, pediatric preventive services, and services for children subject to child support enforcement (CSE beneficiaries). At the time of GAO's review,

- Officials from four of the nine selected states reported having fully implemented the changes for prenatal care services, which were required to be implemented starting in February 2018. Officials from the remaining five states were discussing the changes internally, researching how to implement the changes in their Medicaid payment systems, or waiting for additional guidance from the Centers for Medicare & Medicaid Services (CMS), the federal agency responsible for overseeing states' Medicaid programs.

- None of the nine states had implemented the changes to pediatric preventive services and services for CSE beneficiaries, which must be implemented starting in October 2019. Officials from six states told GAO that they were in the early stages of exploring how they would make the changes, while the remaining three states had not developed such plans.

GAO found that guidance issued by CMS in June 2018 to assist states in implementing the third-party liability changes contains information inconsistent with the law. For example, CMS's guidance incorrectly informs states that providers do not need to seek third-party payments before the state pays for some prenatal services. In addition, CMS has not determined the extent to which states are meeting third-party liability requirements. CMS officials stated that they expect states to comply with current law for Medicaid third-party liability and that they do not verify whether states have implemented the required third-party liability changes unless the agency is made aware of non-compliance. However, this approach is inconsistent with CMS's Medicaid oversight responsibilities, including its responsibility to ensure federal funds are appropriately spent.

Medicaid experts and other stakeholders told GAO that the third-party liability changes could affect some health care providers in ways that could result in decreased beneficiary access to care, because some providers might be less willing to see Medicaid patients. According to stakeholders, this could occur for two primary reasons.

1. The changes may increase administrative requirements for providers by requiring them to identify sources of coverage, obtain insurance information, and submit claims to third-party insurers before submitting them to Medicaid.
2. The changes may result in providers waiting longer to receive Medicaid payment for certain services to the extent that states require providers to seek third-party payments before paying the providers' claims.

August 9, 2019

The Honorable Chuck Grassley
Chairman

The Honorable Ron Wyden
Ranking Member
Committee on Finance
United States Senate

The Honorable Frank Pallone
Chairman

The Honorable Greg Walden
Ranking Member
Committee on Energy and Commerce
House of Representatives

With few exceptions, Medicaid is considered the payer of last resort, meaning that when beneficiaries have another source of health care coverage—such as private health insurance provided through an employer—that source, to the extent of its liability, should generally pay for services before Medicaid does. This concept is referred to as "third-party liability." When a third party pays for its share of an individual's Medicaid costs, savings can accrue to the federal government and the states.

The Bipartisan Budget Act of 2018 made changes to the procedures state Medicaid agencies must follow when they receive certain claims for which a third party might be liable, among other things.[1] Specifically, the act changed states' responsibilities for processing claims for three types of services: prenatal care services, pediatric preventive services, and services for children for whom child support enforcement (CSE) is being carried out by the state (also known as CSE beneficiaries).[2] The changes pertaining to prenatal care services went into effect in February 2018; the changes related to pediatric services and services for CSE beneficiaries go into effect in October 2019. Before the act, in the case of these three services, states were generally required to pay providers for services delivered to Medicaid beneficiaries and then obtain any payments from liable third parties—a process known as "pay and chase." The Congressional Budget Office estimated that the Bipartisan Budget Act of 2018 third-party liability changes would result in approximately $4 billion in federal savings from 2018 through 2027.

The Bipartisan Budget Act of 2018 includes a provision for GAO to study the impact or potential future impact of these third-party liability changes on both Medicaid beneficiaries and providers. In this chapter we

1. describe the status of selected states' implementation of third-party liability changes for state Medicaid programs;

---

[1] See Pub. L. No. 115-123, § 53102, 132 Stat. 64 (codified as amended at 42 U.S.C. § 1396a(a)(25)).

[2] In this chapter, we refer to these statutory changes as the "third-party liability changes," although the Bipartisan Budget Act of 2018 made other changes to the Medicaid third- party liability statute that are not the focus of this chapter. CMS defines "pediatric preventive services" to include all services covered under the Medicaid early and periodic screening, diagnosis and treatment benefit. 42 C.F.R § 433.139(b)(3)(i) (2018). CMS provides definitions of prenatal care services, which it defines to include, at state option, pregnancy-related services (i.e., labor, delivery, and postpartum care services) in section 3904.4 of the State Medicaid Manual, but indicates that states have the option to define these terms more broadly, such as to include preexisting conditions that are likely to affect the pregnancy. In this chapter, we use the term "CSE beneficiary" to refer to a Medicaid beneficiary on whose behalf child support enforcement is being carried out by the state.

2. evaluate CMS's implementation and oversight of third-party liability changes for state Medicaid programs; and
3. describe stakeholders' views on the possible effects of third-party liability changes and the methods state Medicaid program officials could use to monitor these changes.

To describe the status of states' implementation of third-party liability changes, we judgmentally selected nine states: Connecticut, Florida, Illinois, Kentucky, Nevada, New Jersey, Tennessee, Texas, and Utah. We selected these states to include a range of characteristics such as the delivery systems of their Medicaid programs (e.g., fee-for-service verses managed care), Medicaid spending, percentage of births financed by Medicaid, and third-party liability collections, and while also taking into consideration recommendations from background experts and national provider associations.[3] We conducted semi-structured interviews with relevant officials from each state's Medicaid agency between November 2018 and March 2019. We also conducted interviews with stakeholders from state chapters of the American Academy of Pediatrics and the American College of Obstetricians and Gynecologists, with two providers, with Medicaid managed care organizations (MCO) in three of our selected states, and with three groups advocating for the needs of Medicaid beneficiaries.[4] Throughout this chapter, we use the term "stakeholders" to refer collectively to officials from state Medicaid agencies and Medicaid MCOs, background experts, beneficiary advocates, provider associations, and providers. To evaluate CMS's implementation and oversight of third-party liability changes for state Medicaid programs, we reviewed relevant laws and available guidance, including relevant regulations, CMS's Coordination of Benefits and Third-Party Liability (COB/TPL) in Medicaid handbook, and an informational bulletin released on June 1, 2018, concerning CMS's implementation of federal third-party liability requirements and agency oversight responsibilities regarding Medicaid state plans and state plan amendments. We also conducted interviews with officials from CMS and obtained written responses from CMS officials.

To describe stakeholders' views on the possible effects of the third-party liability changes and the methods state Medicaid officials could use to monitor the potential

---

[3] During the course of interviews with background experts and national provider associations, we asked which states they recommended we review regarding this topic. Background experts we interviewed included two individuals with experience in Medicaid policy, as well as officials from the National Health Law Program, the Medicaid and CHIP Payment and Access Commission, the Center on Budget and Policy Priorities, the National Association of Medicaid Directors, and Medicaid Health Plans of America. The national provider associations we interviewed included the American Academy of Pediatrics and the American College of Obstetricians and Gynecologists.
Some of these stakeholders suggested states based on factors such as the number of children and women served by a state's Medicaid program and the perceived effectiveness of the Medicaid agency within a state, among other things.

[4] Medicaid managed care organizations (MCO) are organizations with which states may contract to provide a specific set of Medicaid-covered services to beneficiaries. States pay MCOs a set amount per beneficiary to provide these services, typically per month.

effects on providers and beneficiaries, we conducted interviews with state Medicaid agency officials in the nine selected states. During these interviews, we asked officials about what potential effects they anticipated these changes having on beneficiaries and providers and how states could monitor the effects of the third-party liability changes. We also conducted interviews with other relevant stakeholders—including individuals and organizations with expertise in Medicaid (identified through interviews), national provider associations (e.g., the American Academy of Pediatrics and the American College of Obstetricians and Gynecologists), state chapters for provider associations, and organizations representing beneficiaries—during which we asked about the potential effects the third-party liability changes would have on affected beneficiaries and providers.[5] We conducted this performance audit from April 2018 to August 2019 in accordance with generally accepted government auditing standards. Those standards require that we plan and perform the audit to obtain sufficient, appropriate evidence to provide a reasonable basis for our findings and conclusions based on our audit objectives. We believe that the evidence obtained provides a reasonable basis for our findings and conclusions based on our audit objectives.

BACKGROUND

Overview of Medicaid Expenditures and Oversight

Medicaid expenditures are financed jointly by the federal government and the states. In order to receive federal matching funds for Medicaid expenditures, states must adhere to a broad set of federal requirements and administer their programs consistent with individual state plans approved by CMS. These plans are agreements between a state and the federal government that describe how states will administer their Medicaid programs, including how the state will administer Medicaid third- party liability procedures. When states make changes to their Medicaid programs or policies, including when necessary to comply with a change in federal law, they must submit a state plan amendment to CMS. CMS reviews and approves state Medicaid plans and state plan amendments.

The federal government matches each state's Medicaid expenditures for services according to a statutory formula called the Federal Medical Assistance Percentage. This formula provides for a match that is no lower than 50 percent of a state's Medicaid expenditures and no higher than 83 percent.[6] States can receive a 90 percent federal

[5] We interviewed officials from organizations that have expertise in Medicaid, including the National Association of Medicaid Directors, the Center on Budget and Policy Priorities, the Medicaid and CHIP Payment and Access Commission, and the National Health Law Program.

[6] Adjustments may apply to certain populations or services, however. For example, for certain Medicaid enrollees, states receive a higher federal match based on whether the state expanded Medicaid, as provided for under the Patient Protection and Affordable Care Act. See Pub. L. No. 111-148, § 2001(a)(3), 124 Stat. 119, 272 (2010) (codified as amended at 42 U.S.C. § 1396d(y)).

match for the costs associated with the development of each state's Medicaid Management Information System (MMIS), a claims processing and retrieval system supporting the administration of the state's Medicaid program.[7] States also receive a 75 percent match for the costs associated with ongoing MMIS maintenance and operations.[8] States use their MMIS systems to process provider claims, including claims for prenatal care services, pediatric preventive services, and services provided to CSE beneficiaries.

The Medicaid program is administered at the state level and overseen at the federal level by CMS, which, among other things, ensures that funds are used appropriately and beneficiaries have access to covered services. Medicaid allows significant flexibility for states to design and implement their programs. Within broad federal parameters, states have discretion in, among other things, setting Medicaid eligibility standards and provider payment rates; determining the amount, scope, and duration of covered benefits; and developing their own administrative structures.

States may also decide how Medicaid-covered services provided to beneficiaries will be delivered. For example, states may pay health care providers for each service they provide—fee-for-service—or contract with MCOs to provide a specific set of Medicaid-covered services to beneficiaries and pay them a set amount per beneficiary, typically per month. While most states use both delivery systems, the percentage of beneficiaries served through MCOs has grown in recent years, and represented nearly 70 percent of all Medicaid beneficiaries in 2016.[9]

Federal Third-Party Liability Requirements

Medicaid beneficiaries across various eligibility categories may have access to private health insurance or other sources of third-party coverage. For example, some adult beneficiaries may be covered by employer-sponsored private health insurance even though they also qualify for Medicaid. Children, similarly, may be eligible for Medicaid, while also being covered as a dependent on a parent's private health plan.[10] As such, federal law requires states to perform various activities to ensure that Medicaid is the

---

[7] See 42 C.F.R. § 433.111(b) (2018).

[8] See 42 U.S.C. §§ 1396b(a)(3)(A)(i), (B).

[9] See Centers for Medicare & Medicaid Services, Medicaid Managed Care Enrollment and Program Characteristics, 2016 (Spring 2018).

[10] Third parties are not limited to health insurers. Rather, they include any individual, program, or entity legally responsible—liable—for payment for all or part of a claim for a health care item or service. Such third parties may include private health insurance, medical support from non-custodial parents, automobile insurance, workers' compensation, probate-estate recoveries, and public programs, among others—unless excluded by federal statute. See 42 U.S.C. § 1396a(a)(25)(A); 42 C.F.R. § 433.136 (2018) (definition of a third party); CMS, State Medicaid Director Letter #06-026 (Dec. 15, 2006).
Because children are generally not permitted to enroll in a State Children's Health Insurance Program (CHIP) if they have another source of health care coverage, the existence of third-party liability in CHIP is rare. However, if a child enrolled in CHIP were to obtain private health insurance or another source of coverage (such as court-ordered medical support from a non-custodial parent) during the course of an eligibility period, third-party liability requirements would apply.

payer of last resort, including taking all reasonable measures to identify Medicaid beneficiaries' other potential sources of health coverage and their legal liability.[11] Specifically, states must ensure that the following steps, among others, are taken.

1. Coverage identification. To identify beneficiaries with third-party health coverage, states are required to request coverage information from potential Medicaid beneficiaries at the time the agency makes any determination or redetermination of eligibility. States are also required to obtain and use information pertaining to third-party liability, for example, by conducting data matches with state wage information agencies, Social Security Administration wage and earning files, state motor vehicle accident report files, or state workers' compensation files.
2. Coverage verification. When other health coverage is identified, states often verify the information, including the services covered through the other insurance and the dates of eligibility.
3. Cost avoidance payment procedures. As a general rule, federal law requires states to apply cost avoidance payment procedures to claims for most Medicaid items and services. Under cost avoidance procedures, the state must reject claims for which a third party is or is probably liable, and the agency instructs the provider to collect from the third party.[12] Once the provider determines the amount of the third party's liability, the provider submits a claim to the state Medicaid agency for any remaining balance, up to the maximum amount allowed under the state's payment schedule.[13] States are then required to make timely payment to the provider, generally within 30 days from the date the claim for the balance is filed.[14]
4. Pay-and-chase payment procedures. The Consolidated Omnibus Budget Reconciliation Act of 1985 made an exception to cost avoidance procedures for three types of services: prenatal care services, pediatric preventive services, and services provided to CSE beneficiaries.[15] It required states to pay such claims

[11] See 42 U.S.C. § 1396a(a)(25)(A). CMS requires such activities to include the measures specified in sections (b) through (k) of 42 C.F.R. § 433.138 unless waived. See 42 C.F.R. § 433.138(a) (2018). States may delegate these responsibilities to entities such as a contractor or managed care organization.

[12] See 42 C.F.R. § 433.139(b)(1) (2018) (requiring states to reject, but not deny, such claims under cost avoidance procedures). See also, CMS, State Medicaid Manual, § 3904.1.

[13] Once the amount for which a third party is liable is known, the state Medicaid agency must then pay the claim to the extent, and in the amount, that Medicaid payment for the particular claim exceeds the amount of the third party's payment. See 42 C.F.R § 433.139(b)(1) (2018).

[14] Specifically, states are required to make timely payments within 30 days for 90 percent of clean claims—those for which no additional information from the provider or a third party is necessary to process the claim. See 42 C.F.R. §§ 447.45(b), (d) (2018).

[15] See Pub. L. No. 99-272, § 9503, 100 Stat. 82, 205 (1986). The conference report accompanying the act notes that prenatal care and preventive pediatric services were excepted from the application of cost avoidance procedures so that third-party collections would be pursued by the state, not by the provider. The conferees expressed a concern that the administrative burdens associated with third-party collection efforts should not discourage provider participation in Medicaid. The conference report also notes that the intent of the conferees

without regard to the liability of the third party, a procedure CMS calls "pay and chase." Under the pay-and-chase payment procedure, the state Medicaid agency is generally required to make a timely payment to the provider within 30 days, and then the state, instead of the provider, will seek to recover payment from any potentially liable third parties within 60 days.[16] According to CMS, cost avoidance does not apply to these claims because there is a risk some providers might not participate in Medicaid to avoid dealing with the administrative burden of cost avoidance.[17] (See Figure 1.)

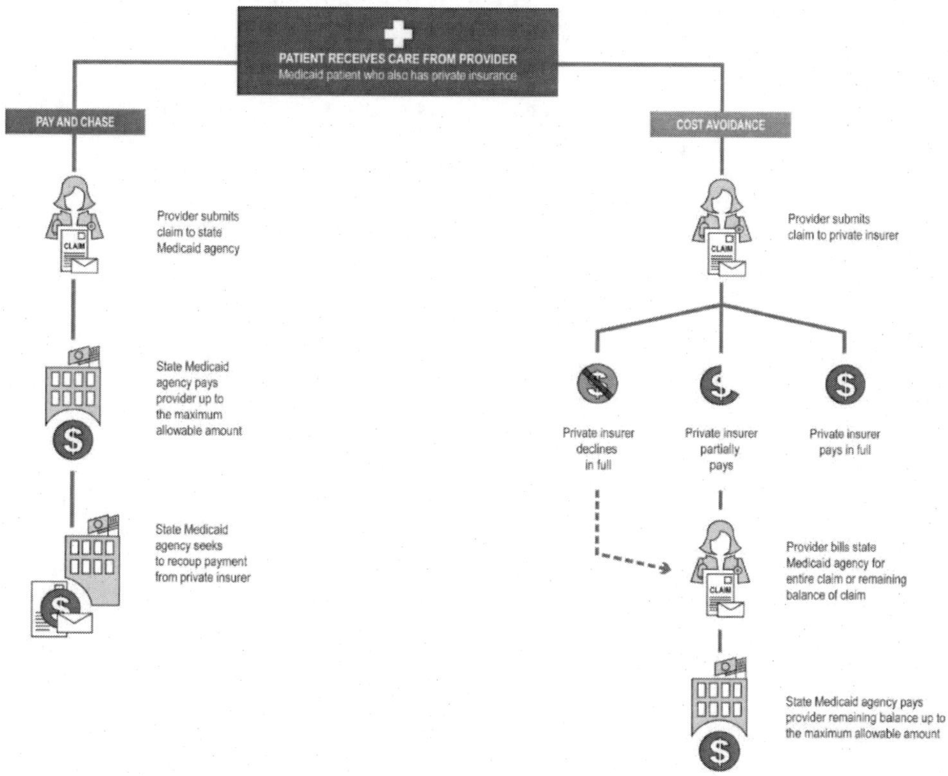

Source: GAO analysis. | GAO-19-601

Note: With few exceptions, Medicaid is considered the payer of last resort, meaning that when beneficiaries have another source of health care coverage—such as private health insurance provided through an employer—that source, to the extent of its liability, should pay for services before Medicaid does. This concept is referred to as "third-party liability."

Figure 1. Third-Party Liability Payment Processes for Medicaid Claims with Probable Private Insurer Liability.

---

in excepting services provided to CSE beneficiaries was to protect the custodial parent from pursuing collections from the non-custodial parent's employer, insurer, or other funding sources. See H.R. Rep. No. 99-453, at 544 (1985) (Conf. Rep.).

[16] States may request initial and continuing waiver of the requirement to recover payments, and may suspend or terminate such recovery efforts, if the state determines it would not be cost-effective to pursue recovery. See 42 C.F.R. §§ 433.139(e), (f) (2018).

[17] Center for Medicaid and CHIP Services Informational Bulletin (June 1, 2018), p. 1.

The Bipartisan Budget Act of 2018 amended various sections of the Medicaid third-party liability statute, including the required processes states must follow when paying claims with probable third-party liability for the following three types of services:

- Prenatal care services. The Bipartisan Budget Act of 2018 eliminated, effective February 2018, the statutory exception for prenatal care services that had required states to apply pay-and- chase procedures to such claims.[18] Thus, under the amended statute, states must apply cost avoidance procedures to claims for prenatal care services when it is apparent that a third party is or may be liable at the time the claim is filed.[19] Additionally, to the extent states had opted under CMS regulations to apply pay-and-chase procedures to claims for labor, delivery, or postpartum care services—which CMS calls "pregnancy-related services"—states must now apply cost avoidance procedures to those as well.[20]
- Pediatric preventive services. Beginning in October 2019, under federal law as amended by the Bipartisan Budget Act of 2018, states are no longer required to pay claims for pediatric preventive services immediately.[21] While states will still have the option to apply pay-and- chase procedures to these claims, a state may instead choose—if it determines doing so is cost-effective and will not adversely affect access to care—to require the provider to first submit the claim to the third party and wait 90 days for payment by the third party before seeking Medicaid payment. For purposes of this chapter, we refer to such a 90-day period as a "wait-and-see period."
- Services provided to CSE beneficiaries. Beginning in October 2019, states must make payment for a CSE beneficiary's claim if the third party has not paid the provider's claim within a 100-day wait-and-see period.[22] However, the state may

[18] See Pub. L. No. 115-123, § 53102(a)(1) (codified at 42 U.S.C. § 1396a(a)(25)(E)).

[19] See 42 U.S.C. § 1396a(a)(25)(A).

[20] CMS regulations issued in 1985 permitted states to apply either cost avoidance or pay- and-chase procedures to claims for labor, delivery, and postpartum care services, excluding any costs associated with an inpatient hospital stay. See 42 C.F.R. § 433.139(b)(2) (2018). In section 3904.4 of the State Medicaid Manual, CMS explained its view that the statutory prenatal care services exception permitted states to apply pay-and-chase procedures broadly to "pregnancy-related services," reasoning that obstetricians frequently bundled these claims with prenatal care services.

[21] These statutory requirements initially appeared in the Bipartisan Budget Act of 2013, but the effective date was delayed by subsequent legislation, most recently by the Bipartisan Budget Act of 2018. See Pub. L. No. 113-67, § 202, 127 Stat. 1165, 1177 (2013) and Pub. L. No. 115-123, § 53102(b)(2), 132 Stat. 64, 298 (2018), codified as amended at 42 U.S.C. § 1396a note.

[22] The Bipartisan Budget Act of 2018 provided for a 90-day wait-and-see period for claims for CSE beneficiaries with probable third-party liability; however, subsequently enacted legislation extended it to 100 days. See Medicaid Services Investment and Accountability Act of 2019, Pub. L. No. 116-16, § 7, 133 Stat. 852. The Congressional Budget Office estimates that the additional 10 days of the wait-and-see period, which is optional for states, would save $60 million over 10 years. See Congressional Budget Office, *Cost Estimate: H.R. 1839, Medicaid Services Investment and Accountability Act of 2019,* (Washington, D.C.: Mar. 22, 2019), accessed July 3, 2019, https://www.cbo.gov/system/files/2019-03/hr1839_0.pdf.)

instead choose—if the state determines doing so is cost-effective and necessary to ensure access to care—to make payment within 30 days.[23] (See Table 1.)

Table 1. Pre- and Post-Bipartisan Budget Act of 2018 Requirements for State Medicaid Payment of Certain Claims with Probable Third-Party Liability

Type of claim	Pre-Bipartisan Budget Act of 2018	Post-Bipartisan Budget Act of 2018	Effective date
Prenatal care services (including pregnancy-related services)[a]	Pay-and-chase. State must make timely payment to provider and then seek payment from third party.[b]	Cost-avoidance. State must reject claim until the provider bills the third party. If balance remains after provider bills third party or if third party denies claim, provider can submit claim to state for balance.	Feb. 2018
Pediatric preventive services	Pay-and-chase. State must make timely payment to provider and then seek payment from third party.	State option. State must pay-and-chase or, upon determination of cost-effectiveness and access, reject claim for up to 90 days before making timely payment.	Oct. 2019
Services for children subject to child support enforcement	State option. State must pay-and-chase or reject a claim for up to 30 days before making timely payment.	State option. State must reject claim for up to 100 days or, upon determination of cost-effectiveness and access, make payment within 30 days.	Oct. 2019

Source: GAO analysis of the Bipartisan Budget Act of 2018 and related legislation. | GAO-19-601

Note: See Pub. L. No. 115-123, § 53102, 132 Stat. 64, 298 (codified as amended by the Medicaid Services Investment and Accountability Act of 2019, Pub. L. No. 116-16, § 7, 133 Stat. 852, at 42 U.S.C. §§ 1396a(a)(25), note).

[a] We use the term "pregnancy-related services" to refer to labor, delivery, and postpartum care services, excluding any costs associated with an inpatient hospital stay. Under Centers for Medicare & Medicaid Services (CMS) regulations, states had the option to treat these services the same as prenatal care services. See 42 C.F.R. § 433.139(b)(2) (2018). Under current law as amended by the Bipartisan Budget Act of 2018, states must apply cost avoidance to all prenatal care and pregnancy- related services. See 42 U.S.C. § 1396a(a)(25)(A).

[b] We use the term "timely payment" to refer to a payment made within the timeframe required by CMS under its prompt payment regulation, 42 C.F.R. § 447.45(d) (2018), which requires states to pay 90 percent of clean claims—those for which no additional third party information is necessary—within 30 days of the date such claims are filed with the state agency and to pay 99 percent of clean claims within 90 days of that date. See 42 C.F.R. § 447.45(b) (2018) (definition of a clean claim).

Once the third-party liability changes in the Bipartisan Budget Act of 2018 are fully implemented, states will have authority to require providers to wait longer to receive Medicaid payments in certain circumstances.[24] For example,

- Prenatal care services claims, which were previously paid within 30 days under pay-and-chase procedures, are now subject to cost avoidance. This could potentially result in providers waiting indefinitely to receive payment, depending on whether the provider is able to resolve the third-party liability (i.e., submit a

[23] CMS has not announced whether a state that chooses to make payment within 30 days will continue to have the option of requiring providers to certify that they have waited 30 days for third-party payment before filing the claim with the state or whether the state will be required to pay right away under pay-and-chase procedures. Under current regulations, states have both options and must specify the state's procedures in their state Medicaid plans. See 42 C.F.R. § 433.139(b)(3)(ii) (2018).

[24] Although states are required to implement some of the third-party liability changes, such as the requirement to apply cost-avoidance procedures to prenatal care services, the changes applicable to pediatric preventive services claims and claims for services for CSE beneficiaries provide the state with options.

claim for payment to the third party and determine the amount of the third-party liability), which must occur before the state may make payment under cost avoidance.

- Pediatric preventive services claims, which are generally paid within 30 days under pay-and-chase procedures, could be subject to a 90-day wait-and-see period beginning in October 2019 if a state decides to implement one. This could result in providers waiting 120 days to receive payment (90 days to wait and see if the liable third party pays, and then another 30 days for the state to make timely payment on any remaining balance).
- Claims for services for CSE beneficiaries, which are currently subject to pay-and-chase procedures or a 30-day wait-and-see period at state option, may be subject to either a 30-day or 100-day wait-and- see period beginning in October 2019, depending on which option the state chooses. This could result in providers waiting 130 days to receive payment (up to 100 days to wait and see if the liable third party pays, and then another 30 days for the state to make timely payment on any remaining balance).

Some Selected States Have Implemented Third-Party Liability Changes for Prenatal Care Services; Most of the States Were in the Early Stages of Planning for Other Changes

Officials from four of the nine selected states we reviewed reported having implemented the required third-party liability changes for prenatal care services. The changes were required to be implemented in February 2018. For the third-party liability changes affecting pediatric preventive services and services provided to CSE beneficiaries, which are due to take effect October 2019, Medicaid officials from six of the nine selected states noted that they were in the very early stages of planning how they might implement the changes.

Four of Nine Selected States have Implemented Required Third-Party Liability Changes for Prenatal Care Services

Officials from four of the nine selected states we reviewed stated that their state Medicaid agency had implemented the mandated third-party liability changes for prenatal care services, which required states to implement cost avoidance payment procedures for claims for these services beginning in February 2018.[25] Officials from three of the four states that have implemented the third-party liability changes for prenatal care services told us that changing from pay-and-chase to cost avoidance procedures involved identifying all the applicable service codes for prenatal care and making the necessary changes in their systems to ensure that any new claims were subject to cost avoidance procedures. They said it also involved communicating the need for such changes to the MCOs in their state.[26]

State Medicaid officials from the remaining five states generally noted that they were discussing the changes internally, researching how to implement the changes in their MMIS, assessing the likely impact of these changes on MMIS, or waiting for additional guidance from CMS.[27] For example:

- Officials from several states noted that they were undertaking activities, such as identifying the prenatal care codes in their data systems that would need to be switched to cost avoidance payment procedures, or researching the best way to implement these changes.
- Officials from one state said they were in the process of assessing what the likely impact of these changes on beneficiaries and providers would be, and would only subject claims for prenatal care services to cost avoidance if they determined that doing so was the best course of action.[28]
- Officials from one state indicated that they were waiting to determine whether it was more cost effective to implement these changes in their legacy MMIS, or wait and implement the changes in the new MMIS they are planning to roll out in the future.

State Medicaid officials also described other efforts that they would need to undertake as they implemented these changes to third-party liability. These included staff retraining and communicating the changes to providers in their states.

Beyond state Medicaid programs, officials from the five Medicaid MCOs we interviewed all stated that their organizations had not yet implemented the prenatal care third-party liability changes. The MCO officials stated that they were waiting for

---

[25] Under the new law, the state must reject any provider's claim for prenatal care services when it is apparent that a third party may be liable for those services. Once the provider determines the amount of the third party's liability, the state Medicaid agency may pay any remaining balance up to the maximum allowed under the state's payment schedule.

[26] Officials from two states said that they had already been applying cost avoidance procedures to claims for prenatal care services, even though the law in effect prior to the Bipartisan Budget Act of 2018 required states to apply pay-and-chase payment procedures to these claims.

[27] Although CMS issued initial guidance to states regarding the third-party liability changes on June 1, 2018, the statutory requirement applicable to prenatal care services went into effect in February 2018. See Center for Medicaid and CHIP Services, Informational Bulletin (June 1, 2018).

[28] While federal law allows states certain options in processing claims for pediatric preventive services and services provided to CSE beneficiaries, it does not allow states to apply any procedures other than cost avoidance for prenatal care claims.

additional instructions on how to implement the third-party liability changes or for revised contract language from their state Medicaid agencies. Officials from one of the MCOs noted they were not aware of the third-party liability changes until we reached out to them for an interview. Officials from two MCOs we interviewed generally agreed that the third-party liability changes for prenatal care services would require changes to claims processing systems and internal processes, but would not be significant. Several MCO officials noted that these changes would likely result in some cost-savings to MCOs in the future.

Most Selected States Were in Early Stages of Planning Implementation of Third-Party Liability Payment Changes for Pediatric Preventive Services and Services to CSE Beneficiaries

Medicaid officials from six of the nine selected states noted that they were in the very early stages of planning whether—or how—they would implement the wait-and-see periods for pediatric preventive services and services to CSE beneficiaries.[29] For example, some Medicaid officials from these six states described how they were assessing what changes would need to be made to their MMIS, deciding whether to implement the wait-and-see periods, or exploring how to assess the potential impact of these changes. Some Medicaid officials also expressed uncertainty regarding how such changes would affect Medicaid beneficiaries or the amount of effort required by their agency to implement the third-party liability changes. Officials from one state noted that they had begun discussions about implementing the third-party liability changes for both pediatric preventive services and services for CSE beneficiaries in June 2018, and were in the process of identifying the necessary system changes needed to implement third-party liability changes by the October 2019 effective date. Officials from two of these states stated that they do not believe their state will implement the wait-and-see periods for pediatric preventive services or CSE beneficiaries when the changes go into effect. Officials from the remaining three states noted at the time of our interviews they had not yet developed plans for assessing implementation of these changes. Table 2 summarizes the status of selected states' implementation of the third-party liability changes.

[29] During a wait-and-see period, the state must reject a claim with probable third-party liability while the provider attempts to collect payment from the third party. The Bipartisan Budget Act of 2018 gives states the option of implementing a 90-day wait-and-see period for pediatric preventive services if states determine that implementing a wait-and-see period would be cost-effective and would not adversely affect beneficiaries' access to care. In addition, the Bipartisan Budget Act of 2018 gives states the option of not extending the wait-and-see period for child support enforcement beneficiaries to 100 days if the state determines that not extending the wait-and-see period would be cost-effective and necessary to ensure access to care. See Pub. L. No. 115-123, § 53102(b)(2), 132 Stat. 64, 298 (2018), as amended by Medicaid Services Investment and Accountability Act of 2019, Pub. L. No. 116-16, § 7, 133 Stat. 852 (codified as amended at 42 U.S.C. § 1396a note).

Table 2. Status of Selected States' Implementation of Bipartisan Budget Act of 2018 Medicaid Third-Party Liability Changes

State	Prenatal care changes (effective February 2018)	Pediatric preventive and child support enforcement beneficiaries' changes (effective October 2019)
#1	Not implemented	No plans developed
#2	Not implemented	Has plans to implement (will implement if they determine it is the best course of action)
#3	Not implemented	No plans developed
#4	Not implemented	Has plans to implement
#5	Implemented	In discussions on the advantages and disadvantages and exploring wait-and-see periods
#6	Not implemented	No plans developed at this time
#7	Implemented	Evaluating the changes and the approach they might take for implementing these changes
#8	Implemented	Has plans to implement. In process of identifying what system and process changes are needed
#9	Implemented	Has plans to implement

Source: GAO interviews with officials from nine selected state Medicaid agencies. | GAO-19-601

Note: Under the Bipartisan Budget Act of 2018 and subsequently-enacted legislation, state Medicaid programs were required to use cost avoidance, as opposed to pay and chase, payment procedures when processing claims for prenatal care and pregnancy-related services for which a third party may be liable beginning in February 2018. This law also gives states the option to establish 90-day and 100-day wait-and-see periods for claims for pediatric preventive services and services for CSE beneficiaries. During a wait-and-see period, the state must reject a claim with potential third party liability while the provider attempts to collect payment from the third party. These pediatric changes will go into effect in October 2019. See Pub. L. No. 115-123, § 53102(a)-(b), 132 Stat. 64, 298 (2018), as amended by Medicaid Services Investment and Accountability Act of 2019, Pub. L. No. 116-16, § 7, 133 Stat. 852 (codified as amended at 42 U.S.C. §§ 1396a(a)(25), note).

For pediatric preventive services, state Medicaid officials generally noted that the third-party liability changes would involve identifying the relevant codes and making changes to their MMIS to ensure those claims were subject to a wait-and-see period, if implemented. Several state Medicaid officials characterized this effort as "significant" or "difficult." For services delivered to CSE beneficiaries, officials from several state Medicaid agencies speculated that making the third-party liability changes to their MMIS would necessitate having some sort of indicator in their system to identify which claims were for the CSE beneficiaries and, therefore, should be subject to a wait-and-see period, if implemented. Some state Medicaid agency officials said that this would require obtaining the information from another state agency responsible for administering CSE agreements.

Several of the state Medicaid officials we interviewed expressed concerns regarding how to implement the wait-and-see periods for pediatric preventive services and services for CSE beneficiaries. Specifically, these officials noted that—within their MMIS—it is not possible to capture on a Medicaid claim when a provider has billed a third party, waited a specified amount of time, and not received payment. As a result, officials from one state noted that additional guidance from CMS on how to implement and track provider billing of third parties—including wait-and-see periods and providers' collection of payment—would be necessary before moving forward with implementing the third-party liability changes. Officials from two states said that the administrative burden associated with these changes would possibly make them not cost-effective to implement. However, MCO officials we interviewed generally acknowledged that while these changes would require changes to their claims processing systems and internal processes, they were not significant and could potentially result in some cost-savings to their MCO in the future.

The third-party liability change affecting all Medicaid services provided to CSE beneficiaries was a particular concern for officials from three state Medicaid agencies and three MCOs. Specifically, these officials said there is currently no way to identify CSE beneficiaries in their MMIS or claims processing systems, which could potentially make this change difficult, if not impossible, to implement. Officials from one state described how setting up a system to receive this information would involve a significant effort, potentially necessitating new hardware and system modifications, as well as a data sharing agreement with the state entity maintaining the CSE information. Officials from one MCO noted that the third-party liability changes affecting CSE beneficiaries was a particular concern, because those changes would potentially require additional administrative work and changes to their processes in order for providers in their network to track down insurance information from a non-custodial parent.

CMS HAS ISSUED IMPLEMENTING GUIDANCE WITH INFORMATION INCONSISTENT WITH FEDERAL LAW AND HAS NOT OVERSEEN STATES' IMPLEMENTATION OF THIRD-PARTY LIABILITY CHANGES

CMS's Implementing Guidance Contains Information Inconsistent with Provisions of Federal Law Related to Medicaid Third-Party Liability

After enactment of the Bipartisan Budget Act of 2018 in February 2018, CMS issued guidance in the form of an informational bulletin to states on June 1, 2018, to facilitate states' implementation of the key provisions of the Bipartisan Budget Act of 2018 related to third-party liability in Medicaid. However, CMS's June informational bulletin is missing some key information and contains information that is inconsistent with the federal law. This is inconsistent with CMS's responsibility for ensuring states' compliance with federal requirements. In particular,

- Pregnancy-related claims. Under federal law, states must apply standard cost avoidance procedures to all non-pediatric claims, including claims for prenatal services beginning in February 2018.[1] However, CMS guidance indicates that a state need not apply cost avoidance procedures to claims for labor and delivery services if those claims can be differentiated from prenatal services.[2] The guidance also provides that, effective October 1, 2019, states will have 90 days to pay claims related to labor, delivery, and postpartum care claims. As a result, CMS's guidance is inconsistent with federal law, which requires states to reject any such claim under cost avoidance procedures until the third-party liability is resolved, regardless of how many days that might take.[3]
- Pediatric preventive claims. Under federal law, states must generally apply pay-and-chase procedures to pediatric preventive services. However, beginning in October 2019, states are permitted to implement a 90-day wait-and-see period before making payment for these services if the state determines that it would be cost-effective and would not adversely affect access to care to do so.[4] However, CMS guidance simply provides that states will have 90 days to pay such claims, suggesting that states need not make the cost- effectiveness or access determinations required by statute.[5]

---

[1] See 42 U.S.C. § 1396a(a)(25)(A) (requiring standard cost avoidance procedures for all Medicaid claims with probable third-party liability under subsection (A) except for certain pediatric claims identified in subsections (E) and (F)).

[2] See Center for Medicaid and CHIP Services, Informational Bulletin (June 1, 2018), p. 2.

[3] See 42 U.S.C. § 1396a(a)(25)(A).

[4] See 42 U.S.C. § 1396a note.

[5] See Center for Medicaid and CHIP Services, Informational Bulletin (June 1, 2018), p. 2.

- CSE beneficiary claims. Under federal law, beginning in October 2019, for claims for services to CSE beneficiaries, states may choose to make payment within 30 days (as opposed to implementing a 100- day wait-and-see period), if the state determines doing so is cost-effective and necessary to ensure access to care.[6] If the state does not make such a determination, the statute would require the state to avoid making payment for such services for up to 100 days to allow third parties to make payment first. However, CMS guidance does not identify this as an option for states. Instead, CMS guidance simply provides states with the option of implementing the wait-and-see period, omitting the option for states to make payment within 30 days.

CMS officials told us that the Bipartisan Budget Act of 2018 did not change state responsibilities related to cost-effectiveness and access to care, and CMS does not intend to issue additional guidance on this issue. However, prior to enactment of the Bipartisan Budget Act of 2018 in February 2018, federal third-party liability law did not authorize states to apply cost avoidance procedures to preventive pediatric claims or pediatric services provided to CSE beneficiaries.[7]

Furthermore, other CMS guidance documents, such as the third-party liability handbook and CMS regulations on third-party liability, are out of date and not a reliable source of information for states to use in implementing the new federal third-party liability requirements. In particular, the third-party liability handbook was last revised in 2016 and does not reflect the Bipartisan Budget Act of 2018 changes. Additionally, CMS regulations implementing federal requirements for state payment of claims for prenatal care, labor and delivery services, postpartum care, preventive pediatric services, and services to CSE beneficiaries were last amended in 1997 and, accordingly, do not reflect current statutory requirements, including the Bipartisan Budget Act of 2018 requirement to cost avoid prenatal and other non-pediatric claims beginning February 2018.[8]

CMS officials told us the agency is in the process of updating its third- party liability handbook and anticipates issuing the updated document in September 2019. Agency officials also told us they plan to revise the agency's regulations regarding pay-and-chase and release the revised regulations in early 2020. However, federal law requires state Medicaid plans to provide for proper third-party liability procedures, which states often carry out through references to federal regulation, according to CMS officials. Without updated third-party liability guidance that is timely, complete, and consistent with federal

[6] See 42 U.S.C. § 1396a note.

[7] Under CMS regulations, states are permitted to request a waiver of cost avoidance or recovery of reimbursement requirements if the state determines that such a requirement is not cost-effective. See 42 C.F.R. § 133.139(e) (2018). However, this cost-effectiveness determination for purposes of the waiver does not involve a determination of access to care or permit a state to waive pay-and-chase requirements. According to CMS officials, no waivers are currently in effect.

[8] Compare 42 C.F.R. § 433.139 (2018) with 42 U.S.C. §§ 1396a(a)(25)(A), (E), (F), note.

law, states may lack the necessary information to update their state Medicaid plans so that they comply with these requirements.

CMS Has Not Overseen States' Implementation of Third- Party Liability Changes

CMS has not taken steps to determine the extent to which state Medicaid agencies are meeting the third-party liability requirements, and therefore CMS officials were unaware of whether states were meeting the new requirements. In particular, CMS officials did not know the extent to which the selected states in our review had implemented the required third-party liability changes. In our interviews with nine selected state Medicaid agencies conducted between November 2018 and March 2019, we learned that five states continued to apply pay-and-chase procedures to prenatal care claims, despite the federal requirement to implement cost avoidance since February 2018.[9]

During our interviews, we also learned that CMS had not monitored state Medicaid agencies' third-party liability approaches prior to the Bipartisan Budget Act of 2018. For example, officials from one of the selected states told us that they had been using cost avoidance for most claims for pediatric preventive care, rather than applying pay-and-chase procedures, as required by law.[10] We also learned from an official from another selected state that the state had been applying cost avoidance procedures to claims for prenatal care services well in advance of the enactment of the Bipartisan Budget Act of 2018, despite the federal requirement to apply pay-and-chase procedures to such claims from 1986 to 2018.

CMS's failure to monitor the implementation of the third-party liability changes in the Bipartisan Budget Act of 2018 is inconsistent with the agency's responsibilities for oversight of the Medicaid program, including ensuring that federal funds are appropriately spent. We have previously recommended that, given the significant federal Medicaid outlays, the federal government has a vested financial interest in further increasing states' third-party liability cost savings, and that CMS should play a more active leadership role in monitoring, understanding, supporting, and promoting state third-party liability efforts.[11]

However, CMS officials stated that they expect states to comply with current law for Medicaid third-party liability, and that they do not verify whether states have

---

[9] Federal law requires Medicaid state plans to provide for the cost avoidance of prenatal care claims effective February 9, 2018. See 42 U.S.C. § 1396a(a)(25)(A) (as amended by the Bipartisan Budget Act of 2018, Pub. L. No. 115-123, § 53102(a), 132 Stat. 64, 298).

[10] Officials from the state noted that they apply pay-and-chase procedures to claims for pediatric immunizations and apply cost avoidance procedures to all other pediatric services.

[11] See GAO, *Medicaid: Additional Federal Action Needed to Further Improve Third-Party Liability Efforts*, GAO-15-208 (Washington, D.C.: Jan. 28, 2015).

implemented the required third-party liability changes unless the agency is made aware of non-compliance. When asked how CMS ensures that states apply pay-and-chase procedures required under federal law, such as for pediatric preventive claims, CMS officials stated that it is the agency's expectation that states comply with current law. According to agency officials, if a state has difficulty complying and reaches out to CMS for technical assistance, the agency will work with that state to come into compliance. CMS officials told us that CMS plans to review all state Medicaid plans and provide technical assistance for any necessary action only after the agency has updated its regulations related to third-party liability.[12] As of May 2019, CMS anticipated that it would release updated regulations in early 2020.

Because CMS has not monitored states' compliance with federal third- party liability requirements, the agency does not know whether states have applied the federally required third-party liability procedures to certain Medicaid claims as required by federal law. In the case of prenatal care services claims, the failure to implement cost avoidance payment procedures could result in unnecessary Medicaid expenditures, to the extent that Medicaid pays providers for services for which a third party is liable. To the extent that states are not properly applying pay-and-chase procedures to pediatric preventive service claims, children's access to such services could be impacted.

STAKEHOLDERS ANTICIPATE THIRD-PARTY LIABILITY CHANGES COULD AFFECT BENEFICIARY ACCESS TO CARE; SELECTED STATES DISCUSSED USING EXISTING METHODS TO ASSESS EFFECTS OF CHANGES

Most Stakeholders Anticipate Increased Administrative Requirements for Providers and a Possible Decrease in Beneficiary Access to Care

According to most of the stakeholders we interviewed, Medicaid providers—especially prenatal care and rural providers—could face increased administrative requirements or delays in payments for services as a result of the third-party liability payment changes to the three service categories in the Bipartisan Budget Act of 2018. Several stakeholders agreed that the tasks associated with identifying sources of third-party liability and attempting to collect from third parties would shift from state Medicaid agencies to providers as a result of the payment changes, although opinions differed on the extent to which this shift would affect providers.

---

[12] However, CMS officials noted in response to our identification of specific state compliance concerns that the agency would follow up with the identified states directly.

- Several stakeholders said that the third-party liability changes could increase administrative requirements for providers, because obtaining accurate information on third-party liability sources for Medicaid beneficiaries and resubmitting claims that result from incorrect or outdated third-party liability information can be resource intensive and time consuming. One provider and officials from one state Medicaid agency noted that providers may lack the administrative resources or claims-processing expertise to deal with these changes. Officials from one state Medicaid agency, two state provider associations, and an organization advocating for Medicaid beneficiaries also noted that providers may encounter Medicaid beneficiaries who may be unaware or may not disclose that they have other insurance policies; for example, children who are covered under multiple insurance policies by custodial and non-custodial parents or experience insurance transitions following birth. These issues may increase the amount of time and resources providers spend on processing and resubmitting claims.
- Other stakeholders were less certain that the added requirements would cause difficulties for providers. Officials from one state Medicaid agency and one MCO said that the payment changes would not be difficult to implement, because providers were familiar with billing third parties for medical services for other beneficiaries. Officials from four state Medicaid agencies and two MCOs noted that providers may prefer to submit claims to commercial insurers, because these insurers pay at a higher rate compared with state Medicaid programs.

Several stakeholders we interviewed agreed that providers could wait longer periods of time for payment as they track down third-party insurers or wait up to 100 days for potential payment from these insurers before seeking payment from the state Medicaid agency. According to one provider and officials from two provider associations and one MCO, these delays could put providers at risk of not receiving payments for services or not having enough cash on hand to sustain operations. Additionally, officials from three provider associations noted that payment delays would affect pediatric providers in particular, because the majority of the services that pediatricians provide are preventive care—which would be affected by the third-party liability changes.

According to several stakeholders we interviewed, smaller or independent providers and those located in rural areas could be more affected by the third-party liability changes compared with providers affiliated with managed care systems or those located in urban areas. Officials from one state Medicaid agency, two provider associations, and one MCO noted that smaller or rural-based providers generally have fewer staff and resources to deal with the larger volume of administrative paperwork and delays in payment for services that could result from the payment changes.

Most of the stakeholders we interviewed said that providers might be less willing to serve Medicaid beneficiaries due to the administrative and payment issues, potentially reducing access to care or delaying services for children and pregnant women.[13] However, some other stakeholders said that the third-party liability changes would have little to no effect on Medicaid beneficiaries. Officials from one state Medicaid agency and one MCO noted that third-party liability payment practices for other Medicaid populations and services have been in place for many years, and providers would already be familiar with processing claims with third-party liability.

Several stakeholders said that providers may opt to reduce or eliminate the number of Medicaid beneficiaries they serve, because of actual or perceived increase in administrative requirements or payment delays. Officials from three state provider associations speculated that the potential for additional delays in payment for services could be the "final straw" in providers' decision to stop serving Medicaid beneficiaries. Other stakeholders, including a Medicaid expert, one provider, and officials from one state provider association noted that providers may decide to see fewer Medicaid beneficiaries, but are unlikely to stop seeing them entirely, because some providers are reluctant to deny care to these beneficiaries.

Payment delays could also lead to delays in beneficiaries receiving time- sensitive services, such as immunizations, as well as reduced access to specialists, such as midwives or mental health professionals, according to several stakeholders. Officials from one national provider association and an organization advocating for Medicaid beneficiaries noted that providers may seek to identify sources of third-party liability before providing services to beneficiaries. In addition, officials from one state Medicaid agency, a state provider association, and an organization advocating for Medicaid beneficiaries expressed concern that the third-party liability changes had the potential to reduce access to care for populations, such as children and pregnant women, that already faced challenges in accessing adequate, timely, or quality health care.

Selected States Discussed Using Existing Methods for Assessing Provider Availability and Beneficiary Access to Care Once Payment Changes are Implemented

Medicaid officials we interviewed from seven of the nine selected states said that their agencies will—or could—use existing methods to assess the effects of the third-party liability changes on provider availability and beneficiary access to prenatal care services, pediatric preventive services, and services for CSE beneficiaries. Officials from

[13] Providers may not refuse to see a Medicaid beneficiary on the basis of their potential third-party liability, although a provider may reduce or stop their participation in the Medicaid program. 42 U.S.C. § 1396a(a)(25)(D).

the remaining two states did not discuss or provide information on how they could assess the effects of the changes.

Medicaid officials provided examples of existing methods that could be used to assess the effects of payment changes:

- Tracking beneficiary access by comparing a set of access-to-care measures for a state's Medicaid population with its non-Medicaid, commercially insured population, as well as carrying out customer satisfaction surveys with Medicaid beneficiaries,
- Using a third-party liability hotline to track patient issues and conducting secret shopper calls to monitor if providers are accepting new patients,
- Contracting with a state university to evaluate Medicaid beneficiary access for prenatal and pediatric services.

In addition, one state has an independent health advocacy agency that monitors and seeks to resolve provider availability and beneficiary access issues on behalf of the state's Medicaid population.

However, one state Medicaid official and a Medicaid expert agreed that measuring any possible effects of the third-party liability changes—such as a decline in provider availability or beneficiary access—would be difficult without baseline data. According to officials from two state Medicaid agencies and a Medicaid expert, many other factors could potentially affect provider availability and beneficiary access, making it difficult or impossible to pinpoint if a decline in provider availability or beneficiary utilization of services was the result of the third-party liability changes or something else—such as changes in the managed care market or levels of private coverage among beneficiaries.

We found other evidence suggesting that it might be challenging for some states to assess the effects of the third-party liability changes. Specifically, Medicaid officials from eight of the nine selected states did not readily identify the number of beneficiaries in their state that had third- party liability and would be affected by the changes. Moreover, officials from two states noted that obtaining this data would require a "significant" effort.

- Officials from five states shared information on the number of children, pregnant women, or births covered by Medicaid in their state, but did not specify how many of these beneficiaries had other insurance coverage.
- Seven of the nine selected states had no data readily available on CSE beneficiaries who were also covered by Medicaid. In several cases, officials noted that their MMIS or other data systems had no way to track whether a child was a CSE beneficiary.

CONCLUSION

Omissions and inaccuracies in CMS's guidance to states on third-party liability changes from the Bipartisan Budget Act of 2018 have the potential to adversely affect the extent to which Medicaid expenditures are being used to pay for services for which a third party is liable, as well as states' compliance with federal requirements. Furthermore, CMS has not assessed whether state Medicaid agencies are complying with federal third-party liability requirements, under which states must change how they pay claims for certain services as a result of the Bipartisan Budget Act of 2018 and subsequently enacted legislation. In the absence of CMS overseeing states' compliance, the agency cannot ensure that federal funds are being spent properly and that states are complying with current federal statute.

RECOMMENDATIONS

We are making the following two recommendations to CMS:

- The Administrator of CMS should ensure the agency's Medicaid third- party liability guidance is consistent with federal law related to
    - the requirement for states to apply cost avoidance procedures to claims for labor, delivery, and postpartum care services,
    - the requirement for states to make payments without regard to potential third-party liability for pediatric preventive services unless the state has made a determination related to cost-effectiveness and access to care that warrants cost avoidance for 90 days, and
    - state flexibility to make payments without regard to potential third- party liability for pediatric services provided to child support enforcement beneficiaries. (Recommendation 1)
- The Administrator of CMS should determine the extent to which state Medicaid programs are meeting federal third-party liability requirements and take actions to ensure compliance as appropriate. Such actions can include ensuring that state plans reflect the law. (Recommendation 2)

AGENCY COMMENTS

We provided a draft of this chapter to the Department of Health and Human Services for comment. In its written comments, which are reprinted in appendix I, HHS concurred with our recommendations and indicated a commitment to providing states with accurate guidance on the third-party liability changes in the Bipartisan Budget Act of 2018. The agency noted that it is in the process of updating its guidance and third-party liability handbook to reflect the changes and ensure that such guidance is consistent with federal law. The agency also noted that it will determine the extent to which state Medicaid programs are meeting federal third- party liability requirements and will take actions to ensure compliance. We are sending copies of this chapter to the appropriate congressional committees, the Secretary of Health and Human Services, and other interested parties.

Carolyn L. Yocom
Director, Health Care

APPENDIX I: COMMENTS FROM THE DEPARTMENT OF HEALTH AND HUMAN SERVICES

DEPARTMENT OF HEALTH & HUMAN SERVICES

OFFICE OF THE SECRETARY

Assistant Secretary for Legislation
Washington, DC 20201

JUL 3 0 2019

Carolyn Yocom
Director, Health Care
U.S. Government Accountability Office
441 G Street NW
Washington, DC 20548

Dear Ms. Yocom:

Attached are comments on the U.S. Government Accountability Office's (GAO) report entitled, "*Medicaid Payment: CMS Has Not Overseen States' Implementation of Changes to Third-Party Liability*" (GAO-19-601).

The Department appreciates the opportunity to review this report prior to publication.

Sincerely,

for

Sarah Arbes
Acting Assistant Secretary for Legislation

GENERAL COMMENTS FROM THE DEPARTMENT OF HEALTH & HUMAN SERVICES ON THE GOVERNMENT ACCOUNTABILITY OFFICE'S DRAFT REPORT ENTITLED - MEDICAID PAYMENT: CMS HAS NOT OVERSEEN STATES' IMPLEMENTATION OF CHANGES TO THIRD-PARTY LIABILITY (GAO-19-601)

The Department of Health and Human Services (HHS) appreciates the opportunity to review and comment on this draft report. HHS is committed to working with states to ensure compliance with all Medicaid statutory and regulatory requirements.

Third Party Liability refers to the legal obligation of third parties (for example, certain individuals, entities, insurers, or programs) to pay part or all of the expenditures for medical assistance furnished under a Medicaid state plan. By law, all other available third party resources must meet their legal obligation to pay claims before the Medicaid program pays for the care of an individual eligible for Medicaid. States are required to take all reasonable measures to ascertain the legal liability of third parties to pay for care and services that are available under the Medicaid state plan.

There are certain circumstances under which a State Medicaid Agency may pay a claim and then seek to recover payment from the liable third party. This is required when there is a risk that if the State Medicaid Agency were to cost avoid claims, or not pay until a liable third party had paid, providers might choose not to participate in the Medicaid program in order to avoid dealing with the administrative burden associated with Medicaid cost-avoidance claims processing requirements. Previously, the law provided third party liability exceptions for prenatal services, pediatric preventive services, and pediatric services for children subject to child support enforcement. These exceptions permitted states to make payments for these services, and if a third party was found to be liable and it was cost-effective to recover payment, seek reimbursement after payment was made.

However, the Bipartisan Budget Act of 2018 included several provisions, which modify third party liability rules related to the special treatment of these services and payment.[1] Specifically, it removed the third party liability exception for prenatal services effective upon enactment. In addition, it amended the third party liability exception for pediatric preventive services and pediatric services of children subject to child support enforcement effective October 1, 2019. States are now generally required to pay and seek reimbursement from a third party after payment is made unless they make a determination relating to cost-effectiveness and access to care, in which case they would delay payments for 90 days before making payment.

HHS is committed to providing accurate guidance to states on the Third Party Liability changes from the Bipartisan Budget Act of 2018 and is in the process of updating its guidance and Third Party Liability Handbook to reflect the changes. HHS will continue to provide technical assistance on third party liability via monthly calls with states and will also monitor states' implementation of the Third Party Liability requirements to ensure compliance.

HHS thanks GAO for their efforts on this issue and looks forward to working with GAO on this and other issues in the future.

GAO's recommendations and HHS' responses are below.

[1] https://www.congress.gov/115/bills/hr1892/BILLS-115hr1892eas2.pdf

GAO Recommendation 1

The Administrator of CMS should ensure the agency's Medicaid third party liability guidance is consistent with federal law related to the requirement for states to apply cost avoidance procedures to claims for labor, delivery, and postpartum care services, the requirement for states to make payments without regard to potential third party liability for pediatric preventive services unless the state has made a determination related to cost-effectiveness and access to care that warrants cost avoidance for 90 days, and state flexibility to make payments without regard to potential third party liability for pediatric services provided to child support enforcement beneficiaries.

HHS Response

HHS concurs with GAO's recommendation. HHS will update the third party liability guidance to be consistent with federal law.

GAO Recommendation 2

The Administrator of CMS should determine the extent to which state Medicaid programs are meeting federal third-party liability requirements and take actions to ensure compliance as appropriate. Such actions can include ensuring that state plans reflect the law.

HHS Response

HHS concurs with GAO's recommendation. HHS will determine the extent to which state Medicaid programs are meeting federal third party liability requirements and take actions to ensure compliance.

In: Medicaid: Fraud, Payments and Beneficiaries
Editor: Nadia M. Hedegaard
ISBN: 978-1-53617-666-7

Chapter 4

MEDICAID: ADDITIONAL CMS DATA AND OVERSIGHT NEEDED TO HELP ENSURE CHILDREN RECEIVE RECOMMENDED SCREENINGS*

United States Government Accountability Office

ABBREVIATIONS

CHIP	Children's Health Insurance Program
CMS	Centers for Medicare & Medicaid Services
EPSDT	Early and Periodic Screening, Diagnostic, and Treatment
HHS	Department of Health and Human Services
T-MSIS	Transformed Medicaid Statistical Information System

WHY GAO DID THIS STUDY

The EPSDT benefit is key to ensuring that Medicaid beneficiaries aged 20 and under receive periodic screening services, such as well-child screenings, and diagnostic and treatment services, such as physical therapy and eyeglasses, to correct or ameliorate conditions discovered during a screening.

GAO was asked to examine the extent to which Medicaid beneficiaries aged 20 and under receive health care services under the EPSDT benefit. Among other things, GAO

* This is an edited, reformatted and augmented version of United States Government Accountability Office; Report to Congressional Requesters, Publication No. GAO-19-481, dated August 2019.

examined (1) what is known about the provision of EPSDT services based on CMS-required annual state reporting, and (2) CMS oversight of the EPSDT benefit. To do this, GAO analyzed annual state reporting data from fiscal years 2010 through 2017, the most current year data were available; CMS documentation; and federal internal control standards. GAO also interviewed CMS officials and Medicaid officials from 16 states selected, in part, on the variation in number of beneficiaries and geographic diversity.

What GAO Recommends

GAO is making six recommendations to CMS regarding its oversight of the EPSDT benefit, including collecting appropriate blood lead screening data; taking action, if needed, after assessing the appropriateness of performance measures and targets for EPSDT; and evaluating states' performance in meeting CMS's EPSDT targets. CMS agreed with three recommendations, but disagreed with three others regarding performance measures and targets. GAO maintains that these recommendations are valid, as discussed in this chapter.

What GAO Found

Approximately half of all Medicaid beneficiaries aged 20 and under received screenings and services recommended under the Early and Periodic Screening, Diagnostic, and Treatment (EPSDT) benefit in fiscal year 2017, but nearly as many did not. For example, GAO's analysis of state-reported data found that about 59 percent of all beneficiaries (20.2 million) who should have received at least one recommended well-child screening received one. About 48 percent of beneficiaries aged 1 to 20 (18.3 million) received a preventive dental service in fiscal year 2017. Older beneficiaries tended to have lower rates of screening.

The Centers for Medicare & Medicaid Services (CMS), the agency that oversees Medicaid, including EPSDT, has taken steps to improve the quality of information that states report about the provision of EPSDT services. CMS has also set some EPSDT performance measure targets for states; yet, the agency has not taken other steps to oversee the EPSDT benefit, such as

- collecting the data necessary to evaluate whether states are complying with CMS's policy for beneficiaries to receive a blood lead screening;
- taking action, as needed, based on assessments of the appropriateness of some performance measures, such as well-child screening measures; and

- using state-reported information to regularly evaluate states against CMS's EPSDT targets, or assisting states in planning improvements to meet the targets.

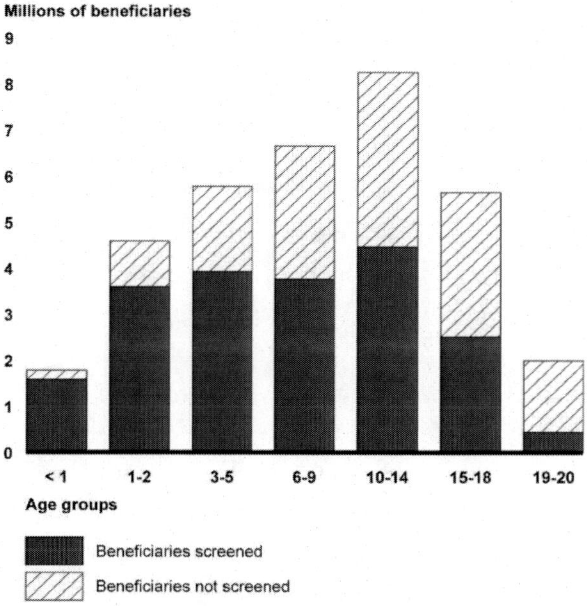

Source: GAO analysis of Centers for Medicare & Medicaid Services Early and Periodic Screening, Diagnostic, and Treatment data for fiscal year 2017. | GAO-19-481

Number of Medicaid Beneficiaries Receiving and Not Receiving Well-Child Screenings in Fiscal Year 2017, by Age Group.

Absent these steps, CMS's oversight is limited and beneficiaries may not be receiving appropriate EPSDT services when they need them.

August 16, 2019

The Honorable Frank Pallone, Jr.
Chairman
Committee on Energy and Commerce
House of Representatives

The Honorable Joseph P. Kennedy,
III House of Representatives

The Early and Periodic Screening, Diagnostic, and Treatment (EPSDT) benefit is key to ensuring that eligible beneficiaries aged 20 and under receive appropriate services under Medicaid, a joint federal-state health care program for low-income and medically needy individuals. The EPSDT benefit is a comprehensive set of covered services for

Medicaid's youngest beneficiaries that includes periodic screening services, such as physical exams, and diagnostic and treatment services, such as physical therapy and eyeglasses, among other services.[1] In fiscal year 2017, approximately 40 million Medicaid beneficiaries were entitled to receive ESPDT services. However, we and the Department of Health and Human Services (HHS) Office of Inspector General have previously found that millions of beneficiaries had not received the services to which they were entitled.[2]

The Centers for Medicare & Medicaid Services (CMS), an agency within HHS, is responsible for overseeing Medicaid at the federal level, including the EPSDT benefit. To help inform its oversight of the EPSDT benefit, CMS relies, in part, on several data sets submitted by states.[3] States are required to report annually on the provision of certain EPSDT services through the Form CMS-416.[4] States may also voluntarily report information to CMS annually on health care services provided to EPSDT beneficiaries, as well as individuals covered under the Children's Health Insurance Program (CHIP) through the Child Core Set.[5] According to CMS, the agency will increasingly rely on the Child Core Set to measure health care outcomes for Medicaid and CHIP beneficiaries, rather than the CMS-416. Finally, as part of a separate effort conducted jointly with states, CMS has sought to improve the quality and usefulness of state- reported Medicaid data through its Transformed Medicaid Statistical Information System (T-MSIS). CMS intends for T-MSIS to provide more information to improve Medicaid oversight and to reduce the number of reports CMS requires states to submit, including the CMS-416 and the Child Core Set.

You asked us to review the extent to which Medicaid beneficiaries aged 20 and under receive health care services under the EPSDT benefit. In this chapter, we examine

1. what is known about the provision of EPSDT services in all states according to what states report on the CMS-416;
2. CMS oversight of the EPSDT benefit; and
3. what is known about the capabilities of T-MSIS data to replace states' CMS-416 and Child Core Set reporting.

---

[1] The EPSDT benefit is defined in federal law to include screening, vision, dental, and hearing services, as well as other necessary services identified in section 1905(a) of the Social Security Act to correct or ameliorate any condition discovered through screening, regardless of whether such service is covered under the state Medicaid plan. 42 U.S.C. § 1396d(r).

[2] See GAO, *Medicaid and CHIP: Reports for Monitoring Children's Health Care Services Need Improvement*, GAO-11-293R (Washington, D.C.: April 5, 2011); and HHS Office of Inspector General, *Most Medicaid Children in Nine States Are Not Receiving All Required Preventive Screening Services*, OEI-05-08-00520 (Washington, D.C.: May 2010).

[3] For the purpose of our report, "states" refers to the 50 states and the District of Columbia.

[4] Guam and Puerto Rico also submitted CMS-416 data in some years from fiscal year 2010 through 2017, but we did not include them in our analysis.

[5] CMS also oversees CHIP, a joint federal-state health care program for uninsured low- income individuals aged 18 and under, whose household income exceeds the limits for Medicaid eligibility.

Our report also describes state practices to promote and facilitate the delivery of EPSDT services. (See app. I.)

To examine what is known about the provision of EPSDT services in all states according to what states report on the CMS-416, we analyzed data states reported to CMS through the CMS-416 from fiscal year 2010, the year in which the current reporting template was implemented, through 2017, the most recent year of data available at the time of our reporting. Specifically, we analyzed data on the three primary ESPDT services reported on the CMS-416: (1) well-child screenings, (2) preventive dental services, and (3) blood lead screenings.[6] For our analysis, we calculated the following, both nationally and for each state, using the fiscal years and age groups that CMS uses for oversight:[7]

- the number and percent of beneficiaries recommended to receive at least one well-child screening who received at least one screening from fiscal years 2010 through 2017, both overall and for each of the seven age groups reported on the CMS-416;[8]
- the number and percent of beneficiaries aged 1 to 20 who received preventive dental services from fiscal years 2011 through 2017; and
- the number of screenings conducted for blood lead levels for beneficiaries aged 12 through 24 months in fiscal year 2017 using the 1 to 2 age group on the CMS-416.[9]

We did not independently verify the accuracy of state-reported CMS-416 data; however, we checked those data for obvious errors and omissions, compared analysis results with CMS's publicly reported data about EPSDT services, and communicated with CMS officials to resolve any identified discrepancies. We also reviewed written guidance and documents from CMS and interviewed CMS officials about the collection

---

[6] At a minimum, well-child screenings include a comprehensive health and developmental history, including both physical and mental health development assessments; physical exams; age-appropriate immunizations; appropriate vision and hearing tests; dental exams; laboratory tests, including blood lead level assessments at certain ages; and health education, including anticipatory guidance.
The CMS-416 also includes information on the provision of dental treatment, dental diagnostic, and oral health services. The CMS-416 does not include information on provision of other EPSDT services, such as hearing and vision services.

[7] CMS focuses on certain age groups based on its policy and guidance, as well as clinical guidelines from nationally recognized medical organizations. For example, CMS focuses on preventive dental services to beneficiaries aged 1 year and older based on American Academy of Pediatric Dentistry guidelines, which state that beneficiaries should begin to receive dental care no later than age 1. We used fiscal year 2011 for our analysis of CMS-416 data on dental services to align with a CMS initiative to improve EPSDT beneficiaries' access to dental services, the Oral Health Initiative.

[8] The age groups reported in CMS-416 are younger than age 1, ages 1 to 2, ages 3 to 5, ages 6 to 9, ages 10 to 14, ages 15 to 18, and ages 19 to 20. For the purposes of our analyses, we rounded percentages to the nearest percentage point.

[9] We also calculated the number of screenings conducted for blood lead levels for beneficiaries aged 3 through 5 in fiscal year 2017 as reported on the CMS-416.

and reliability of CMS-416 data. On this basis, we determined that these data were sufficiently reliable for the purpose of our reporting objective. To examine CMS oversight of the EPSDT benefit, we reviewed guidance from CMS to states on the EPSDT benefit, CMS's process for reviewing EPSDT data on the CMS-416 and Child Core Set, and CMS summary reports about EPSDT performance measures.[10] We also interviewed CMS officials about their oversight activities, including reviewing data, setting and monitoring EPSDT-related performance measure targets, and assisting states with meeting EPSDT targets. We compared these efforts to best practices for results-oriented management as identified in previous GAO work, and assessed them against federal standards for internal control.[11] We also selected a non-generalizable sample of 16 states and interviewed Medicaid officials in these states to obtain information on data reporting and reliability, communications with CMS about EPSDT oversight, and leading practices officials identified for providing EPSDT services in their states.[12] To obtain state variation, the 16 states were selected on the basis of (1) the high and low number of Medicaid beneficiaries aged 20 and under, (2) the high and low number of and percent of beneficiaries recommended to receive at least one well- child screening who receive at least one screening, (3) variation in the way they deliver EPSDT services, (4) variation in whether they participated in a program with CMS to report EPSDT information through T-MSIS, and (5) their geographic diversity.[13]

To examine what is known about the capabilities of T-MSIS data to replace states' CMS-416 and Child Core Set reporting, we interviewed CMS officials about T-MSIS data accuracy and completeness, and CMS's plans for using T-MSIS data to replace state reporting of the CMS-416 and the Child Core Set. We also reviewed the results of two sets of pilot studies CMS conducted to assess the extent to which T-MSIS could be used to replicate certain parts of the CMS-416 and the Child Core Set.[14] In addition, we interviewed knowledgeable Medicaid officials in our selected states regarding T-MSIS data quality and their interactions with CMS about T-MSIS. We assessed CMS's efforts

---

[10] CMS officials said that activities that the agency has undertaken to improve health care services for children in Medicaid generally are efforts to improve states' delivery of EPSDT services. For the purposes of our report, we focused on CMS's activities related to select EPSDT services reported through the CMS-416 and Child Core Set.

[11] GAO, *Executive Guide: Effectively Implementing the Government Performance and Results Act*, GAO/GGD-96-118 (Washington, D.C.: June 1, 1996); *Veterans Justice Outreach Program: VA Could Improve Management by Establishing Performance Measures and Fully Assessing Risks*, GAO-16-393 (Washington, D.C.: Apr. 28, 2016); *Performance Measurement and Evaluation: Definitions and Relationships*, GAO-11-646SP (Washington, D.C.: May 2, 2011); and *Managing for Results: Enhancing Agency Use of Performance Information for Management Decision Making*, GAO-05-927 (Washington, D.C.: Sept. 9, 2005).
See GAO, *Standards for Internal Control in the Federal Government*, GAO-14-704G (Washington, D.C.: Sept. 10, 2014). Internal control is a process effected by an entity's oversight body, management, and other personnel that provides reasonable assurance that the objectives of an entity will be achieved.

[12] The 16 states we selected are California, Delaware, Hawaii, Illinois, Iowa, Louisiana, Mississippi, Missouri, Nebraska, New Hampshire, New Jersey, Pennsylvania, Rhode Island, Tennessee, Texas, and Virginia.

[13] States provide EPSDT services through various delivery models, such as fee-for-service and managed care.

[14] The two sets of pilot studies included three studies on the CMS-416, which included 11 sample states, and one study on the Child Core Set, which included 6 sample states.

to develop a timeline with interim milestones for when T-MSIS will replace state reporting of the CMS-416 or Child Core Set against federal standards for internal control.

We conducted this performance audit from March 2018 to August 2019 in accordance with generally accepted government auditing standards. Those standards require that we plan and perform the audit to obtain sufficient, appropriate evidence to provide a reasonable basis for our findings and conclusions based on our audit objectives. We believe that the evidence obtained provides a reasonable basis for our findings and conclusions based on our audit objectives.

BACKGROUND

EPSDT Benefit

Federal law specifies that the EPSDT benefit covers screening, vision, dental, and hearing services, as well as other Medicaid coverable services that are necessary to correct or ameliorate any conditions discovered through screening.[15] The EPSDT benefit generally entitles beneficiaries to these services regardless of whether such services are covered in a state's Medicaid state plan and regardless of any restrictions that the state may impose on coverage for adult services.[16] The EPSDT screening component includes a wide range of preventive services, such as comprehensive child health assessments known as well-child screenings and age-appropriate blood lead screenings. Because EPSDT covers any medically necessary service that could be covered for adults in addition to the specified preventive screenings, the EPSDT benefit is generally more comprehensive than the benefits provided for adult beneficiaries.

The federal government and states jointly share responsibility for implementing the EPSDT benefit. CMS, as part of its Medicaid oversight responsibilities, approves state Medicaid plans, which describe how the state administers its Medicaid program, including components related to the provision of EPSDT services. CMS also develops and issues general guidance to states about the EPSDT benefit, such as explanations of covered services and strategies for providing those services.[17]

---

[15] See 42 U.S.C. § 1396d(r).

[16] The EPSDT benefit is a mandatory benefit for all categorically eligible individuals aged 20 and under covered under the state plan and may be provided at state option to other individuals eligible for Medicaid or CHIP. See 42 U.S.C. §§ 1396a(a)(10)(A), 1396d(a)(4)(B).

[17] In addition, agency officials cited working with affinity groups that bring officials and experts together to address such topics as school based health and antipsychotic drug use in children; quality demonstration grants to states; and technical advisory groups, webinars, and publications on various topics, such as improving immunization rates.

Table 1. CMS Performance Measures that have Associated Targets to Guide State Implementation of the EPSDT Benefit

EPSDT service	Performance measure	Performance measure target	Year established
Well-child screening[a]	Participant ratio: Percentage of beneficiaries recommended to receive at least one well-child screening—based on the state's periodicity schedule[b]—who receive at least one screening.	Eighty percent of beneficiaries receive screening.	1990
Well-child screening[a]	Screening ratio: Ratio of the total number of screenings provided to the expected number of screenings, based on the state's periodicity schedule.	Eighty percent of screenings are provided.	1990
Dental services[c]	Percentage of beneficiaries aged 1 to 20 who receive a preventive dental service.	(1) At least 10 percentage point improvement over a 5-year period in each state.[d] (2) 52 percent nationally in fiscal year 2015.	2010
Blood lead screening[e]	Percentage of beneficiaries who receive a blood lead test.	All beneficiaries (100 percent) are required to receive a test at 12 months and 24 months of age. Beneficiaries between 24 and 72 months of age must receive a blood lead screening if they have not been previously screened for lead.[f]	1998

Source: GAO analysis of information from the Centers for Medicare & Medicaid Services (CMS). | GAO-19-481

Note: CMS developed the performance measure targets to carry out statutory requirements, quality improvement efforts, and agency policy.

[a] The Omnibus Budget Reconciliation Act of 1989 required the Secretary of Health and Human Services to establish Early and Periodic Screening, Diagnostic, and Testing (EPSDT) participation goals for each state. See Pub. L. No. 101-239, § 6403(c), 103 Stat. 2106, 2263 (codified as amended at 42 U.S.C. § 1396d(r)). Participant and screening ratios are defined in section 5360 of CMS's State Medicaid Manual.

[b] A periodicity schedule sets the frequency by which certain services should be provided and will be covered.

[c] Dental services performance measures and performance measure targets were set as part of CMS's Oral Health Initiative. CMS began the Oral Health Initiative to improve access to dental services under the EPSDT benefit for Medicaid beneficiaries' aged 1 to 20, with an emphasis on prevention. These services included preventive dental services and sealants on permanent molar teeth for beneficiaries aged 6 to 9. CMS officials reported that in March 2016 they informed states that CMS no longer planned to use the target for measuring states' performance on the sealant performance measure.

[d] Though CMS originally set a 5-year time frame (fiscal years 2011 through 2015) for meeting the 10 percentage point improvement targets for the dental service performance measures set as part of the Oral Health Initiative, agency officials said in March 2019 that the time frame is now open-ended.

[e] See CMS, State Medicaid Manual, Section 5123.2.D.1.

[f] In 2012, CMS announced an option for states to request approval from CMS to implement a targeted lead screening program. According to CMS officials as of 2019, one state has an approved targeted lead screening policy, and all other states are subject to the universal screening policy.

Additionally, CMS has developed a goal for EPSDT, which is to assure that beneficiaries get the health care they need when they need it: the right care to the right child at the right time in the right setting.[18] Further, CMS established performance measures, some with associated targets, to guide states' implementation of EPSDT.[19] For

[18] See CMS, *EPSDT – A Guide for States: Coverage in the Medicaid Benefit for Children and Adolescents* (Washington, D.C.: June 2014).

[19] Performance measurement is the ongoing monitoring and reporting of program accomplishments, particularly progress toward pre-established goals. It involves identifying performance goals and measures, including establishing performance baselines by tracking performance over time; identifying quantifiable, numerical targets for improving performance; and measuring progress against those targets.

example, CMS set performance measures and performance measure targets as part of its Oral Health Initiative.[20] CMS developed the performance measure targets to carry out statutory requirements, quality improvement efforts, and agency policy. (See Table 1 for EPSDT performance measures that have associated targets.)

States have flexibility, within federal parameters, to determine how EPSDT services are provided. For example, states are required to ensure that Medicaid-eligible beneficiaries and their families are aware of the EPSDT benefit and have access to required services, but states can choose whether to administer the benefit themselves or to oversee managed care organizations that are contracted to provide the benefit. States may also determine the frequency of screening services and communicate them through periodicity schedules that meet federal requirements.[21]

EPSDT Reporting

CMS uses various sources of information to oversee the EPSDT benefit, such as the CMS-416, the Child Core Set, and the Medicaid and CHIP Scorecard.

CMS-416 and Child Core Set

States report information about the provision of select ESPDT services to CMS annually through the CMS-416 and measures on the Child Core Set.[22] The CMS-416 provides CMS with basic information about EPSDT services, such as the participant ratio and number of beneficiaries receiving a preventive dental service.[23] It includes the information necessary for CMS to assess states' performance on the participant ratio and the screening ratio, among other things.[24] The agency then can compare performance on the two ratios with the agency's ESPDT performance measure targets. The Child Core Set provides CMS with information about the quality of health care provided to Medicaid

[20] CMS began the Oral Health Initiative in April 2010 to improve Medicaid beneficiaries' aged 1 to 20 access to dental services under the EPSDT benefit, with an emphasis on prevention. These services included preventive dental services and sealants on permanent molar teeth for beneficiaries aged 6 to 9. CMS set performance measure targets for both services, but CMS officials reported that in March 2016 they informed states that CMS no longer planned to use the target for measuring states' performance on the sealant performance measure. The officials said the performance measure and target were removed when the agency identified issues with calculating the measure.

[21] States must establish reasonable standards, known as periodicity schedules, for medical, vision, hearing, and dental screening services in consultation with recognized medical and dental child health organizations. Periodicity schedules set the frequency by which certain services should be provided and will be covered.

[22] States are required by law to report annually to HHS the number of children provided child health screening services, the number of children referred for corrective treatment, the number of children receiving dental services, and states' results in attaining EPSDT participation goals established by the department. States must submit data to CMS by April 1 for the prior fiscal year's reporting. See 42 U.S.C. § 1396a(a)(43)(D).

[23] The participant ratio is the percentage of Medicaid beneficiaries aged 20 and under who received at least one recommended well-child screening, based on the state's periodicity schedule.

[24] In April 2011, we recommended that the Administrator of CMS work with states to identify additional improvements that could be made to reporting about the provision of EPSDT services. See GAO-11-293R. CMS agreed with our recommendation; however, as of March 2019, we consider the recommendation open.

and CHIP beneficiaries, and supports state efforts to improve health care quality and health outcomes.[25] Child Core Set reporting becomes mandatory on an annual basis beginning with the state reports on fiscal year 2024. As of 2019, the Child Core Set included performance measures related to the provision of EPSDT services, such as well-child visits in the first 15 months of life. Because reporting is currently voluntary, states vary in the number of performance measures they choose to report. In fiscal year 2017, for example, 50 states and the District of Columbia voluntarily reported on at least one of the 27 Child Core Set performance measures, with states reporting a median of 18 Child Core Set performance measures.[26] (See app. II for the information reported in the CMS-416 and Child Core Set.) As shown in Table 2, there are both similarities and differences between the CMS-416 and Child Core Set.

Table 2. Selected Features of the Form CMS-416 and Child Core Set

Characteristic	CMS-416	Child Core Set
Population reported	Medicaid beneficiaries aged 20 and under	Medicaid beneficiaries aged 20 and under Children's Health Insurance Program (CHIP) beneficiaries aged 18 and under[a]
Enrollment requirements for inclusion in population	Beneficiaries enrolled in Medicaid for 90 continuous days[b]	Varies by measure
Year reporting began	1990	2011
Reporting required or voluntary	Required	Voluntary[c]
Information reported	Basic information regarding the number of eligible beneficiaries Primary care access and preventive care Dental and oral health services	Basic information regarding the number of eligible beneficiaries, by measure Primary care access and preventive care Maternal and perinatal health Care of acute and chronic conditions Behavioral health care Dental and oral health services Experience of care
Comparability of state information	Not comparable, data affected by states' periodicity schedules[d]	Comparable

Source: GAO analysis of information from the Centers for Medicare & Medicaid Services (CMS) CMS-416 and Child Core Set. | GAO-19-481

[a] CMS prefers that states combine reporting of Child Core Set performance measures for beneficiaries enrolled in Medicaid and CHIP, whenever possible.

[b] States also report the total number of beneficiaries eligible for Early and Periodic Screening, Diagnostic, and Treatment (EPSDT) services at any point during the fiscal year. However, this is not used in calculating any of the other information reported on the CMS-416.

[c] Child Core Set reporting is mandatory beginning with the annual state report for fiscal year 2024. Because reporting is voluntary until then, states vary in the number of performance measures they choose to report. In fiscal year 2017, for example, 50 states and the District of Columbia voluntarily reported on at least one of the 27 Child Core Set performance measures, with states reporting a median of 18 Child Core Set performance measures. We used fiscal year 2017 data, because it is the most recent year for which data were available.

[d] A periodicity schedule sets the frequency by which certain services should be provided and will be covered.

---

[25] The CHIP Reauthorization Act of 2009 required HHS to identify and publish a core set of children's health care quality measures for voluntary use by state Medicaid and CHIP programs. See Pub. L. No. 111-3, § 401, 123 Stat. 8, 72 (codified as amended at 42 U.S.C. § 1320b-9a).

[26] We used fiscal year 2017 data, because it is the most recent year for which data were available.

Since the Child Core Set performance measures include CHIP beneficiaries who may not be entitled to the EPSDT benefit, data from the Child Core Set are not directly comparable with reporting on the CMS-416.[27] In addition, CMS-416 data cover a longer period of time, as they are available from 1995, while Child Core Set data are available from 2011. CMS officials said that having more years of CMS-416 data helps identify trends in the provision of EPSDT services over a longer period of time than possible with the Child Core Set. On the other hand, CMS officials said it is difficult to compare states' performance using the CMS-416, because some performance measures are based on periodicity schedules, which vary state-to-state and over time. In contrast, the Child Core Set allows for more consistency in comparing data across states, because each state is expected to calculate performance measures in the same way.

Medicaid and CHIP Scorecard

In June 2018, CMS published the first Medicaid and CHIP Scorecard, which includes performance measures about the provision of services to Medicaid and CHIP beneficiaries.[28] The scorecard includes 17 performance measures related to the provision of EPSDT services, six of which are performance measures from the Child Core Set—and one of these six measures is derived from the CMS-416.[29] In January 2019, CMS officials reported that the scorecard will be used to provide increased transparency about state Medicaid program administration and beneficiary health outcomes, and drive health care quality improvement across states.

According to CMS officials, CMS envisions that the scorecard will be strengthened as state reporting of data through T-MSIS becomes more timely, accurate, and complete. CMS has been working since 2011 to implement T-MSIS as a replacement for some current reporting to improve and increase states' reporting of Medicaid and CHIP data.[30] CMS intends for T-MSIS to provide a national data repository to support federal and state Medicaid and CHIP program management, among other things. T-MSIS includes data

---

[27] States can administer CHIP through a separate CHIP program, an expanded Medicaid program, or a combination of the two. CMS-416 captures data for beneficiaries enrolled in CHIP through Medicaid expansion, because they are entitled to ESPDT coverage, but does not capture data for beneficiaries enrolled in separate CHIP programs. States may, but are not required to, provide EPSDT coverage to beneficiaries in separate CHIP programs.

[28] The scorecard also includes performance measures about how states and the federal government work together to administer Medicaid and CHIP.

[29] The remaining performance measures come from the Adult Core Set and a nationwide adult Medicaid Consumer Assessment of Healthcare Providers and Systems survey. The preventive dental service performance measure on the Child Core Set is derived from the CMS-416.

[30] We and others have reported insufficiencies in available Medicaid data, including Medicaid Statistical Information System data. See GAO, *Medicaid: Program Oversight Hampered by Data Challenges, Underscoring Need for Continued Improvements*, GAO-17-173 (Washington, D.C.: Jan. 6, 2017). See also HHS, Office of Inspector General, *Office of Inspector General's FY 2015 Top Management and Performance Challenges Facing the Department of Health and Human Services*, accessed October 3, 2017, https://oig.hhs.gov/reports-and-publications/top-challenges/2015/challenge01.asp. CMS has acknowledged the need for improved Medicaid data, and T-MSIS is CMS's primary effort, conducted jointly with states, to improve the collection of Medicaid data and replace the current Medicaid Statistical Information System.

not previously reported by states and is intended to improve Medicaid and CHIP program efficiency, in part, by allowing states to compare their data with other states' data.[31] T-MSIS includes data that can measure the provision of EPSDT services. According to CMS officials, T-MSIS also includes aspects designed to improve the accuracy of available state data. For example, states' T-MSIS submissions undergo approximately 2,800 automated quality checks, which provide states with feedback on data format and consistency. As of January 2019, all 50 states and the District of Columbia were submitting data monthly, according to CMS, but T-MSIS data were not being used to create the CMS-416, Child Core Set, or the scorecard. Agency officials said research-ready files are in development and T-MSIS data are improving in quality over time with historical state resubmissions.

CMS Reports Indicate that Approximately Half of Beneficiaries Received Recommended Screenings and Services in 2017, but Nearly as Many Did Not

According to our analysis of CMS-416 data for fiscal year 2017, millions of Medicaid beneficiaries received recommended EPSDT well-child screenings and preventive dental services. However, nearly as many eligible beneficiaries did not receive the various recommended screenings and services, and few states met CMS's performance measure targets for EPSDT services. Additionally, while available data show that millions of blood lead screenings were performed, the total number of beneficiaries receiving blood lead screenings is unknown, because the data are incomplete.

Well-Child Screenings

In fiscal year 2017, 20.2 million (59 percent) of the 34.2 million beneficiaries who should have received at least one recommended well- child screening received that screening, known as the participant ratio, according to our analysis of state-reported CMS-416 data.[32] Additionally, our analysis indicates that the national participant ratio has declined 5 percentage points since fiscal year 2010.

[31] We have previously recommended that CMS expedite efforts to obtain complete information from all states on unreported T-MSIS data elements and use such data for program oversight. See GAO, *Medicaid: Further Action Needed to Expedite Use of National Data for Program Oversight*, GAO-18-70 (Washington, D.C.: Dec. 8, 2017).

[32] The number of beneficiaries recommended to receive a screening (34.2 million) is less than the total number of beneficiaries (40.1 million), because of differences in states' periodicity schedules, which set the frequency of

Three states met CMS's participant ratio target of 80 percent in fiscal year 2017, as shown in Figure 1. Our analysis also indicates that no more than four states met CMS's participant ratio target in any one fiscal year from 2010 through 2017. (See app. III, Table 6, for participant ratios in each state and nationally from fiscal years 2010 through 2017.)

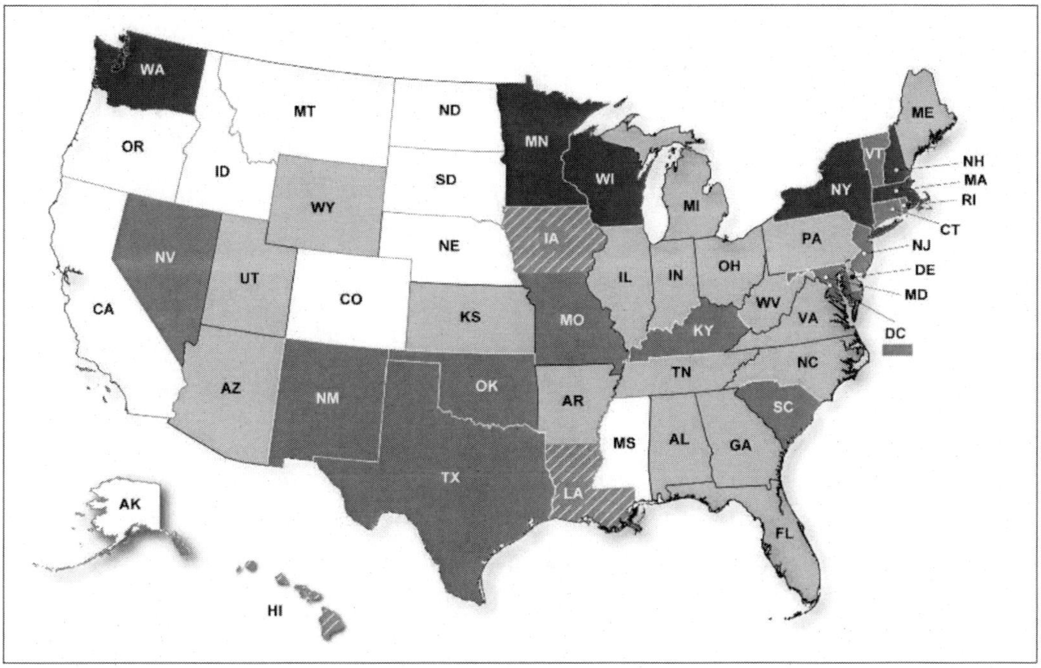

Participant ratio[a]	Number of states
Less than 50 percent	10
50-59 percent	19
60-69 percent	13
70-79 percent	6
80 percent or greater[b]	3

Source: GAO analysis of Centers for Medicare & Medicaid Services (CMS) Form CMS-416 data for fiscal year 2017; Map Resources (map). | GAO-19-481

[a] The participant ratio is the percentage of Medicaid beneficiaries aged 20 and under who received at least one recommended well-child screening, based on the state's periodicity schedule, which sets the frequency of screening services.

[b] State met CMS's participant ratio target of 80 percent.

Figure 1. Participant Ratios for Medicaid Well-Child Screenings in Fiscal Year 2017, By State.

screening services. For example, some older beneficiaries are not recommended to receive screenings every year.

Our analysis also indicates that as beneficiaries age, they tend to receive fewer recommended well-child screenings, which results in lower participant ratios. (See Figure 2 for participant ratios and numbers of beneficiaries receiving and not receiving well-child screenings for each CMS-416 age group in fiscal year 2017.) CMS has issued a guide on serving older eligible beneficiaries, stating that regular preventive care visits can lead to early identification of health issues. CMS officials said the agency included measures focusing on these beneficiaries on the Child Core Set and Medicaid and CHIP Scorecard to recognize the importance of addressing these beneficiaries and to encourage states to focus on this population. CMS officials noted that some states have already taken steps to increase the number of well-child screenings that older eligible beneficiaries receive, for example, by partnering with schools.

Dental Services

In fiscal year 2017, 18.3 million (48 percent) of the 38.3 million Medicaid beneficiaries aged 1 to 20 received a preventive dental service, according to our analysis of CMS-416 data. This is an increase from the 42 percent of beneficiaries receiving preventive dental services in 2011—the baseline year for measuring state progress toward CMS's Oral Health Initiative targets—but less than CMS's 52 percent national performance measure target. Our analysis also shows that from fiscal years 2011 through 2017, nine states met CMS's performance measure target of a 10 percentage point increase in each state's percentage of beneficiaries aged 1 to 20 receiving a preventive dental service.[33] (See Figure 3 and Table 8 in app. III for the percentage of beneficiaries aged 1 to 20 that received preventive dental services in each state and nationally from fiscal years 2011 through 2017.)

Blood Lead Screenings

Available data on blood lead screenings in the CMS-416 are incomplete and, as a result, do not provide information necessary to determine how many beneficiaries received the screenings. According to CMS's November 2016 guidance, CMS-416 data do not accurately represent the number of beneficiaries receiving blood lead screenings.

[33] Though CMS originally set a 5-year time frame (fiscal years 2011 through 2015) for meeting the 10 percentage point improvement targets for the dental service performance measures set as part of the Oral Health Initiative, agency officials said in March 2019 that the time frame is now open-ended for the preventive dental service performance measure. Therefore, we analyzed data through fiscal year 2017—the most recent year of data available at the time of our reporting.

- The CMS-416 data capture screenings paid for by Medicaid, but not those performed using funding from other sources, such as the Centers for Disease Control and Prevention. This could under-count the number of screenings performed.
- In addition, the blood lead screening data reported on the CMS-416 show how many screenings were performed, but do not identify the number of beneficiaries who received a blood lead screening.

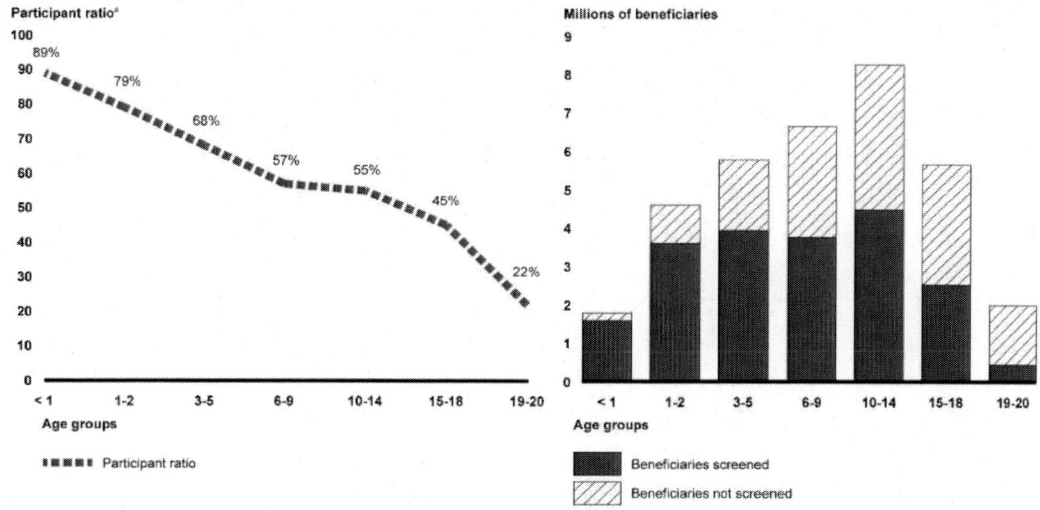

Source: GAO analysis of Centers for Medicare & Medicaid Services (CMS) Form CMS-416 data for fiscal year 2017. | GAO-19-481

Note: Includes data for 50 states and the District of Columbia. Age groups are based on those reported in CMS-416 data.

[a] The participant ratio is the percentage of Medicaid beneficiaries aged 20 and under who received at least one recommended well-child screening, based on the state's periodicity schedule, which sets the frequency of screening services.

Figure 2. Participant Ratio and the Number of Medicaid Beneficiaries Who Did and Did Not Receive Well-Child Screenings in Fiscal Year 2017, by Age Group.

Our analysis of available CMS-416 data shows that in fiscal year 2017 states reported 2.0 million blood lead screenings for beneficiaries aged 12 through 24 months, and there were 4.6 million beneficiaries aged 12 through 24 months.[34]

[34] Beneficiaries are required to receive a blood lead screening at 12 months and 24 months of age. States reported these blood lead screenings in the 1 to 2 age group on the CMS-416. Additionally, beneficiaries between 24 and 72 months of age must receive a blood lead screening if they have not been previously screened for lead. In fiscal year 2017, states reported 0.9 million blood lead screenings for these beneficiaries. States reported these blood lead screenings in the 3 to 5 age group on the CMS-416.

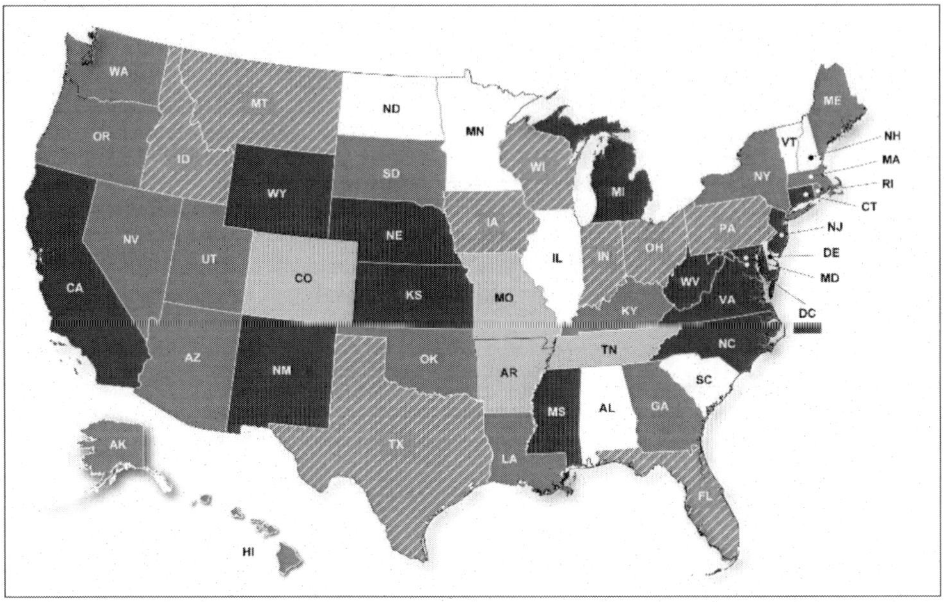

Percentage point change	Number of states
Percentage point reduction	8
No percentage point change	4
1 to 4 percentage point increase	16
5 to 9 percentage point increase	14
10 percentage point increase or greater[a]	9

Source: GAO analysis of Centers for Medicare & Medicaid Services (CMS) Form CMS-416 data for fiscal year 2011 and 2017; Map Resources (map). | GAO-19-481

Note: CMS set a 5-year time frame (fiscal years 2011 through 2015) for states to meet the 10 percentage point improvement targets for the dental service performance measures set as part of the Oral Health Initiative. CMS officials said in March 2019 that the time frame is now open-ended for the preventive dental service performance measure.

[a] State met CMS's performance measure target for preventive dental services.

Figure 3. Changes in Percentage of Medicaid Beneficiaries Aged 1 to 20 Receiving Preventive Dental Services from Fiscal Year 2011 through Fiscal Year 2017, By State.

CMS Has Improved EPSDT Data Quality; Additional Actions Are Needed to Improve Oversight of EPSDT Services, Particularly Blood Lead Screening Data

CMS is Improving EPSDT Data, yet Does Not Regularly Take Action Based on Assessing the Appropriateness of the CMS-416 for Oversight

CMS has regularly taken actions to use both the CMS-416 and the Child Core Set to improve the quality of information about the provision of EPSDT services. These actions have made the data reported about EPSDT services more complete and reliable. For example, CMS collects data annually from states on performance measures for both the CMS-416 and the Child Core Set. (See Table 3.) Additionally, CMS annually reviews the Child Core Set measures to determine whether measures need to be added, deleted, or revised. CMS also regularly provides technical assistance to states about data reliability, such as through its monthly Quality Technical Advisory Group.[35] For example, during one group meeting, states shared challenges with reporting information about developmental screenings on the Child Core Set and suggestions for how to overcome these challenges. These actions are generally consistent with federal internal control standards regarding information and communication, which specify that management should use quality information to achieve the entity's objectives.[36]

While CMS has taken actions to improve the quality of information about EPSDT, and agency officials said they regularly assess whether the information CMS collects on the CMS-416 is appropriate and useful for EPSDT oversight, CMS has not taken action, as needed, based on such assessments. For example, CMS has not added, removed, or amended any performance measures on the CMS-416 since 2010, even though officials acknowledge limitations in these measures.[37]

- The participant ratio, for example, is dependent, in part, on a state's chosen periodicity schedule, which means that the measure is not consistently defined across states.
- The screening ratio reflects the extent to which beneficiaries received the recommended number of well-child screenings during the year, but this information is aggregated and therefore cannot be used to determine whether individual beneficiaries received the recommended number of well-child screenings.

Although federal law requires collecting certain information about the provision of EPSDT services, it provides the agency with flexibility to determine the form and manner in which data are collected and to set performance measures.[38]

---

[35] The Quality Technical Advisory Group involves monthly meetings between CMS and representatives from state Medicaid agencies where states can share information with CMS and with other states on Medicaid quality issues.

[36] See GAO-14-704G.

[37] In the 2010 reporting year, the CMS-416 was revised to provide more information on dental sealants and oral health services provided by clinicians other than dentists. CMS officials said that the agency has not prioritized any further substantive changes to the CMS-416 in order to allow states to focus their resources on reporting of T-MSIS data and Child Core Set measures.

[38] Beginning in 1990, the Omnibus Budget Reconciliation Act of 1989 required state Medicaid programs to annually report to HHS information on EPSDT services including the number of children provided child health screening services, the number of children referred for corrective treatment, the number of children receiving dental services, and states' results in attaining EPSDT participation goals established by the department. Pub. L. No. 101-239, § 6403, 103 Stat. 2106, 2262-64 (codified as amended at 42 U.S.C. § 1396a(a)(43) (D)).

Table 3. Examples of CMS Actions to Collect and Improve Information about the Provision of EPSDT Services Using the Form CMS-416 and Child Core Set

Oversight activity standard		CMS-416	Child Core Set
Establish performance measures for ESPDT services, regularly assess performance measures and ensure their relevance, and communicate performance measures to the states	Actions taken	• Established well-child performance measures in 1990. • Established performance measures for dental services in 2010 as part of its Oral Health Initiative.[a] • Provides publicly available instructions to help states complete the CMS-416. • Issued guidance to states in November 2016 communicating the blood lead screening policy. • Assesses whether the information it collects on the CMS-416 is appropriate and useful for EPSDT oversight	• Established performance measures on a range of services, including well-child screenings and dental services, in 2011. • Reviews the Child Core Set annually and identifies ways to improve it.[b] • Issues annual federal notice with changes to the Child Core Set for states.
Establish performance measures for ESPDT services, regularly assess performance measures and ensure their relevance, and communicate performance measures to the states	Actions not taken	• No actions based on assessments of whether the information it is gathering is appropriate or useful for EPSDT oversight. For example, no additions, removals, or amendments of any performance measures on the CMS-416 since 2010, despite acknowledged limitations.	no significant deficiencies in actions
Collect performance measure data from states	Actions taken	• Collects performance data annually from states.	• Collects performance data annually from states.[c]
Collect performance measure data from states	Actions not taken	no significant deficiencies in actions	no significant deficiencies in actions
Ensure data reliability	Actions taken	• Reviews states' CMS-416 submissions and performs logical validation checks before accepting and publishing final yearly data. • Convenes affinity groups that bring officials and experts together to address different topics, such as school-based health, and technical advisory groups, and provides technical assistance upon request, such as issuing guidance in November 2016 about how to improve reporting of blood lead screenings.	• Works with states to increase number of performance measures reported and the number of states reporting each measure, as well as the accuracy of the performance measures. • Provides technical assistance to improve the extent of reporting on Child Core Set measures.
	Actions not taken	no significant deficiencies in actions	no significant deficiencies in actions

Source: GAO comparison of federal internal control standards for information and communication to Centers for Medicare & Medicaid Services (CMS) information. | GAO-19-481

NOTE: A dash (—) reflects no significant deficiencies in actions taken under a given oversight activity for a given data set.

[a] CMS began the Oral Health Initiative to improve Medicaid beneficiaries' aged 1 to 20 access to dental services under the Early and Periodic Screening, Diagnostic, and Treatment (EPSDT) benefit, with an emphasis on prevention. These services include preventive dental services and sealants on permanent molar teeth for beneficiaries aged 6 to 9. CMS officials reported that in March 2016 they informed states that CMS no longer planned to use the target for measuring states' performance on the sealant performance measure.

[b] The CHIP Reauthorization Act of 2009 directed the Secretary of Health and Human Services to establish a pediatric quality measures program to improve core set measures on an ongoing basis, among other things. The Secretary is required to recommend updates to the core measures annually, which CMS carries out in partnership with the National Quality Forum, which is a nonprofit organization that fosters agreement on national standards for measurement and public reporting of health care performance data. See Pub. L. No. 111-3, § 401, 123 Stat. 8, 72 (codified as amended at 42 U.S.C. § 1320b-9a).

[c] State reporting on the Child Core Set is voluntary until reports on fiscal year 2024, so not all states report all measures.

For example, CMS could change the way states are required to calculate the participant ratio or the screening ratio, and could examine ways to do so to address the limitations that the agency has identified and improve the quality of information about the provision of EPSDT services.

Because CMS has not taken action, as needed, based on assessments of the appropriateness of its CMS-416 performance measures, the agency cannot be sure that it has the information it needs to oversee state implementation of EPSDT. This is inconsistent with federal internal control standards regarding information and communication, which specify that management should identify information requirements in an iterative and ongoing manner and ensure information remains relevant.[39] We have previously reported that results-oriented organizations set performance goals to define desired program outcomes and develop performance measures that are clearly linked to these performance goals and outcomes.[40]

CMS Has Set Some Performance Measure Targets, yet Does Not Consistently Evaluate States' Performance against These Targets

CMS has taken steps to develop, assess, and use CMS-416 information to improve states' performance in providing EPSDT services. For example, CMS has set performance measure targets for participant and screening ratios reported on the CMS-416, and CMS publishes state-level results of the participant and screening ratios. In addition, after identifying issues with calculating the performance measure and target for the permanent molar sealants, CMS removed them from the Oral Health Initiative. CMS also convenes affinity groups and technical advisory groups to provide assistance to states in improving performance, often centered on specific services, such as dental services.

However, CMS and state Medicaid officials told us that CMS does not consistently (1) communicate CMS-416 performance measure targets to states, (2) evaluate state performance against performance measure targets, or (3) provide states with assistance in reaching performance measure targets. While it has not done so across all performance measure targets, CMS did take these actions regarding targets for preventive dental services as part of its Oral Health Initiative. For example, CMS

- communicated with states about the preventive dental service performance measure target after it developed the Oral Health Initiative;
- disseminated a national oral health strategy and published a review of eight states identifying innovative approaches in providing preventive dental services; and

[39] See GAO-14-704G.
[40] See GAO-05-927.

- provided targeted outreach to states with the lowest performance on the preventive dental service performance measure.

Improvements in the provision of dental services occurred in many states. For example, in 2013, CMS met with state Medicaid officials in Florida about improving the provision of preventive dental services. Five years later, the percentage of beneficiaries receiving preventive dental services had increased 18 percentage points.

CMS has not taken action in other areas. For example:

- CMS does not communicate the participant and screening ratio targets. Officials from CMS and from each of our 16 selected states told us that CMS does not mention these targets in communications with states, including discussions related to performance improvement.
- CMS has not evaluated state performance in meeting the participant and screening ratio targets, nor has it provided focused assistance to states to resolve gaps in states' performance in reaching these targets comparable to the assistance provided for the preventive dental screening performance measure as part of the Oral Health Initiative.
- CMS did not provide formal written notification to states when in March 2016 the agency informed participants in two meetings that CMS no longer planned to use the target for measuring states' performance on the permanent molar sealants performance measure.[41] The notification was not provided through an official policy document, such as an agency informational bulletin distributed to all states. Despite removing the target, CMS issued a technical assistance brief in March 2018 that referenced it, which could have led to confusion among state officials.

With regard to the Child Core Set, CMS has not established any performance measure targets and agency officials were not able to provide information about plans for setting targets. CMS officials said that the CMS-416 will remain a part of its EPSDT oversight. However, because its information is not standardized across states, CMS plans to increasingly rely on the standardized Child Core Set data to assess and improve states' performance on the provision of EPSDT services. CMS officials noted that it publishes median, top quartile, and bottom quartile information for each state for all the Child Core Set measures that are publicly reported. Officials further reported in June 2019 that CMS and states use these as performance benchmarks, with an aim of reaching the national median on these measures if not the top quartile.

---

[41] CMS officials said that they clarified to states through presentations at the National Association of Medicaid Directors and the Oral Health Technical Advisory Group in 2016 that due to issues with the performance measure, the agency had dropped that performance measure and target from the Oral Health Initiative.

Reporting these data is an important step in ensuring better oversight of EPSDT. However, CMS has not developed fixed targets that explicitly track states' progress in increasing beneficiaries' receipt of EPSDT screenings and services. Using a median to assess states' performance ensures that half the states will not meet this target, regardless of their individual performance. Further, CMS officials have not provided plans or timelines for when the Child Core Set would be used to help states achieve performance measure targets.

CMS's inaction regarding using the CMS-416 and Child Core Set to improve performance on the provision of EPSDT services limits the agency's oversight and is inconsistent with federal internal control standards for monitoring, and practices of leading organizations. Federal internal control standards specify that management should (1) set performance measure targets in measureable, numeric terms; (2) communicate necessary information to achieve performance targets; (3) evaluate progress toward desired targets; and (4) take action to resolve identified issues.[42] Without regularly using the CMS-416 and Child Core Set to improve the provision of EPSDT services, CMS is unable to identify whether state or federal efforts and policies are increasing the number of beneficiaries receiving EPSDT services. As a result, CMS's oversight is limited and beneficiaries may not be receiving appropriate EPSDT services when they need them—CMS's stated goal for EPSDT. (See Table 4 for examples of actions CMS has and has not taken regarding using the CMS-416 and Child Core Set for improving the provision of EPSDT services.)

CMS Has Taken Limited Actions to Improve Data on the Number of Blood Lead Screenings, which are Critical to Identifying Harmful Lead Exposure

CMS is unable to determine whether all eligible EPSDT beneficiaries are receiving blood lead screenings in accordance with CMS policy. As previously noted, CMS-416 data are incomplete, because they only include blood lead screenings paid for by Medicaid, and the form reports the number of screenings performed instead of the number of beneficiaries receiving screenings.[43]

---

[42] See GAO-14-704G; and GAO, *Military Bands: Military Services Should Enhance Efforts to Measure Performance*, GAO-17-657 (Washington, D.C.: Aug. 10, 2017).

[43] CMS officials said that all EPSDT services reported on the CMS-416 are limited to those paid for by Medicaid, and not just blood lead screenings. However, blood lead screenings are the only EPSDT service reported on the CMS-416 that is required for all beneficiaries, unless the state has implemented a targeted lead screening program.

Table 4. Examples of CMS Actions to Improve Performance on Provision of EPSDT Services Using Form CMS-416 and Child Core Set

Oversight activity standard	Oversight activity standard	CMS-416	Child Core Set[a]
Set targets for states to achieve on performance measures, regularly assess targets, and communicate those targets to the states	Actions taken	• Established participant ratio and screening ratio performance measure targets in 1990 and communicated to states through the State Medicaid Manual. • Established performance measure targets for preventive dental services and permanent molar sealants as part of the Oral Health Initiative in 2010 and communicated to states through a n oral health strategy document • CMS removed the permanent molar sealants performance measure and target when it identified problems with calculating the performance measure. • Established performance measure targets for beneficiaries receiving blood lead screenings in 1998 and communicated to states through the State Medicaid Manual. • Issued bulletin in November 2016 reminding states of targets for beneficiaries receiving blood lead screenings. • In January 2019, CMS officials said that they plan to evaluate the performance measure targets developed as part of the Oral Health Initiative for preventive dental services by the end of 2019.	• None
Set targets for states to achieve on performance measures, regularly assess targets, and communicate those targets to the states	Actions not taken	• CMS does not remind states about participant and screening ratio targets. • CMS officials described limitations of the participant and screening ratios in August 2018. Yet, CMS has not adjusted the participant ratio or screening ratio performance measure targets since 1990. • In March 2016, CMS informed participants in two meetings that the agency no longer planned to use the target for measuring states' performance on the permanent molar sealants performance measure; however, CMS did not provide formal written notification to states.	• No performance targets set or plans for future targets available as of March 2019.
Conduct regular evaluations comparing states' performance to the established targets	Actions taken	• CMS issued a bulletin in July 2014 comparing states' performance with performance measure targets for preventive dental services.	• None
Conduct regular evaluations comparing states' performance to the established targets	Actions not taken	• CMS does not compare states' performance with participant ratio and screening ratio performance measure targets. • Since its July 2014 bulletin, CMS has not issued subsequent bulletins comparing states' performance with performance measure targets for preventive dental services.	• No evaluations conducted directly comparing performance on Child Core Set measures with targets, nor plans to conduct such evaluations in the future, as of March 2019; no performance targets set or plans for future targets available as of March 2019.

Oversight activity standard	Oversight activity standard	CMS-416	Child Core Set[a]
Assist states with planning and implementing needed improvement to address performance gaps	Actions taken	• CMS convenes affinity groups and technical advisory groups, and provides technical assistance upon request, such as its Oral Health Technical Advisory Group. • CMS has provided focused technical assistance to several states to improve provision of preventive dental services. • CMS issued a bulletin in July 2014 with technical support for states to improve provision of preventive dental services and permanent molar sealants.	• CMS provides technical assistance and analytic support to support states' efforts to measure and improve the quality of health care for children and adults enrolled in Medicaid and CHIP. Specific topics include: collecting, reporting, and using the Child Core Set; assessing data quality to improve completeness and accuracy of state reporting of the Child Core Set measures; and designing and implementing quality improvement initiatives focused on the Child Core Set measures. • Eighteen states participated in the CHIP Reauthorization Act Quality Demonstration grant program. The goal of this grant program is to provide staff resources to states to strengthen the quality of and access to children's health care through a variety of health care delivery models, provider and patient-level interventions, and measurement approaches.
Assist states with planning and implementing needed improvement to address performance gaps	Actions not taken	• CMS does not provide focused technical assistance on improving the provision of well-child screenings to meet performance measure targets. • CMS has not developed affinity groups on the provision of well-child services associated with the participant ratio and screening ratio performance measure targets.	• No technical assistance provided to improve performance on provision of EPSDT services relative to performance measure targets, since no performance targets set or plans for future targets available as of March 2019.

Source: GAO comparison of federal internal control standards for information and communication to Centers for Medicare & Medicaid Services (CMS) information. | GAO-19-481

[a] State reporting on the Child Core Set is voluntary until reports on fiscal year 2024, so not all states report all measures.

CMS has stated that screenings are important for identifying beneficiaries with elevated blood lead levels at as young an age as possible, because lead exposure can harmfully affect nearly every system of the body and cause developmental delays. According to a presidential task force on environmental health and safety risks to children, co-chaired by HHS, early identification of developmental delays allows providers and communities to intervene earlier to improve health outcomes.[44] The presidential task force issued goals in December 2018 to reduce lead exposure and associated harms, including a goal to identify lead-exposed individuals and improve their health outcomes.

[44] See President's Task Force on Environmental Health Risks and Safety Risks to Children, *The Federal Action Plan to Reduce Childhood Lead Exposures and Associated Health Impacts* (Washington, D.C.: December 2018).

State Examples of Collecting Blood Lead Screening Data

Nebraska

Medicaid officials said that the state has developed a database with the Nebraska Health Information Initiative containing laboratory testing data. Treating providers and managed care organizations can access the database to determine whether a Medicaid beneficiary has received a blood lead screening.

New Jersey

Medicaid officials said that it can be difficult to track blood lead screenings that are performed using funding from sources other than Medicaid; for example, those performed by the state health department. Officials said that they have been building a lead registry to capture data on lead screenings performed, regardless of how they are funded. New Jersey Medicaid officials said they collect data every 6 months on screenings not paid for by Medicaid and enter the data into the state's blood lead registry.

Source: GAO interviews with Medicaid officials in selected states. | GAO-19-481

Without complete information about blood lead screenings, CMS cannot identify the number of beneficiaries who have not received blood lead screenings. As a result, the agency may be unaware of beneficiaries with unidentified lead exposures. CMS issued guidance in 2016 to states on improving blood lead screening reporting, including correcting reporting errors and partnering with providers to ensure beneficiaries receive blood lead screenings. (See sidebar for examples of efforts states have taken to improve available data about blood lead screenings.) However, as of February 2019, the screening data remained incomplete, according to agency officials. CMS officials also told us they are currently in discussions with the Centers for Disease Control and Prevention about how to capture more complete information about Medicaid beneficiaries who are receiving blood lead screenings through programs funded by that agency. However, as of February 2019, CMS officials had not identified specific actions to gather this data. The lack of data is inconsistent with federal internal control standards, which specify that management should obtain relevant data from reliable sources based on identified information requirements, and use such data for effective monitoring.[45]

[45] See GAO-14-704G.

CMS Replicated Some CMS-416 and Child Core Set Information Using T-MSIS, but Lacks Time Frames and Interim Milestones for Using T-MSIS Data to Streamline State Reporting

According to CMS, the results of recent pilot studies indicate that T-MSIS data can be used to replicate some information on the CMS-416 and Child Core Set.[46] CMS officials said that the results also suggest that CMS may eventually be able to use T-MSIS data to produce the CMS-416 and Child Core Set data, thus eliminating the need for states to report this information themselves separately. As previously noted, CMS intends for T-MSIS to both reduce the number of reports CMS requires states to submit and to provide more information to improve Medicaid oversight.

CMS officials said that they were encouraged that the pilot studies to replicate portions of the CMS-416 and Child Core Set generally yielded positive results. For example, CMS was able to use T-MSIS to replicate the total number of Medicaid beneficiaries aged 20 and under eligible for EPSDT from the CMS-416 within 5 percent of state-reported values for eight of nine pilot states—which CMS officials viewed as a positive result.[47] CMS officials noted some concerns with inaccurate state Medicaid eligibility data; for example, multiple dates of birth reported through T-MSIS for the same beneficiary. However, CMS officials believe the accuracy and completeness of T-MSIS data has improved since the pilot studies, which were conducted using data from 2015 and 2016.[48] Regarding the Child Core Set, CMS was able to use T-MSIS to replicate some of the information, such as adolescent well-care visits, but not other information, such as emergency department visits.

While CMS found generally positive results from the pilots, the agency has not developed a plan with time frames and interim milestones for when it will use state-reported T-MSIS data to produce the CMS-416 and Child Core Set data sets instead of states separately producing both T- MSIS data and the two data sets. In April 2019, CMS officials said that they were planning additional pilots beginning in fiscal year 2019 to replicate portions of the CMS-416 and the Child Core Set.

---

[46] CMS conducted two sets of pilot studies in 2017 and 2018 in separate samples of states selected based on the agency's assessment of the completeness and quality of states' T- MSIS data. The two sets of pilot studies included three studies on the CMS-416 and one study on the Child Core Set. An 11-state sample was initially selected for the CMS-416 pilot studies, while a 6-state sample was initially selected for the Child Core Set pilot study.

[47] Eleven states were initially included in the sample. CMS identified data reliability issues in two states, which were removed from the pilot study.

[48] CMS used state-reported T-MSIS data from calendar years 2015 and 2016 to replicate portions of the sample states' CMS-416, and T-MISIS data from calendar year 2015 to replicate portions of the sample states' Child Core Set.

However, CMS officials were unable to provide planned next steps, including time frames and interim milestones, for using T-MSIS data to replace the CMS-416 and Child Core Set. This is inconsistent with federal internal control standards related to using and communicating quality information to achieve objectives. Without a specific plan with time frames with interim milestones, CMS may miss opportunities to use T-MSIS data to streamline state reporting and better oversee states' provision of EPSDT services. This limitation is similar to one we reported in December 2017 about the initial steps CMS had taken for using T-MSIS data.[49] We found CMS was limited in using T-MSIS for its broader oversight efforts of state Medicaid programs, in part, due to the absence of an articulated plan and time frames.

CONCLUSION

Under EPSDT, millions of Medicaid's youngest beneficiaries received well-child screenings and dental services in fiscal year 2017; however, nearly as many of them did not. Further, existing data on blood lead screenings are incomplete and inaccurate, leaving CMS unaware of beneficiaries with unidentified lead exposures that can cause developmental delays. The EPSDT data collected—whether via the CMS-416, Child Core Set, or T-MSIS—have the potential to improve CMS oversight of beneficiaries' receipt of necessary services and screenings. However, CMS has not taken sufficient steps to help ensure the appropriateness of its state data collection, evaluations, and assistance; and its plans for new reporting, including time frames and interim milestones, are lacking.

RECOMMENDATIONS FOR EXECUTIVE ACTION

We are making the following six recommendations to CMS:

- The Administrator of CMS should work with states and relevant federal agencies to collect accurate and complete data on blood lead screening for Medicaid beneficiaries in order to ensure that CMS is able to monitor state compliance with its blood lead screening policy, and assist states with planning improvements to address states' compliance as needed. (Recommendation 1)
- The Administrator of CMS should regularly assess the appropriateness of performance measures and targets for the EPSDT benefit, and take any necessary

[49] See GAO-18-70. CMS concurred with our recommendation to articulate a specific plan and associated time frames for using T-MSIS data for oversight. As of April 2019, the recommendation remains open.

actions to ensure their relevance and use, including adding, changing, or removing measures, or targets, and regularly communicating performance measures and targets to states. (Recommendation 2)

- The Administrator of CMS should conduct regular evaluations of state performance by comparing states' performance measurement data with CMS's EPSDT targets to identify gaps in states' performance and areas for improvement. (Recommendation 3)
- The Administrator of CMS should assist states with planning needed improvements, including providing focused assistance, to resolve gaps in states' performance in meeting CMS's EPSDT targets. (Recommendation 4)
- The Administrator of CMS should develop a plan with time frames and interim milestones for using T-MSIS data to generate the necessary data from the CMS-416 to improve EPSDT oversight and streamline state reporting. (Recommendation 5)
- The Administrator of CMS should develop a plan with time frames and interim milestones for using T-MSIS data to generate the necessary data from the Child Core Set to improve EPSDT oversight and streamline state reporting. (Recommendation 6)

AGENCY COMMENTS AND OUR EVALUATION

We provided a draft of this chapter to HHS for comment, and its comments are reprinted in appendix IV. HHS also provided us with technical comments, which we incorporated in the report as appropriate. Overall, HHS concurred with three recommendations and did not occur with three recommendations.

HHS concurred with our first recommendation that CMS should work with states and relevant federal agencies to collect accurate and complete data on blood lead screening for Medicaid beneficiaries and assist states with planning improvements to resolve gaps in states' performance as needed. However, HHS stated that it would not be possible to obtain complete data on blood lead screenings, because some screenings are not paid for by Medicaid. In our report, we noted some state and CMS efforts to improve available data on blood lead screenings. We continue to believe CMS needs to take additional actions to collect accurate and complete data to oversee whether eligible EPSDT beneficiaries are receiving blood lead screenings in accordance with CMS policy.

HHS did not concur with our second recommendation, which stated that CMS should regularly assess the appropriateness of performance measures and targets for the EPSDT benefit, and take any necessary actions to ensure their relevance and use.

- HHS noted that it assesses the appropriateness of Child Core Set measures annually and may update existing measures based on that assessment, including measures on the CMS-416. We acknowledge CMS's actions to assess the appropriateness of Child Core Set measures annually and update those measures as appropriate, and we found these actions generally consistent with federal internal control standards regarding information and communication. However, CMS has not taken action, as needed, related to any assessments of the CMS-416 performance measures, even though officials acknowledge limitations in these measures, such as the participant and screening ratios.
- HHS also stated that it may set targets in key areas as appropriate, and has done so as part of the Oral Health Initiative, but that HHS does not believe it would be productive at this time to set targets for every measure. We are encouraged that HHS agreed that it may set targets in key areas as appropriate. This is consistent with our recommendation for CMS to regularly assess the appropriateness of its targets. Our recommendation does not assume that targets should be set for every measure—rather, that CMS needs to regularly assess the appropriateness of performance measures and targets for the EPSDT benefit and communicate them to states.

HHS did not concur with our third recommendation, which stated that CMS should conduct regular evaluations of state performance by comparing states' performance measurement data with CMS's EPSDT targets.

- HHS stated that it offers a wide range of technical assistance on quality improvement to help states address performance goals. HHS commented that it believes this is the most effective method of helping states identify and address areas for potential improvement. We acknowledge that CMS has provided states with technical assistance and individual state snapshots of selected Child Core Set measures over time. However, regular evaluations of states' performance against appropriate EPSDT targets are necessary to help identify gaps in states' performance and areas for improvement.
- HHS noted that states recently received snapshots about their performance on publicly reported Child Core Set measures for the past 5 years, through fiscal year 2017. According to HHS, the snapshots include information about a state's performance on each measure relative to other states' performance and highlights significant changes in a state's performance for each measure. However, these snapshots include descriptions of all states' performance—using medians, and top and bottom quartiles—which are subject to change over time. Moreover, because the median is the midpoint of all states' performance, this target ensures that half of states will not meet it, regardless of their individual performance. A

fixed target—or targeted improvement goal, such as the one developed as part of the Oral Health Initiative—would provide states with the opportunity to measure performance over prior years' results, which is a more meaningful measure that all states can strive to achieve.

HHS did not concur with our fourth recommendation, which stated that that CMS should assist states with planning needed improvements to resolve gaps in states' performance in meeting EPSDT targets.

- HHS stated that it has developed national and state-specific improvement goals for children enrolled in Medicaid with respect to receipt of at least one preventive dental service and provided targeted technical assistance to the lowest performing states. In this chapter, we noted states' progress in meeting targets once CMS developed a performance measurement target for preventive dental services, including actions to improve state performance. Developing additional targets on performance measures critical to beneficiaries' health and well-being could help improve oversight of EPSDT.
- HHS also described other examples of targeted technical assistance to remedy gaps in states' performance, which included working with states on improving their performance on certain Child Core Set measures and improving access to EPSDT services by better leveraging schools as settings for care. Such technical assistance could be valuable for CMS to provide to states after identifying gaps in states' performance relative to EPSDT targets. Doing so would allow CMS to share additional strategies to help states plan and implement needed improvements.

HHS concurred with our fifth and sixth recommendations that CMS should develop a plan with time frames and interim milestones for using T-MSIS data to generate the necessary data from the CMS-416 and Child Core Set to improve EPSDT oversight and streamline state reporting.

As agreed with your office, unless you publicly announce the contents of this chapter earlier, we plan no further distribution until 30 days from the report date. At that time, we will send copies to the Secretary of Health and Human Services, the Administrator of the Centers for Medicare & Medicaid Services, and other interested parties.

Carolyn L. Yocom
Director, Health Care

Appendix I: Selected States' Practices for Delivering Early and Periodic Screening, Diagnostic, and Treatment Services

Selected states used several types of practices to promote and facilitate the delivery of Early and Periodic Screening, Diagnostic, and Treatment (EPSDT) services, according to Medicaid officials in the 16 selected states we interviewed and profiles of these states created by the American Academy of Pediatrics. The practices selected states used included outreach and education, financial incentives, collaboration in EPSDT administration, and EPSDT service delivery initiatives, as shown in Figure 4.

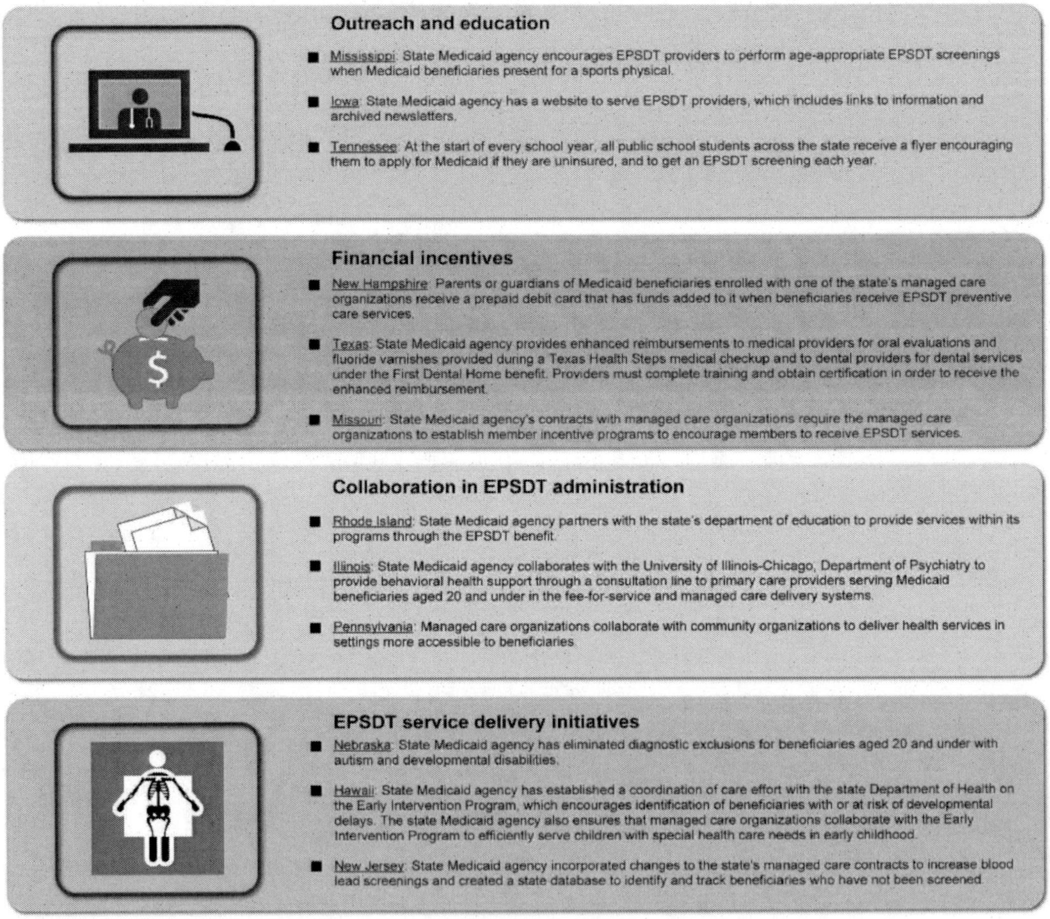

Source: GAO analysis of interviews with Medicaid officials in 16 selected states and American Academy of Pediatrics state profiles regarding the Early and Periodic Screening, Diagonostic and Treatment (EPSDT) benefit. | GAO-19-481

Figure 4. Selected States' Practices for Promoting and Facilitating the Delivery of EPSDT Services, as Reported by States and the American Academy of Pediatrics.

APPENDIX II: INFORMATION REPORTED ON FORM CMS-416 AND CHILD CORE SET

States annually report information about Early and Periodic Screening, Diagnostic, and Treatment (EPSDT) services to the Centers for Medicare & Medicaid Services (CMS), through the Form CMS-416 and the Child Core Set. The CMS-416 provides basic information about EPSDT for Medicaid beneficiaries aged 20 and under, such as the participant ratio and number of beneficiaries receiving a preventive dental service. The Child Core Set provides CMS with information about the quality of health care provided to Medicaid beneficiaries and individuals aged 18 and under who are covered under the Children's Health Insurance Program. In fiscal year 2024, annual reporting of the Child Core Set will become mandatory. As of 2019, the Child Core Set included performance measures related to the provision of EPSDT services, such as well-child visits in the first 15 months of life. Because Child Core Set reporting is currently voluntary, states vary in the number of performance measures they choose to report. In fiscal year 2017, for example, 50 states and the District of Columbia voluntarily reported on at least one of the 27 Child Core Set performance measures, with states reporting a median of 18 Child Core Set performance measures.[50] Some information is only reported on the CMS-416 or Child Core Set, while other information— well-child visits, preventive dental services, and dental sealants—is reported on both CMS-416 and Child Core Set. (See Table 5 for information reported on the CMS-416, the Child Core Set, or both.)

Table 5. Overview of Measures Reported on Form CMS-416 and Child Core Set

Category of information	Information reported	Reported on CMS-416	Reported on Child Core Set
Participation and eligibility measures	• Total individuals eligible for Early and Periodic Screening, Diagnostic, and Treatment (EPSDT) benefit	yes	
Participation and eligibility measures	• State periodicity schedule	yes	
Participation and eligibility measures	• Period of EPSDT eligibility	yes	
Participation and eligibility measures	• Expected and total number of received screenings	yes	
Participation and eligibility measures	• Total individuals recommended to receive screening	yes	
Participation and eligibility measures	• Total individuals receiving recommended screening	yes	
Participation and eligibility measures	• Participant and screening ratios	yes	
Primary care access and preventive care	• Well-child screenings	yes	yes

[50] We used fiscal year 2017 data, because it is the most recent year for which data were available.

Table 5. (Continued)

Category of information	Information reported	Reported on CMS-416	Reported on Child Core Set
Primary care access and preventive care	• Blood lead screenings	yes	
Primary care access and preventive care	• Referrals for treatment	yes	
Primary care access and preventive care	• Weight assessments		yes
Primary care access and preventive care	• Depression screenings		yes
Primary care access and preventive care	• Chlamydia screenings		yes
Primary care access and preventive care	• Access to primary care practitioners		yes
Primary care access and preventive care	• Immunization status		yes
Maternal and perinatal health[a]	• Prenatal and postpartum care timeliness		yes
Maternal and perinatal health[a]	• Low birth weight		yes
Maternal and perinatal health[a]	• Central line-associated bloodstream infections		yes
Maternal and perinatal health[a]	• Cesarean births		yes
Maternal and perinatal health[a]	• Audiological diagnoses		yes
Maternal and perinatal health[a]	• Contraceptive care		yes
Care of acute and chronic conditions	• Asthma medication		yes
Care of acute and chronic conditions	• Emergency department visits		yes
Behavioral health care	• Attention-Deficit/Hyperactivity Disorder medication		yes
Behavioral health care	• Follow-ups post-hospitalization for mental illness		yes
Behavioral health care	• Use of psychosocial care for beneficiaries on antipsychotics		yes
Behavioral health care	• Use of multiple concurrent antipsychotics		yes
Dental and oral health services	• Preventive dental services	yes	yes
Dental and oral health services	• Dental sealants	yes	yes
Dental and oral health services	• Receipt of any dental service	yes	
Dental and oral health services	• Receipt of dental treatment or diagnostic service	yes	
Experience of care	• Consumer Assessment of Healthcare Providers and Systems survey results		yes

Source: GAO analysis of information from the Centers for Medicare & Medicaid Services (CMS) Form CMS-416 and Child Core Set. | GAO-19-481

[a] According to CMS, the health of a child is affected by a mother's health and the care she receives during pregnancy. When women access the health care system for maternity care, an opportunity is presented to promote services and behaviors to optimize their health and the health of their children.

APPENDIX III: SUMMARY OF SELECTED EARLY AND PERIODIC SCREENING, DIAGNOSTIC, AND TREATMENT DATA

Table 6. Well-Child Screening Participant Ratio for Medicaid Beneficiaries Aged 20 and Under, Fiscal Years 2010 through 2017, by State and Nationally

Percentage											
State	2010	2011	2012	2013	2014	2015	2016	2017	Percentage point change, FY 2010 to FY	Min[a]	Max[b]
Alabama	54	53	53	54	52	52	53	55	1	52	55
Alaska	55	56	38	36	41	40	41	39	(16)	36	56
Arizona	65	64	64	61	54	52	48	50	(15)	48	65
Arkansas	46	47	48	48	48	45	48	50	4	45	50
California	91	88	100	100	52	51	42	49	(42)	42	100
Colorado	N/A[c]	47	51	49	49	47	46	49	2[d]	46	51
Connecticut	53	52	64	65	67	66	69	68	15	52	69
Delaware	59	59	59	60	57	57	53	54	(5)	53	60
District of Columbia	81	81	69	63	63	63	64	66	(15)	63	81
Florida	66	51	59	57	53	57	59	59	(7)	51	66
Georgia	51	49	54	54	55	54	55	56	5	49	56
Hawaii	76	76	77	78	78	82	75	81	5	75	82
Idaho	46	51	51	52	48	47	47	47	1	46	52
Illinois	77	76	74	73	77	54	54	54	(23)	54	77
Indiana	50	47	69	77	55	54	53	52	2	47	77
Iowa	81	81	81	81	70	73	77	82	1	70	82
Kansas	57	58	56	58	58	52	50	53	(4)	50	58
Kentucky	57	58	57	57	57	58	59	60	3	57	60
Louisiana	71	73	66	67	74	76	77	80	9	66	80
Maine	38	51	53	54	93	62	56	53	15	38	93
Maryland	63	63	64	64	65	65	67	66	3	63	67
Massachusetts	75	71	71	71	70	69	71	70	(5)	69	75
Michigan	50	51	50	51	51	51	52	52	2	50	52
Minnesota	72	68	68	71	72	70	72	73	1	68	73
Mississippi	42	42	42	41	43	40	43	43	1	40	43
Missouri	73	75	74	74	70	70	68	66	(7)	66	75
Montana	56	56	59	44	42	38	43	44	(12)	38	59
Nebraska	92	51	47	46	35	43	44	46	(46)	35	92
Nevada	68	67	67	66	67	66	68	65	(3)	65	68
New Hampshire	73	71	62	67	66	65	67	71	(2)	62	73
New Jersey	62	63	63	64	62	61	62	63	1	61	64
New Mexico	71	60	60	62	63	62	61	60	(11)	60	71
New York	61	62	61	72	73	70	67	75	14	61	75
North Carolina	55	57	57	57	58	57	57	58	3	55	58
North Dakota	46	45	44	45	45	42	N/A[e]	42	(4)	42	46
Ohio	57	46	44	30	37	42	49	50	(7)	30	57
Oklahoma	56	55	56	56	60	60	63	61	5	55	63
Oregon	63	64	43	41	40	41	46	48	(15)	40	64
Pennsylvania	55	61	63	58	58	66	79	58	3	55	79

Table 6. (Continued)

Percentage State	2010	2011	2012	2013	2014	2015	2016	2017	Percentage point change, FY 2010 to FY 2017	Min[a]	Max[b]
Rhode Island	61	58	57	57	N/A[f]	62	62	60	(1)	57	62
South Carolina	62	63	63	61	61	60	63	64	2	60	64
South Dakota	51	52	48	54	48	33	35	35	(16)	33	54
Tennessee	64	64	58	59	58	55	54	57	(7)	54	64
Texas	65	64	62	65	66	70	71	68	3	62	71
Utah	61	59	57	56	57	57	57	57	(4)	56	61
Vermont	52	56	57	51	54	53	58	60	8	51	60
Virginia	73	62	50	73	74	55	56	55	(18)	50	74
Washington	64	65	65	67	71	71	72	73	9	64	73
West Virginia	46	44	52	54	53	56	60	54	8	44	60
Wisconsin	74	74	74	71	76	76	78	79	5	71	79
Wyoming	51	45	44	45	44	43	47	50	(1)	43	51
U.S. total	**64**	**61**	**62**	**63**	**59**	**58**	**58**	**59**	**(5)**	**58**	**64**

Source: GAO analysis of the Centers for Medicare & Medicaid Services (CMS) Form CMS-416 data for fiscal years (FY) 2010 through 2017. | GAO-19-481

Note: The participant ratio is the percentage of Medicaid beneficiaries aged 20 and under who received at least one recommended well-child screening, based on the state's periodicity schedule, which sets the frequency of screening services.

[a] The lowest participant ratio for Medicaid beneficiaries aged 20 and under from FY 2010 through FY 2017.

[b] The highest participant ratio for Medicaid beneficiaries aged 20 and under from FY 2010 through FY 2017.

[c] Colorado did not report the necessary information to calculate the participant ratio in FY 2010.

[d] Since Colorado did not report the necessary information to calculate the participant ratio in FY 2010, the percentage point change is calculated from FY 2011 to FY 2017.

[e] North Dakota did not report this information for FY 2016.

[f] Rhode Island did not report information for beneficiaries under age 1 in FY 2014.

Tables 6 through 8 present annual state-reported data from the Centers for Medicare & Medicaid Services' (CMS) Form CMS-416 on the provision of selected Early and Periodic Screening, Diagnostic, and Treatment (EPSDT) services by state and nationally. Well-child screenings are presented from fiscal year 2010, the year in which the current reporting template was implemented, through fiscal year 2017, the most recent year for which data were available at the time of our review. Preventive dental services data are presented from fiscal year 2011, the baseline year for measuring states' progress toward CMS's Oral Health Initiative targets, through fiscal year 2017, the most recent year for which data are available.[51]

[51] CMS began the Oral Health Initiative in April 2010 to improve Medicaid beneficiaries' aged 1 to 20 access to dental services under the EPSDT benefit, with an emphasis on prevention. These services included preventive dental services and sealants on permanent molar teeth for beneficiaries aged 6 to 9. CMS officials said that in March 2016 they informed states that CMS no longer planned to use the target for measuring states' performance on the sealant performance measure.

Table 7. Well-Child Screening Participant Ratio for Medicaid Beneficiaries Aged 20 and Under in Fiscal Year 2017, by Age Group, by State, and Nationally

Percentage							
State	**Younger than 1**	**1 to 2**	**3 to 5**	**6 to 9**	**10 to 14**	**15 to 18**	**19 to 20**
Alabama	76	77	65	48	51	40	16
Alaska	91	64	51	26	33	29	7
Arizona	95	73	60	45	48	38	16
Arkansas	94	71	60	65	40	33	4
California	71	68	68	47	47	36	14
Colorado	94	78	62	43	45	34	13
Connecticut	96	88	82	64	67	58	34
Delaware	100	79	66	50	48	38	19
District of Columbia	91	80	73	66	66	57	33
Florida	94	83	73	54	54	43	21
Georgia	95	81	69	48	50	37	12
Hawaii	96	82	73	94	85	85	27
Idaho	96	75	56	38	40	28	17
Illinois	91	79	69	42	52	41	28
Indiana	93	79	61	44	47	39	18
Iowa	93	81	77	91	83	88	41
Kansas	93	75	67	44	46	37	18
Kentucky	96	80	68	81	49	35	26
Louisiana	96	82	66	91	85	86	39
Maine	34	84	60	55	53	42	21
Maryland	93	85	78	62	63	55	36
Massachusetts	75	83	81	72	70	64	44
Michigan	92	76	60	46	47	39	24
Minnesota	91	77	67	83	72	66	40
Mississippi	97	76	55	32	33	23	12
Missouri	92	70	52	75	64	67	47
Montana	98	76	56	32	39	29	8
Nebraska	93	74	58	30	39	31	12
Nevada	83	71	57	73	65	58	22
New Hampshire	92	86	76	100	61	50	26
New Jersey	93	84	74	59	61	54	32
New Mexico	93	74	66	87	60	35	15
New York	77	82	80	100	67	60	32
North Carolina	96	90	73	49	52	39	16
North Dakota	85	59	46	31	36	30	10
Ohio	92	76	65	41	43	39	17
Oklahoma	92	71	53	67	59	49	20
Oregon	95	77	59	41	42	34	17
Pennsylvania	94	81	68	54	54	48	26
Rhode Island	86	79	68	58	58	51	32
South Carolina	92	73	54	72	65	57	20
South Dakota	87	60	44	21	27	20	9
Tennessee	94	82	70	52	52	40	23
Texas	96	85	77	65	65	53	23

Table 7. (Continued)

Percentage							
State	**Younger than 1**	**1 to 2**	**3 to 5**	**6 to 9**	**10 to 14**	**15 to 18**	**19 to 20**
Utah	94	77	61	77	40	34	14
Vermont	96	89	74	58	58	48	24
Virginia	93	83	74	46	48	38	15
Washington	93	81	64	88	75	65	29
West Virginia	93	81	71	50	47	39	17
Wisconsin	95	81	66	97	80	77	46
Wyoming	96	74	57	53	34	26	8
U.S. total	**89**	**79**	**68**	**57**	**55**	**45**	**22**

Source: GAO analysis of the Centers for Medicare & Medicaid Services (CMS) Form CMS-416 data for fiscal year 2017. | GAO-19-481

Note: The participant ratio is the percentage of Medicaid beneficiaries aged 20 and under who received at least one recommended well-child screening, based on the state's periodicity schedule, which sets the frequency of screening services.

Table 8. Percentage of Medicaid Beneficiaries Aged 1 to 20 Receiving Preventive Dental Services, Fiscal Years 2011 through 2017, by State and Nationally

Percentage										
State	**2011**	**2012**	**2013**	**2014**	**2015**	**2016**	**2017**	**Percentage point change, FY 2011 to FY**	**Min[a]**	**Max[b]**
Alabama	51	51	52	50	49	49	49	(2)	49	52
Alaska	43	44	42	46	46	46	46	4	42	46
Arizona	46	44	45	46	47	43	48	2	43	48
Arkansas	48	49	50	51	50	48	48	0	48	51
California	37	36	37	38	37	36	45	8	36	45
Colorado	51	51	50	51	49	51	51	0	49	51
Connecticut	57	59	60	60	59	63	63	6	57	63
Delaware	44	46	46	47	48	48	42	(2)	42	48
District of Columbia	50	48	50	53	54	53	56	6	48	56
Florida	14	19	25	27	33	36	37	24	14	37
Georgia	48	50	50	51	52	52	52	4	48	52
Hawaii	41	41	44	44	49	63	46	4	41	63
Idaho	49	53	56	50	47	59	65	17	47	65
Illinois	49	50	52	51	45	42	45	(4)	42	52
Indiana	29	28	38	48	48	45	45	16	28	48
Iowa	40	45	49	49	50	51	52	12	40	52
Kansas	41	42	46	48	47	46	46	5	41	48
Kentucky	44	38	43	43	45	47	48	4	38	48
Louisiana	47	48	48	48	47	47	49	2	47	49
Maine	32	34	40	40	38	38	36	4	32	40
Maryland	50	52	53	53	53	54	55	5	50	55
Massachusetts	51	53	54	53	52	55	54	3	51	55
Michigan	36	37	40	40	40	42	43	6	36	43

Table 8. (Continued)

Percentage										
State	**2011**	**2012**	**2013**	**2014**	**2015**	**2016**	**2017**	**Percentage point change, FY 2011 to FY**	**Min[a]**	**Max[b]**
Minnesota	38	30	38	38	37	37	37	(2)	30	38
Mississippi	45	47	48	50	47	50	51	6	45	51
Missouri	32	34	35	35	36	34	33	0	32	36
Montana	36	41	47	43	40	30	53	18	30	53
Nebraska	47	48	52	52	53	54	54	7	47	54
Nevada	40	38	45	37	38	43	43	3	37	45
New Hampshire	56	55	56	50	55	55	54	(2)	50	56
New Jersey	43	44	47	48	48	49	50	7	43	50
New Mexico	47	51	51	47	52	53	53	6	47	53
New York	39	39	41	43	43	44	40	1	39	44
North Carolina	45	49	49	49	50	51	51	6	45	51
North Dakota	29	29	29	29	29	N/A[c]	27	(1)	27	29
Ohio	25	37	21	33	34	35	35	10	21	37
Oklahoma	44	46	47	48	48	48	49	4	44	49
Oregon	39	40	40	35	37	39	41	2	35	41
Pennsylvania	36	37	40	43	44	46	47	11	36	47
Rhode Island	43	43	41	44	44	47	47	4	41	47
South Carolina	53	54	51	51	48	50	50	(3)	48	54
South Dakota	44	45	41	40	36	45	45	1	36	45
Tennessee	47	48	49	48	48	48	47	0	47	49
Texas	56	54	53	53	66	67	68	12	53	68
Utah	48	50	52	47	53	53	50	3	47	53
Vermont	58	59	59	62	54	54	55	(3)	54	62
Virginia	47	48	48	49	50	50	53	6	47	53
Washington	53	54	55	55	56	56	56	3	53	56
West Virginia	42	45	46	45	47	50	48	6	42	50
Wisconsin	25	26	25	26	27	30	39	15	25	39
Wyoming	40	40	41	43	42	47	49	9	40	49
U.S. total	**42**	**42**	**43**	**44**	**45**	**46**	**48**	**6**	**42**	**48**

Source: GAO analysis of the Centers for Medicare & Medicaid Services (CMS) Form CMS-416 data for fiscal years (FY) 2011 through 2017. | GAO-19-481

Note: Percentages in parentheses represent a negative number. The reported percentage point change from FY 2011 to FY 2017 does not equal the difference between FY 2011 and FY 2017 percentages in some states due to rounding.

[a] The lowest percentage of Medicaid beneficiaries aged 1 through 20 receiving preventive dental services from FY 2011 through FY 2017.

[b] The highest percentage of Medicaid beneficiaries aged 1 through 20 receiving preventive dental services from FY 2011 through FY 2017.

[c] North Dakota did not report this information for FY 2016.

APPENDIX IV: COMMENTS FROM THE DEPARTMENT OF HEALTH AND HUMAN SERVICES

DEPARTMENT OF HEALTH & HUMAN SERVICES OFFICE OF THE SECRETARY

Assistant Secretary for Legislation
Washington, DC 20201

JUN 0 7 2019

Carolyn Yocom
Director, Health Care
U.S. Government Accountability Office
441 G Street NW
Washington, DC 20548

Dear Ms. Yocom:

Attached are comments on the U.S. Government Accountability Office's (GAO) report entitled, "*Medicaid: Additional CMS Data and Oversight Needed to Help Ensure Children Receive Recommended Screenings*" (GAO-19-481).

The Department appreciates the opportunity to review this report prior to publication.

Sincerely,

Matthew D. Bassett
Assistant Secretary for Legislation

GENERAL COMMENTS OF THE DEPARTMENT OF HEALTH AND HUMAN SERVICES (HHS) ON THE GOVERNMENT ACCOUNTABILITY OFFICE'S DRAFT REPORT ENTITLED: MEDICAID: ADDITIONAL CMS DATA AND OVERSIGHT NEEDED TO HELP ENSURE CHILDREN RECEIVE RECOMMENDED SCREENINGS (GAO-19-481)

The Department of Health and Human Services (HHS) appreciates the opportunity to review and comment on this draft report. HHS is committed to ensuring that children in Medicaid receive screening and other services they are entitled to under the Early Periodic Screening, Diagnostic, and Treatment benefit (EPSDT).

HHS currently collects information on EPSDT services through mandatory reporting on the Form CMS-416 and voluntary reporting on the Child Core Set. The Child Core Set, in particular, allows HHS to evaluate state performance using a wide array of evidence-based quality metrics which are reviewed annually through a rigorous stakeholder engagement process to ensure that they are meaningful for the Medicaid and Children's Health Insurance Program (CHIP) beneficiary populations. As GAO notes in its report, these efforts are generally consistent with federal internal control standards specifying that management should use quality information to achieve the entity's objectives.

HHS releases information on state reporting of Form CMS-416 data each year. HHS also annually releases state progress in reporting the Child Core Set quality measures and assesses state-specific performance for measures that are reported to CMS by at least 25 states and meet CMS standards for data quality. The annual reports include information on median performance for all publicly reported measures, as well as the top and bottom quartiles of performance. HHS has also developed a Medicaid and CHIP Scorecard to increase transparency about the programs' administration and outcomes. The Scorecard includes six of the Child Core Set measures as a tool to increase visibility on state health system performance and encourage performance improvement.

HHS does not have the authority to establish binding targets for states on either the Child Core Set measures or the Form CMS-416. However, when appropriate and resources allow, HHS has developed initiatives to improve performance on specific areas of concern identified through quality reporting. The Oral Health Initiative is one example of how HHS has used state-reported data to develop national and state-specific benchmarks for quality improvement using the preventive dental service measure on the Child Core Set. In Fiscal Year (FY) 2011, 42 percent of children enrolled in Medicaid received at least one preventive dental service. In response, HHS developed national and state-specific 10 percentage point improvement goals for this measure, identified states performing below the national average, and provided targeted technical assistance to the lowest performing states. As of FY 2017, 9 states have met HHS's performance targets, with 39 states demonstrating some level of improvement on this measure over that time period. As a result, the national rate of children enrolled in Medicaid who have received at least one preventive dental service in a year has climbed to 48 percent.

In addition, in late 2018, HHS sent each state an individualized trend snapshot which includes the state's performance on publicly reported Child Core Set measures through FY 2017, information about a state's performance on each measure relative to other states' performance, and highlights significant changes in a state's performance for each measure. This tool is designed to enable states to easily identify how their performance compares to their state peers and whether their performance has trended in a positive direction. HHS believes the trend snapshots will, spur quality improvement efforts by encouraging states to think about their Core Set measure performance over time and not simply at any given point in time.

HHS also regularly analyzes this data to identify states that are outperforming their peers and develop technical assistance resources like learning collaboratives, toolkits, and issue briefs to help disseminate the lessons they learned and share best practices with other states.

HHS believes efforts described above to improve the quality of data being reported in the Child Core Set, set targets in key areas, and provide technical assistance to states to improve their performance on key quality measures strike an appropriate balance between developing quality information, performing monitoring activities, evaluating issues, and remediating deficiencies.

HHS is also working with states to improve the quality of data in the Transformed Medicaid Statistical Information System (T-MSIS). All states, the District of Columbia, and all participating territories have begun submitting T-MSIS data. T-MSIS is a critical source of data for key eligibility, enrollment, program, utilization and expenditure data for the Medicaid and CHIP. The enhanced data available from T-MSIS will support improved program and financial management, robust evaluations of demonstration programs, improve program integrity and efficiency, and will reduce burden on states for reporting requirements. Specific analyses that will be possible with T-MSIS data include assessing beneficiary access to and quality of care, evaluating the impact of different types of delivery system models, and examining important enrollment and service utilization trends. Beginning in July 2017, HHS has identified 12 Top Priority Items (TPIs) for T-MSIS data quality. States have been focused on addressing these 12 TPIs as they are CMS's highest priority T-MSIS data issues. States have made significant progress addressing these TPIs.

In 2019, HHS is beginning to expand its TPIs to include an additional 11 focus areas in support of continuous improvement in T-MSIS data quality. Six focus areas were released in April and the next five TPIs will be released this summer. The guidance on the T-MSIS Coding Blog provides a description of all 23 TPIs.[1] Through a one-on-one state technical assistance effort, HHS reviews a state's data quality issues in these areas and works with the state on addressing them. HHS will also begin to share and use T-MSIS data publicly in 2019.

As noted by GAO, HHS has conducted pilot studies to determine the feasibility of using T-MSIS data to compute EPSDT metrics currently collected through Form CMS-416 and the Child Core Set. As T-MSIS data quality continues to improve, HHS will develop ways to use this data to improve EPSDT oversight and streamline state reporting.

GAO's recommendations and HHS' responses are below.

GAO Recommendation

---

[1] https://www.medicaid.gov/medicaid/data-and-systems/macbis/tmsis/tmsis-blog/?entry=51423

Work with states and relevant federal agencies to collect accurate and complete data on blood lead screening for Medicaid beneficiaries in order to ensure that CMS is able to monitor state compliance with its blood lead screening policy and take corrective action as needed.

HHS Response
HHS concurs with GAO's recommendation.

However, many blood lead screening tests for Medicaid children are paid for by sources other than Medicaid. Therefore, obtaining complete data on blood lead screenings for children enrolled in Medicaid will not be possible. HHS has and will continue to provide guidance to states on the importance of blood lead screening and share best practices on approaches they can take to increase those screening rates.

GAO Recommendation
Regularly assess the appropriateness of performance measures and targets for the EPSDT benefit and take any necessary actions to ensure their relevant use, including adding, changing, or removing measures or targets, and regularly communicating performance measures and targets to states.

HHS Response
HHS does not concur with GAO's recommendation.

HHS assesses the Medicaid and CHIP Child and Adult Core Sets on an annual basis through a rigorous stakeholder engagement process. Through this annual review, HHS updates the existing measures, as appropriate, and assesses whether any measures should be added or deleted, including from the CMS Form 416.

HHS may also set targets in key areas as appropriate. As noted in the report, HHS established a non-binding target for the preventive dental quality measure in the Child Core Set as part of the Oral Health Initiative. Additionally, we provide information to states on whether their performance on publicly-reported Core Set measures is above the median or in the top or bottom quartiles, thus providing performance benchmarks for states.

In conversations with GAO following the release of the draft report, it became clear that this recommendation is requesting targets for all EPSDT measures. HHS does not believe it would be productive at this time to set targets for every measure.

GAO Recommendation
Conduct regular evaluations of state performance by comparing states' performance measurement data with CMS's EPSDT targets to identify gaps in states' performance and areas for improvement.

HHS Response
HHS does not concur with GAO's recommendation.

HHS does not believe it would be productive at this time to set targets for every EPSDT measurement and therefore cannot evaluate states' performance against those targets. As mentioned above, HHS recently sent each state an individualized trend snapshot that provided a state-specific summary of performance on publicly reported Child Core Set measures through FY 2017. The snapshots include a state's performance on publicly reported Child Core Set measures for five years, information about a state's performance on each measure relative to other states' performance, and highlights significant changes in a state's performance for each measure. In addition, HHS offers a wide range of quality improvement technical assistance to help states address performance goals. HHS believes this is the most effective method of helping states identify and address areas for potential improvement.

GAO Recommendation
Assist states with planning needed improvements, including providing focused assistance, to resolve gaps in states' performance in meeting CMS's EPSDT targets.

HHS Response
HHS does not concur with GAO's recommendation.

As mentioned above, HHS has developed initiatives to improve specific areas of concern identified through quality reporting when appropriate and as resources allow. HHS developed national and state-specific improvement goals for children enrolled in Medicaid with respect to receipt of at least one preventive dental service and provided targeted technical assistance to the lowest performing states. Other examples of targeted technical assistance include work with states on improving their performance on the Core Set measure of inappropriate utilization of antipsychotic medication in young children and improving access to EPSDT services by better leveraging schools as settings for care. However, HHS does not believe it is productive at this time to develop similar programs for every EPSDT measurement.

GAO Recommendation
Develop a plan with time frames and interim milestones for using T-MSIS data to generate the necessary data from the CMS-416 to improve EPSDT oversight and streamline state reporting.

HHS Response
HHS concurs with GAO's recommendation.

HHS has conducted pilot studies to determine the feasibility of using T-MSIS data to compute EPSDT metrics currently collected through Form CMS-416 and the Child Core Set. However, not all of the data collected through the CMS-416 can be collected through T-MSIS (for example, state periodicity schedules).

HHS is dependent upon states improving their T-MSIS data submissions in order to generate the EPSDT measures. When the quality of state data is sufficient to reliably generate the EPSDT measures, HHS will produce the applicable EPSDT measures using TMSIS data. As mentioned above, HHS is working with states to improve T-MSIS data quality.

GAO Recommendation
Develop a plan with time frames and interim milestones for using T-MSIS data to generate the necessary data from the Child Core Set to improve EPSDT oversight and streamline state reporting.

HHS Response
HHS concurs with GAO's recommendation.

As mentioned above, HHS is working with states to improve T-MSIS data quality. HHS has conducted pilot studies to determine the feasibility of using T-MSIS data to compute EPSDT metrics currently collected through Form CMS-416 and the Child Core Set. However, not all of the measures on the Child Core Set can be calculated using administrative data from T-MSIS (for example, measures that require electronic health record data).

When the quality of state data is sufficient to reliably generate the EPSDT measures, HHS will produce the applicable EPSDT measures using TMSIS data.

HHS appreciates the work GAO has done, but believes that the current efforts underway to work with states to monitor the EPSDT benefit have not been fully captured in this report. HHS looks forward to future conversations on this issue.

APPENDIX V: ACCESSIBLE DATA

Data Tables

Accessible Data for Number of Medicaid Beneficiaries Receiving and Not Receiving Well-Child Screenings in Fiscal Year 2017, by Age Group

Ages	Total Benes	Beneficiaries Screened	Beneficiaries Not Screened
< 1	1784368	1578479	205889
1-2	4594601	3595722	998879
3-5	5777029	3929859	1847170
6-9	6651672	3762392	2889280
10-14	8255377	4472375	3783002
15-18	5649552	2516835	3132717
19-20	2000416	446236	1554180

Accessible Data for Figure 2. Participant Ratio and the Number of Medicaid Beneficiaries Who Did and Did Not Receive Well-Child Screenings in Fiscal Year 2017, by Age Group

Ages	Total Benes	Beneficiaries Screened	Beneficiaries Not Screened	Participant Ratio
< 1	1784368	1578479	205889	89%
1-2	4594601	3595722	998879	79%
3-5	5777029	3929859	1847170	68%
6-9	6651672	3762392	2889280	57%
10-14	8255377	4472375	3783002	55%
15-18	5649552	2516835	3132717	45%
19-20	2000416	446236	1554180	22%

In: Medicaid: Fraud, Payments and Beneficiaries
Editor: Nadia M. Hedegaard
ISBN: 978-1-53617-666-7

Chapter 5

MEDICAID DISPROPORTIONATE SHARE HOSPITAL (DSH) REDUCTIONS*

Alison Mitchell

The Medicaid statute requires states to make disproportionate share hospital (DSH) payments to hospitals treating large numbers of low-income patients. This provision is intended to recognize the disadvantaged financial situation of those hospitals because low-income patients are more likely to be uninsured or Medicaid enrollees. Hospitals often do not receive payment for services rendered to uninsured patients, and Medicaid provider payment rates are generally lower than the rates paid by Medicare and private insurance. (See CRS Report R42865, Medicaid Disproportionate Share Hospital Payments.)

Whereas most federal Medicaid funding is provided on an open-ended basis, federal Medicaid DSH funding is capped. Each state receives an annual DSH allotment, which is the maximum amount of federal matching funds that each state is permitted to claim for Medicaid DSH payments. In FY2018, federal DSH allotments totaled $12.3 billion.

DSH ALLOTMENT REDUCTION AMOUNTS

The Patient Protection and Affordable Care Act (ACA; P.L. 111-148, as amended) has reduced the number of uninsured individuals in the United States through the health insurance coverage provisions (including the ACA Medicaid expansion). Built on the

* This is an edited, reformatted and augmented version of Congressional Research Service Publication No. IF10422, dated Updated February 26, 2019.

premise that with fewer uninsured individuals there should be less need for Medicaid DSH payments, the ACA included a provision directing the Secretary of the Department of Health and Human Services (HHS) to make aggregate reductions in Medicaid DSH allotments equal to $500 million in FY2014, $600 million in FY2015, $600 million in FY2016, $1.8 billion in FY2017, $5.0 billion in FY2018, $5.6 billion in FY2019, and $4.0 billion in FY2020.

Despite the assumption that decreasing the number of uninsured individuals would reduce the need for Medicaid DSH payments, the ACA was written so that, after the specific reductions for FY2014 through FY2020, DSH allotments would have returned to the amounts that states would have received without the enactment of the ACA. In other words, in FY2021, states' DSH allotments would have rebounded to their pre-ACA-reduced levels, with annual inflation adjustments for FY2014 to FY2021.

Since the ACA, a number of laws have amended the ACA Medicaid DSH reductions by eliminating the reductions for FY2014 through FY2019, changing the reduction amounts, and extending the reductions through FY2025. The specific laws that have amended the Medicaid DSH reductions are

- the Middle Class Tax Relief and Job Creation Act of 2012 (P.L. 112-96),
- the American Taxpayer Relief Act of 2012 (P.L. 112- 240),
- the Bipartisan Budget Act of 2013 (P.L. 113-67),
- the Protecting Access to Medicare Act of 2014 (P.L. 113-93),
- the Medicare Access and CHIP Reauthorization Act of 2015 (P.L. 114-10), and
- the Bipartisan Budget Act of 2018 (BBA 2018; P.L. 115-123).

Under current law, the aggregate reductions to the Medicaid DSH allotments equal $4.0 billion in FY2020 and $8.0 billion for each year from FY2021 through FY2025.

Figure 1 shows estimates of aggregate DSH allotments for FY2012 through FY2028 before the ACA reductions, with the ACA reductions, and under current law. The ACA reductions totaled $18.1 billion, and under current law the DSH allotment reductions total $44.0 billion.

Under current law, the aggregate reductions relative to the Medicaid DSH allotments before the ACA reductions will be an estimated 31% reduction in FY2020 and an estimated 61% reduction in FY2021, and they will phase down to an estimated 55% reduction in FY2025. In FY2026, DSH allotments will rebound to the pre-ACA-reduced levels, with annual inflation adjustments for FY2020 to FY2026.

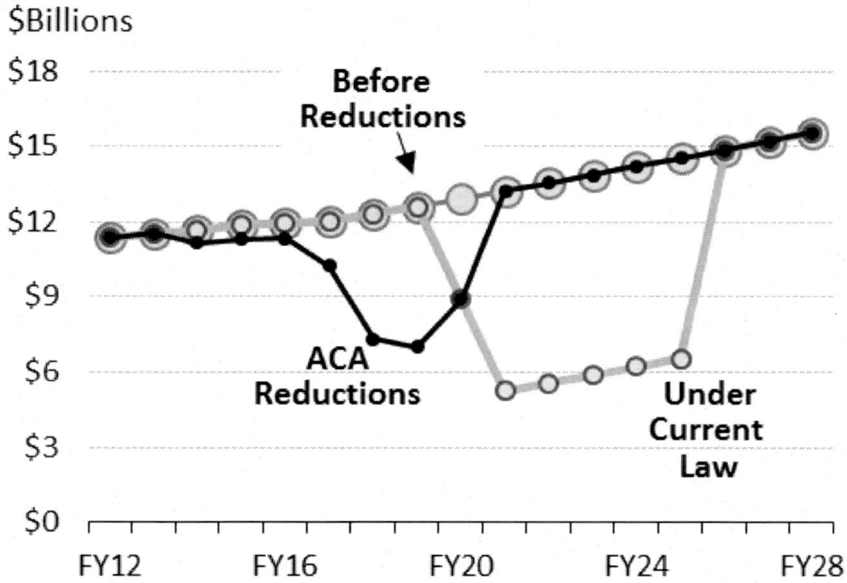

Source: CRS calculation.

Notes: The consumer price index for all urban consumers used to inflate the DSH allotments is based on the factors built into Congressional Budget Office, The Budget and Economic Outlook: Fiscal Years 2018 to 2028, April 2018. DSH allotments are different from DSH expenditures. Allotments reflect the maximum amount of federal DSH funding available to states, and DSH expenditures are the amounts paid to hospitals.

Figure 1. Total DSH Allotments Before the Reductions, with the ACA Reductions, and Under Current Law.

STATUTORY REQUIREMENTS FOR REDUCTIONS TO STATE DSH ALLOTMENTS

Although the aggregate DSH reduction amounts are specified in statute, the Secretary is responsible for determining how to distribute the aggregate DSH reductions among the states using some broad statutory guidelines. The Secretary is required to impose *larger* percentage DSH reductions on states that

- have the lowest percentage of uninsured individuals (determined by the Census Bureau's data, audited hospital cost reports, and other information likely to yield accurate data) during the most recent fiscal year with available data or
- do *not* target their DSH payments to hospitals with high volumes of Medicaid patients and high levels of uncompensated care (excluding bad debt).

The statute also requires the Secretary to impose smaller percentage reductions on low DSH states (i.e., states with total Medicaid DSH payments for FY2000 between 0% and 3% of total Medicaid medical assistance expenditures).

The last specification provided in statute requires the Secretary to take into account the extent to which the DSH allotment for a state was included in the budget neutrality calculation for a coverage expansion approved under a Section 1115 waiver as of July 31, 2009.

Although the statute provides the Secretary with flexibility regarding how to allocate the DSH reductions among the states, in general, states with the lowest percentage of uninsured individuals can be expected to receive relatively larger percentage DSH reductions. In addition, states that do not target their DSH payments to hospitals with the most Medicaid patients and highest levels of uncompensated care can be expected to receive relatively larger percentage DSH reductions. Also, low DSH states should receive relatively smaller percentage DSH reductions. As a result, a non-low DSH state with a low percentage of uninsured individuals that does not target its DSH payments can be expected to receive a relatively larger percentage reduction and a low DSH state with a high percentage of uninsured individuals that targets its DSH payments should receive a relatively smaller percentage DSH reduction.

The magnitude of the Medicaid DSH reductions is such that most states are expected to have DSH allotment reductions. Tennessee is the only state that is not subject to the Medicaid DSH reductions due to the special statutory authority that provides Tennessee with a Medicaid DSH allotment.

PROPOSED METHODOLOGY FOR ALLOCATING DSH REDUCTIONS

On July 28, 2017, prior to passage of BBA 2018, which eliminated the reductions for FY2018 and FY2019, the Centers for Medicare & Medicaid Services (CMS) released a proposed rule regarding the methodology for allocating the DSH reductions. The proposed methodology for allocating the Medicaid DSH reductions begins by splitting the aggregate DSH reduction amount for each year into two separate amounts: one DSH reduction amount for low DSH states and another reduction amount for non-low DSH states.

Then, for each group of states, half of each group's DSH reductions would be allocated according to the uninsured percentage factor and half of the DSH reductions would be allocated according to how states target their DSH funds. As shown in Figure 2, the DSH reductions would be allocated according to the uninsured percentage factor (50%), how states target their DSH funds according to the "high volume of Medicaid inpatient factor" (25%), and how states target their DSH funds according to the "high level of uncompensated care factor" (25%). Each state's reduction would be limited to 90% of the unreduced allotment amount, which preserves at least 10% of each state's DSH allotments.

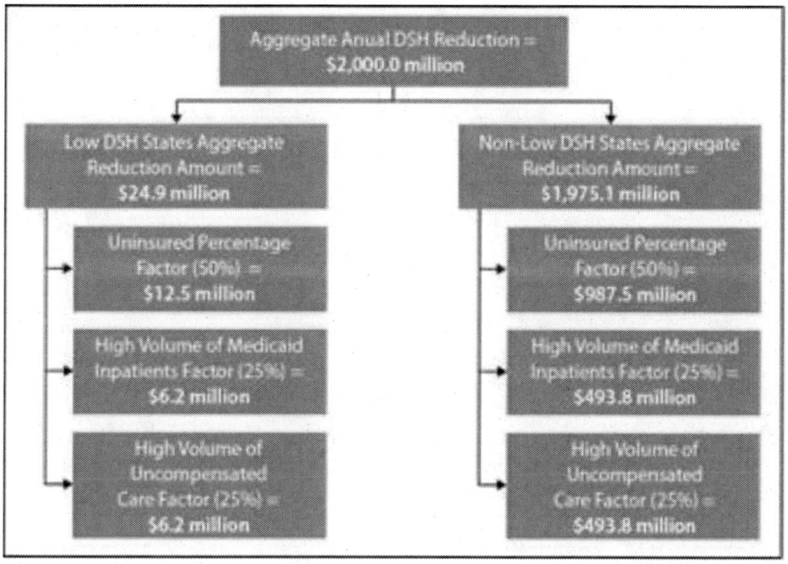

Source: CRS using the illustrative DSH reduction factor weighting allocation from Centers for Medicare & Medicaid Services, "Medicaid Program; State Disproportionate Share Hospital Allotment Reductions," 82 Federal Register 35155, July 28, 2017.

Figure 2. Illustrative Example of Proposed Medicaid DSH Reduction Methodology.

The proposed methodology would not reduce any portion of a state's Medicaid DSH allotment that was included in the budget neutrality calculation for a coverage expansion that was approved under a Section 1115 waiver as of July 31, 2009. This would affect the District of Columbia, Indiana, Maine, Massachusetts, and Wisconsin.

Figure 2 shows CMS's illustrative example of the proposed methodology using a $2.0 billion aggregate Medicaid DSH reduction on FY2017 allotments. Under this example, CMS estimates that low DSH states would have an average allotment reduction of 4.6% and non-low DSH states would have an average allotment reduction of 17.2%.

INDEX

A

B

E

F

G

H

I

K

L

M

N

O

P

Q

R

S